THE BASIS OF
TOXICITY TESTING
SECOND EDITION

Pharmacology and Toxicology: Basic and Clinical Aspects

Mannfred A. Hollinger, Series Editor
University of California, Davis

Forthcoming Titles

Anabolic Treatment for Osteoporosis, James F. Whitfield and Paul Morley
Basis of Toxicity Testing, Second Edition, Donald J. Ecobichon
CNS Injuries: Cellular Responses and Pharmacological Strategies, Martin Berry and Ann Logan
Lead and Public Health: Integrated Risk Assessment, Paul Mushak
Molecular Bases of Anesthesia, Eric Moody and Phil Skolnick
Receptor Characterization and Regulation, Devendra K. Agrawal

Published Titles

Antibody Therapeutics, 1997, William J. Harris and John R. Adair
Muscarinic Receptor Subtypes in Smooth Muscle, 1997, Richard M. Eglen
Antisense Oligodeonucleotides as Novel Pharmacological Therapeutic Agents, 1997, Benjamin Weiss
Drug Delivery Systems, 1996, Vasant V. Ranade and Mannfred A. Hollinger
Experimental Models of Mucosal Inflammation, 1996, Timothy S. Gaginella
Brain Mechanisms and Psychotropic Drugs, 1996, Andrius Baskys and Gary Remington
Receptor Dynamics in Neural Development, 1996, Christopher A. Shaw
Ryanodine Receptors, 1996, Vincenzo Sorrentino
Therapeutic Modulation of Cytokines, 1996, M.W. Bodmer and Brian Henderson
Pharmacology in Exercise and Sport, 1996, Satu M. Somani
Placental Pharmacology, 1996, B. V. Rama Sastry
Pharmacological Effects of Ethanol on the Nervous System, 1996, Richard A. Deitrich
Immunopharmaceuticals, 1996, Edward S. Kimball
Chemoattractant Ligands and Their Receptors, 1996, Richard Horuk
Pharmacological Regulation of Gene Expression in the CNS, 1996, Kalpana Merchant
Human Growth Hormone Pharmacology: Basic and Clinical Aspects, 1995, Kathleen T. Shiverick and Arlan Rosenbloom
Placental Toxicology, 1995, B. V. Rama Sastry
Stealth Liposomes, 1995, Danilo Lasic and Frank Martin
TAXOL®: Science and Applications, 1995, Matthew Suffness

Pharmacology and Toxicology: Basic and Clinical Aspects

Published Titles Continued

SERIES PREFACE

I am pleased to include Dr. Donald Ecobichon's contribution entitled *The Basis of Toxicity Testing*, Second Edition, in the series *Pharmacology and Toxicology: Basic and Clinical Aspects*. Dr. Ecobichon has succeeded at a very difficult task: he has created a comprehensive compendium of practical aspects of toxicity assessment. The breadth of coverage includes traditional aspects of toxicity testing such as acute, subacute, and chronic studies as well as contemporary assays dealing with alternative *in vitro* dermal and ocular irritation studies, and mutagenic and carcinogenic assessment. This is a how-to book that covers both experimental design and data interpretation. Readers, be they graduate student, academician, or industry scientist, interested in the foundation of toxicological investigation will find this book invaluable.

Mannfred A. Hollinger, Ph.D.

Series Editor
Professor
Department of Medical Pharmacology and Toxicology
University of California, Davis

THE BASIS OF
TOXICITY TESTING
SECOND EDITION

Donald J. Ecobichon, Ph.D.

Department of Pharmacology and Therapeutics
McGill University
Montreal, Quebec
Canada

CRC Press
Boca Raton   New York

Library of Congress Cataloging-in-Publication Data

Echobichon, Donald J.
  The Basis of Toxicity Testing, second edition / Donald J. Echobichon
        p. cm. — (CRC Press series in pharmacology and toxicology)
     Includes bibliographical references and index.
     ISBN 0-8493-8554-7
     1. Toxicity testing. I. Title. II. Series
  QR749.H64G78 1997
  616′.0149—dc20   97-21039
                                                                                          CIP

No claim to original U.S. Government works
International Standard Book Number 0-8493-8554-7
Library of Congress Card Number 97-21039
Printed in the United States of America 1 2 3 4 5 6 7 8 9 0
Printed on acid-free paper

Dedication

---

*To the memory of Dr. G. H. Lucas, Professor of Pharmacology
at the University of Toronto and forensic toxicologist who,
as a graduate student's friend, first ignited the spark of interest
in toxicology, and to Werner Kalow, my mentor,
who encouraged and sustained it.*

TABLE OF CONTENTS

PREFACE TO THE SECOND EDITION

The impact of chemicals upon our environment has resulted in an ever-increasing need to monitor, assess, and reevaluate the toxicity data base of many agents. Such toxicity, safety, and risk assessments may be done by individuals at the "action group" level, at municipal, state, or provincial levels, and at the federal levels as well as by various industries involved directly in the manufacture of chemicals or indirectly in the formulation of products using such agents. Naively, one might assume that such assessors have background training and/or experience in toxicology. All too frequently this is not the case, the evaluator having gained experience "on-the-job" without benefit of training.

The fundamental aim of a toxicity study is to obtain biological information that is reproducible, reliable, and can be extrapolated to a potential toxicity situation in humans. Be the toxicant in question a chemical, a physical agent, or a form of energy, toxicological experiments are conducted in a similar manner. Of equal importance is a knowledge of the limitations of such tests, the boundaries beyond which caution and discretion should be exercised in the interpretation of data in risk assessment exercises.

This text has evolved from a course taught over several years to senior undergraduate and graduate students having varied backgrounds, including the spectrum of biological sciences, chemistry, physics, and engineering as well as medical and health sciences, who have or will have the awesome responsibility of evaluation thrust upon them. The text presents fundamental principles and concepts behind the various types of toxicological studies and their design and conduction as well as the interpretation of results and the place of individual studies in the overall toxicological assessment of a chemical.

This edition contains much more information on various "alternative" testing, there being less confusion and better development of various testing protocols than was obvious to this scientist's eye in 1990. The issue of the "Three Rs" (reducing, refining, and replacement of existing animal tests) received a major stimulus by Directives 86/600/EEC and 86/609/EEC which established commitments by the European Community to protect animals in experimentation, replacing such testing if satisfactory alternative tests were available. In the past 5 years, this has led to increased funding, research, and validation of alternative tests, and it is time to take stock on what has been accomplished. Recently, the Sixth Amendment of the Cosmetic Directive 76/768/EEC proposed a 1998 ban in the EEC on the sale of cosmetics for which animal testing was done where nonanimal alternative tests exist. This European initiative precipitated a renewed interest to alternative test development/validation in North America and serious consideration of such test protocols by regulatory agencies.

The modest success of the first edition and the positive comments from many colleagues have encouraged me to heed my editor's entreaties for an updated version. Again I have attempted to present a balanced, informative approach to toxicity studies as well as a concise description of why the studies are done in a particular manner. It is not within the scope of this book to discuss the toxicity of particular agents in depth, though examples will be used to illustrate points and pitfalls. The references with each chapter are not exhaustive but should direct the reader to current or pertinent published literature for a background or overview of a topic. I hope that it is clear to the reader when I am stating facts, conjecture, and/or opinion. If the text can answer some of the queries about toxicological studies and dispel some of the mysticism, then it will have served its purpose.

THE AUTHOR

Donald J. Ecobichon, Ph.D., is Professor of Toxicology in the Department of Pharmacology and Therapeutics, McGill University, Montreal, Quebec, Canada.

Dr. Ecobichon is a graduate of the University of Toronto, having obtained a B.Sc. in Pharmacy and an M.A. and Ph.D. in Pharmacology in 1960, 1962, and 1964, respectively. His research interests have spanned a range of chemicals from drugs through polyhalogenated biphenyls to organophosphorus ester insecticides and tobacco smoke and have involved studies on transplacental and milk acquisition, the biotransformation of chemicals in both adult and perinatal animal models, the subchronic and chronic neurotoxicity of organophosphorus esters, and the biological effects of novel antiviral agents. He has authored and co-authored over 120 research papers in peer-reviewed journals as well as several chapters in books; he has co-edited a monograph on environmental tobacco smoke and co-authored one book entitled *Pesticides and Neurological Disease.* He is an active consultant to industry and governments on toxicological problems.

Dr. Ecobichon has served on expert committees for the National Academy of Sciences/National Research Council, on the pesticide study group for the Task Force on Environmental Cancer and Heart and Lung Diseases, and on a number of expert task groups for the development of environmental health criteria documents for the International Programme on Chemical Safety (IPCS) of the World Health Organization. He lectures on the topics of food toxicology, industrial toxicology, the design of experimental protocols for toxicity testing, medical toxicology, and pharmacokinetics. He serves on the editorial review boards of four toxicological journals.

Dr. Ecobichon is a member of the Society of Toxicology of Canada, the Society of Toxicology, the Pharmacological Society of Canada, the American Society for Pharmacology and Experimental Therapeutics, and the American Association for the Advancement of Science.

Chapter 1

INTRODUCTION

Humans of all ages, domestic livestock, and all forms of wildlife are exposed daily to a myriad of air-, water-, and food-borne toxicants of natural and anthropogenic (man-made) origin. Exposure to contaminants can occur in the environment of the workplace, the home, recreational areas, and even in isolated wilderness regions of the world, such as the Arctic. Public and government concerns about environmental contamination are focused on a vast array of chemicals, ranging from radioactive elements (strontium, cesium, radon), heavy metals (cadmium, mercury, lead), industrial solvents and volatile organic compounds (tri- and tetra-chloroethylene, chlorofluorocarbons, benzene, xylenes, formaldehyde), agrochemicals (fertilizers, pesticides), household products (detergents, cleaners, paints), fuel combustion (nitrogen and sulfur oxides, polycyclic aromatic hydrocarbons, carbon monoxide, carbon dioxide), as well as a plethora of prescription and nonprescription (over-the-counter) drug preparations. The scientific literature and popular press are replete with reports, anecdotes, and terrifying stories of contaminations and poisonings (Whelan, 1985). Such exposures may originate from a *point source* contamination — a localized accidental spill, frequently at high concentration — that can elicit acute toxicity and immediate as well as delayed adverse health effects. Such an incident was the methyl isocyanate (MIC) disaster in Bhopal, India (Varma, 1986). Exposure may also arise from regional or even global low-level chemical contamination, with long-term, insidious acquisition of amounts of toxicant having the potential to cause covert signs and symptoms only after an extended passage of time.

Real and/or perceived hazards are frequently obscured by the commonly held belief that chemicals are either "toxic" or they are "safe," a black-and-white situation with no shades of grey between the two extremes. People cannot understand why, if some degree of toxicity can be demonstrated for a chemical, regulatory agencies permit the presence of low concentrations in foods, etc. Public chemophobia is focused most frequently on what is closest to them: the air they breathe, the water they drink, and the food they eat; these are things to which they are involuntarily exposed and over which they can exert little personal control. However, without much serious thought, we all contribute in our own way to the problems of local and global contamination. While "industry" is blamed for much of the pollution, we are unwilling to live without many of the products and services generated by these industries (automobiles, metal products, plastics, electricity, etc.). We are concerned about pesticides in foods but also demand unblemished, attractive-looking, disease-free, wholesome, nutritious, and, most importantly, inexpensive food. Food preservation is an important aspect of the food industry, but we are frequently more concerned about the chemicals used than about the consequences that would occur in their absence. We rarely pay any attention to natural toxicants in foods, particularly in vegetables (Ames, 1983). We persist in stockpiling toxic waste material from industry, and only recently has recycling begun to address the gigantic problems of the disposable waste of everyday living, our garbage. Everything has become hazardous to our health! Little consideration is ever given to a basic piece of philosophy, stated in the mid 1500s by Philip Theophrastus Bombast von Hohenheim, or Paracelsus: "All substances are poisonous; there is none which is not a poison. Dosage alone determines poisoning," or "the right dose differentiates a poison and a remedy."

Some years ago at a Society of Toxicology meeting in the U.S., a colleague stood up and posed the question "Why do we spend all this time and money studying chemicals? Chemicals never change their properties and always behave in the same manner. It is people that are different; we should be studying them." The audience laughed, appreciating the fact that this well-known toxicologist was an employee of one of the largest chemical manufacturing concerns on the continent. However, he was correct! All chemicals possess a distinctive set of physical and chemical properties which never vary. Frequently, the biological effects observed within or between species of animals reflect these properties *plus* the varying ability and capacity of an organism to store, biotransform, and/or efficiently eliminate the potential toxicant.

Historically, early investigators found that many of the diseases observed in humans could be reproduced faithfully in animals. A classic example involves the astute observation made by Percival Pott in 1775, linking chimney sweeps' cancer with the adherence of soot particles to the epidermal folds of scrotal skin (Pott, 1775). However, his hypothesis was only confirmed almost a century and a half later when the repeated application of coal tar on rabbits' ears (Yamagiwa and Ichikawa, 1918) and mouse skin (Bloch and Dreifuss, 1921) resulted in the induction of localized carcinomas. A more recent illustrative example is the dermatological condition *chloracne*, observed in the Yusho Oil victims in the late 1960s in Japan and, more recently, in Seveso, Italy, in 1976 (Higuchi, 1976; Reggiani, 1978). Considered by the public and the media as a "modern" disease, it should be emphasized that the condition was first described in 1897 by von Bettmann (1901) and was mistakenly named "chlorine acne" by Herxheimer (1899) who associated the condition with occupational exposure to chlorine gas. Using a technique first published in 1941 in which the rabbit ear was used to monitor chemicals causing acneform dermatitis (Adams et al., 1941), Karl Schulz, a dermatologist, finally identified the organic nature of the chlorine-containing, acneogenic agent in chlorophenols as "dioxin" (2,3,7,8-tetrachlorodibenzo-*p*-dioxin or TCDD) (Kimmeg and Schulz, 1957). Descriptions of the "hunt" for this toxic contaminant can be found in Hay (1982) and Gough (1986). The saga continues even today, with interest now being focused at the molecular level, e.g., the interaction of dioxin with the arylhydrocarbon hydroxylase receptor (AhR), dioxin-induced regulation of gene expression, and an approach to chemical-specific risk assessment of carcinogenesis (Gallo et al., 1991). In contrast, the tragic episode of thalidomide-induced congenital malformations in the late 1950s revealed a major defect in relying on animal models as predictors of toxicity in the human: species variability in response to the drug (McBride, 1961; Tuchmann-Duplessis, 1975). While the rat was not susceptible to the dysmorphogenic effects of the agent, treatment of the mouse, rabbit, macaque monkey, and baboon resulted in a high proportion of severe limb deformities (Somers, 1962; Spencer, 1962; Wilson, 1971). Such fortuitous research strengthened the notion that animals could be used as surrogate models to predict problems that might occur in the human if accompanied by a cautious interpretation of the results of such studies. A basic tenet of toxicology is that the more frequently a specific adverse health effect can be measured in different animal species, the greater is the likelihood that, at some dosage, a similar effect might occur in the human.

The 1984 report of the National Research Council, entitled "Toxicity Testing, Strategies to Determine Needs and Priorities," demonstrated that for many commonly used chemicals, the toxicity data base was so limited that complete assessments of the potential hazards to human health could not be conducted (NRC/NAS, 1984). Many of the large-scale production chemicals have never been tested adequately by the methodology in current use. Recognition of these inadequacies and rising concerns about use, misuse, inappropriate disposal and/or destruction, regional pollution, and the seemingly ubiquitous, global, environmental burden of such chemicals has sponsored a plethora of community, provincial/state, national, and international legislation and regulations designed to improve the quality and quantity of toxicity data and to safeguard against the release of chemicals into the environment. Confidence in the current process of regulating chemicals has been shaken repeatedly, resulting in public demands for additional stringent measures for toxicity testing accompanied by the development of new technologies to detect and quantitate trace contaminants and to assess the potential health risks of these extremely low levels. Largely, the thrust of toxicological studies has been diverted from the identification of potentially hazardous agents to the demonstration of "safety" and the establishment of an acceptable level of safety for each perceived adverse health effect.

The key to any assessment of the potential of an agent to pose a hazard to health is based on the toxicity studies conducted and the nature of the multi-science discipline of toxicology. Toxicology may be defined as "the *qualitative* and especially the *quantitative* study of the injurious effects of chemical and physical agents as observed in alterations of structure and response in living systems: it includes the application of the findings of these studies to the evaluation of safety and the prevention of injury to man and all useful forms of life" (Hayes, 1975). The descriptive term "qualitative" in this definition pertains to whether or not a particular agent is toxic and to the concept of relative toxicity of one agent in comparison with the known toxicity of other agents. The term "quantitative" pertains to the relationship between a given concentration (amount) of the agent and some measurable biological effect, i.e., the dose-effect relationship that has become the most important tenet of the discipline of toxicology. It is important to emphasize that, regardless of the nature of the toxicological study being conducted, the objective is to establish a dose-effect relationship between known amounts of agent and biological effects measured in the most susceptible species by sensitive physiological, biochemical, and/or morphological techniques. Most frequently, when the dose-effect relationship has been plotted graphically, a sigmoidal or S-shaped curve will be observed. Imperative to such studies is an examination of: (1) the shape of the dose-effect relationship; (2) the responses at low levels of exposure; (3) the nature of effects at high levels; and (4) the slope of the linear portion, indicative of the order of toxicity, i.e., steep slope, highly toxic; shallow slope, relatively low toxicity (Figure 1.1).

Regardless of the regulatory agency mandated to protect environmental or human well being, three approaches are used to gather the information necessary to assess the hazard(s) to health. First, toxicological studies conducted in suitable animal species provide a vast amount of pertinent information collected under conditions where the dosage (or exposure) can be carefully controlled and adverse health effects can be measured by precise and reproducible methods. The disadvantages of animal studies are two-fold: (1) the inherent problems of extrapolating from animals to the human; and (2) the difficulty of extrapolating from the high dosages required to elicit

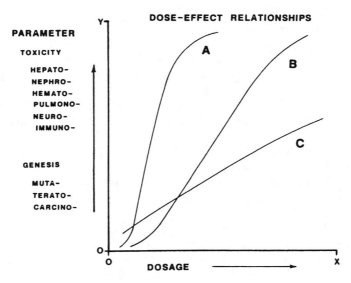

FIGURE 1.1

Graphic displays of possible relationships between measurable adverse physiological, biochemical, or morphological effects (y-axis) on target organs or on functions such as mutagenesis, teratogenesis, or carcinogenesis (causing mutations, birth defects, or cancer, respectively) and the dosage (x-axis) of toxicant administered. The typical S-shaped (sigmoidal) curve usually has a linear portion with a slope (change in response/change in dosage) that is indicative of potency, a small increase in dosage causing a large change in effect (Curve A) or the situation where a large change in dosage is required before marked changes are seen in biological effect(s) (Curve C). In general, only one parameter is plotted against dosage, but all too frequently, a toxicant may elicit effects on more than one target organ, giving rise to dose-effect curves of different configurations.

effects in animal studies to the low level exposures usually encountered by humans. Second, retrospective epidemiological studies, where exposure(s) of humans, domestic animals, or wildlife to toxicants have occurred in the past, are used by regulatory agencies. However, a major disadvantage of such studies is the imprecise determination of the actual levels of exposure, particularly when the concentrations may vary greatly over the years. Additional disadvantages of epidemiological studies include the fact that: (1) adverse health effects must have already occurred as a consequence of exposure; (2) the incidence of the effect must be significant in order to detect it in a randomly sampled, limited population of individuals; and (3) definitive proof of the causality/association of a particular agent is frequently difficult to obtain. However, as in the case of the hexacarbon-induced polyneuropathy in industrial workers and in solvent abuse by inhalation where epidemiological evidence identified the toxicant, similar toxicity elicited in an appropriate animal model provided the means to explore the mechanism(s) of action in the human (Spencer et al., 1980). Third, controlled clinical studies may be used to cautiously explore the toxicity of an agent, exposing a test population to a pollutant under described, controlled conditions and measuring representative biological markers of effects. Advantages of this type of study are that they can be performed with the species (humans, other mammals, fish, birds, etc.) of interest and exposure can vary from acute to chronic, from single doses to repeated, long-term exposures. With humans, the disadvantage is one of ethics in that only short-term and reversible effects can be studied; harmful effects and chronic disease cannot be produced or monitored.

Given the fact that exposure can occur to some 65,000 chemicals in widespread commercial use, one is faced with an almost overwhelming task of health risk and/or

TABLE 1.1

U.S. Code of Federal Regulations Toxicity
Testing Requirements for a Pesticide To Be
Classified For Use on a Terrestrial Food Crop

Acute oral toxicity
Acute dermal toxicity
Acute inhalation toxicity
Primary ocular irritation
Primary dermal irritation
Dermal sensitization
Acute, delayed neurotoxicity
21-d dermal
90-d dermal
90-d feeding study
90-d inhalation
90-d neurotoxicity
Chronic feeding study
Oncogenicity study
Teratogenicity
Reproduction study
Gene mutation
  • structural chromosome aberration
  • other genotoxic effects
General metabolism
Domestic animal safety

From Code of Federal Regulations. Title 40, Part 158,
(40CFR Part 158).

environmental impact assessment (White, 1980; Maugh, 1983). New chemicals being introduced into commerce pose little problem since rigorous premarketing assessments can be demanded contingent to their registration and sale. The concept of "cradle-to-grave" accountability for a chemical has become fashionable for industrial and agricultural chemicals. The major problem is associated with the sheer numbers of older chemicals already "out there," that have been used for decades and have received only very limited toxicological assessment. What is to be done about these agents? An attempt can be made to reassess the potential toxicity, as has occurred for pesticides in the U.S. and Canada, by requesting that new studies be conducted to provide a better data base. Such an exercise was conducted for food additives on the GRAS (generally recognized as safe) list (Anonymous, 1977). An alternative, but unacceptable, pathway is to do nothing and wait for a problem to arise before addressing the issues chemical by chemical.

The demand for more toxicological data for chemicals (both old and new) and physical agents (dust, fibers, noise, light, energy) as well as the expansion of testing protocols to achieve these ends has placed heavy demands on the requirements for research animals (CCAC, 1990; Gad, 1990; Parkinson and Grasso, 1993). One example of a test battery, that of the U.S. EPA for a pesticide, is shown in Table 1.1. While a strong case can be made for the contributions of animal experimentation to biomedical advances over the past 200 years (Figure 1.2), the strategy has become one of reducing, replacing and refining the present *in vivo* tests. Many of the proposed new methods will be *in vitro*, alternative tests involving microorganisms, mammalian cell cultures, tissue slices, whole organs, and embryos. Since these alternative tests cannot identify the effects of an agent on a complex organism with interactive, physiological, and biochemical systems, they will never replace properly designed animal studies. While some investigators see these alternative tests replacing those using animals,

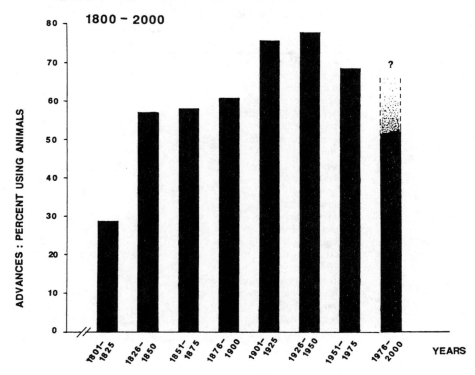

FIGURE 1.2

Major biomedical advances made since 1800, showing the number in which animals made important contributions (Nicoll and Russell, 1991). The trend toward the increasing use of animals may be reversed by the strategy of reducing, replacing, and refining the current, animal-oriented, test systems with *in vitro* screening assays to assess many endpoints of toxicity.

most see these techniques as screening tools to indicate relative toxicity or to explore mechanisms of action, thereby reducing and/or refining the number of *in vivo* studies required. However, it is unrealistic to expect animal use to approach zero.

Toxicology plays a pivotal role in the development of drugs, agrochemicals, food additives, home products, cosmetics, industrial chemicals, etc. An examination of product development reveals that toxicological studies account for some 12 to 15% of the total budget. As is shown in Figure 1.3, toxicity studies begin early in development, almost from the day the new chemical leaves the synthetic chemists' hands. The identification of any adverse health effect during the animal toxicological studies may result in the entire project being abandoned overnight with the chemical being "shelved." It has been estimated that, for one reason or another, only about 1 chemical out of 10,000 tested ever reaches the stage of being marketed as a drug. For agrochemicals, the success rate is 1 chemical in 15,000 agents undergoing assessment and this ratio may decrease even further as regulatory criteria for environmental impact assessments are met.

The results obtained from a toxicological study depends largely upon what efforts are put into the design and conductance of the study. The investigation must be optimized to observe the effects anticipated by a consideration of structure-activity relationships and also those serendipidous observations suggestive of toxicity of an unsuspected nature. The following chapters will attempt to examine the various

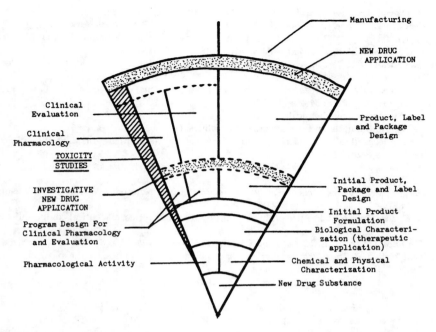

FIGURE 1.3

A schematic diagram showing where the discipline of toxicology impacts on the development of a new therapeutic agent. Initial toxicological screening of the chemical begins early, at a time comparable to when the pharmacological activity and therapeutic application are being explored. The detection of serious adverse biological effects such as mutagenesis or hepatic toxicity may result in (1) cancellation of the development of the drug or (2) a return to basic chemistry to modify the structure to minimize the toxicity. The absence of toxic effects in the initial testing phase will subsequently advance the chemical to more detailed scrutiny in long-term, more labor-intensive, and more costly studies.

designs of different types of toxicological studies in current use, why they are conducted in a certain manner, and their usefulness and limitations in assessing the potential hazard(s) to health.

REFERENCES

Adams, E.M., Irish, D.S., Spencer, H.C., and Rowe, V.K. The response of rabbit skin to compounds reported to have caused acneform dermatitis. *Indus. Med. Indus. Hygiene* Section 2: 1-4 (1941).

Ames, B.H. Dietary carcinogens and anticarcinogens. *Science* 221, 1256-1264 (1983).

Anon. Evaluation of health aspects of GRAS food ingredients: lessons learned and questions unanswered. *Fed. Proc.* 36: 2527-2562 (1977). Report of Select Committee on GRAS substances.

Bettmann, von, S. Chlorakne eine besondere form van professionaller hauterkrankung. *Deutsche. Med. Wochenschr.* 27: 437 (1901).

Bloch, B. and Dreifuss, W. Ueber die experimentelle erzeugung von carcinoma mit lymphdrusen — und lungen metastasen durch teerbestandteile. *Schweiz. Med. Wochenschr.* 51: 1033-1037 (1921).

Canadian Council on Animal Care (CCAC). Research animal use in Canada, 1989. CCAC Resource 15, 1 (1990).

Gad, S.C. Recent developments in replacing, reducing and refining animal use in toxicologic research and testing. *Fund. Appl. Toxicol.* 15, 8-16 (1990).

Gallo, M.A., Scheuplein, R.J., and van der Heijden, K. (Editors). Biological Basis for Risk Assessment of Dioxins and Related Compounds. *Banbury Report* 35. Cold Spring Harbor Laboratory Press, Plainview, N.Y. (1991).

Gough, M. *Dioxin, Agent Orange.* Plenum Press, New York (1986), pp. 27-33.

Hay, A. *The Chemical Scythe. Lessons of 2,4,5-T and Dioxins.* Plenum Press, New York (1982), pp. 89-93.

Hayes, Jr., W.J. *Toxicology of Pesticides.* Williams and Wilkins Company, Baltimore, MD. (1975).

Herxheimer, K. Uber chlorakne. *Munch. Med. Wochenschr.* 46: 278-283 (1899).

Higuchi, K. (Editor). *PCB Poisoning and Pollution.* Kodansha Ltd., Tokyo and Academic Press, New York (1976).

Kimmeg, J. and Schulz, K.H. Occupational acne (so-called chloracne) due to chlorinated aromatic cyclic ethers. *Dermatologica* 115: 540-546 (1957).

Maugh, II, T.H. How many chemicals are there? *Science* 220: 293 (1983).

McBride, W.G. Thalidomide and congenital abnormalities. *Lancet* 2: 1358-1362 (1961).

Nicoll, C.S. and Russell, S.M. Mozart, Alexander the Great and the animal rights/liberation philosophy. *FASEB J.* 5, 2888-2892 (1991).

NRC/NAS. *Toxicity Testing, Strategies to Determine Needs and Priorities.* National Academy Press, Washington, D.C. (1984).

NRC/NAS. *Complex Mixtures. Methods For In Vivo Toxicity Testing.* National Academy Press, Washington, D.C. (1988).

Parkinson, C. and Grasso, P. The use of the dog in toxicity tests on pharmaceutical compounds. *Human Exper. Toxicol.* 12, 99-109 (1993).

Pott, P. *Chirurgical Observations Relative to the Cataract, the Polypus of the Nose, the Cancer of the Scrotum, the Different Kinds of Ruptures and the Mortification of the Toes and Feet.* James, Clarke and Gillins, London (1775).

Reggiani, G. Medical problems raised by the TCDD contamination in Seveso, Italy. *Arch. Toxicol.* 40: 161-188 (1978).

Somers, G.F. Thalidomide and congenital abnormalities. *Lancet* 2: 912-914 (1962).

Spencer, K.E.V. Thalidomide and congenital abnormalities. *Lancet* 2: 100-101 (1962).

Spencer, P.S., Schaumburg, N.H., Sabri, M.I., and Veronesi, B. The enlarging view of hexacarbon neurotoxicity. *CRC Critical Reviews in Toxicology* 7: 279-356 (1980).

Tuchmann-Duplessis, H. Drugs acting on the central nervous system. In *Drug Effects on the Fetus.* ADIS Press, Sydney (1975), pp. 142-146.

Varma, D.R. Anatomy of the methyl isocyanate leak in Bhopal. In *Hazard Assessment of Chemicals.* Vol. 5. J. Saxena (Ed.). Hemisphere Publishers, Washington, D.C. (1986), pp. 233-289.

Whelan, E. *Toxic Terror.* Jameson Books, Ottawa, IL. (1985).

White, G.F. Environment. *Science* 209: 183-190 (1980).

Wilson, E. Use of primates in teratological research and testing. In *Malformations Congenitales des Mammiferes.* H. Tuchmann-Duplessis (Ed.), Masson, Paris (1971), pp. 273-290.

Yamagiwa, K. and Ichikawa, K. Experimental study of the pathogenesis of carcinoma. *J. Cancer Res.* 3: 1-29 (1918).

Chapter 2

PRELIMINARY CONSIDERATIONS

I. INTRODUCTION

Toxicity testing as we know it today began as an outgrowth of the science of biological standardization, the assessment of the potency of drug preparations derived from plant and animal sources by the use of isolated tissues or intact animals to standardize different batches of material to constant biological activities. A survey of the monographs in early editions of the British Pharmacopoeia, the U.S. Pharmacopeia, or the National Formulary will demonstrate the extent to which dose-effect relationships were developed to assess equivalency between a standard formulation and a newly prepared, untested drug. The standardization of Tincture of Digitalis B.P. — using the anesthetized guinea pig into which sufficient digitalis solution was administered by intravenous injection to bring the animal to the brink of arrythmias or cardiac toxicity — is a classical example of such assay procedures (General Medical Council, 1953). With a conscious decision that the harmful effects of chemical and physical agents should be established in animals rather than by trial-and-error in humans, major questions arose. What animal species should be used? How many animals are needed? How long should studies be conducted? Should specific experiments be designed for each toxicological effect? Should an "omnibus approach" be used, where the animals' responses to a battery of standardized clinical and laboratory tests could be employed to "catch" and identify any harmful or undesired effects as they occurred? Early studies demonstrated that while there were many situations when different species behaved in a similar manner when exposed to the same agent, species sensitivity and specificity were strong exceptions to the rules.

The fundamental aim of any toxicological study is to obtain biological (biochemical, physiological, morphological) information indicative of toxicity that is reproducible, reliable, and dose-related and which can be interpreted and/or extended to the assessment of health risks to the human. From the early 1900s, elaborate protocols, partly of the omnibus type and partly specific, have evolved to the point where they have become standardized. They are designed so that high doses of agent are administered over short or prolonged periods of time by various routes to animals that are euthanized at predetermined time intervals to permit necropsy, biochemical and microscopic examination of the organs and comparison with results obtained from animals dying or becoming moribund during the treatment period (Zbinden, 1973). While investigators have tended to treat these regulatory agency-spawned protocols as the gospel, such blanket reliance should not be encouraged. There are a number of preliminary considerations that investigators should resolve prior to embarking on any large-scale experimentation.

II. THE AGENT BEING TESTED

The investigator should have a long discussion with a knowledgeable chemist about the physical and chemical properties of the test agent, including the physical state, the solubility in aqueous or suitable organic vehicles (natural vegetable oils, organic solvents), and the extent or upper limits of solubility in media appropriate for *in vivo* administration. Many agents have only limited water solubility, making it almost impossible to attain concentrations that could elicit toxic effects if the chemical is to be administered intraperitoneally, intravenously, subcutaneously, or via the drinking water. Insolubility in aqueous media will necessitate preparing an emulsion or dissolving the agent in a suitable "inert" organic vehicle, which may limit the routes(s) of administration to oral (gastric lavage) or intraperitoneal techniques.

The chemical stability of the agent in solution or in suspension must be known in order that the investigator will be aware of the frequency with which fresh dosage forms must be prepared. The presence of an abiotic degradation product is disconcerting from the viewpoints that: (1) the biological effects attributed to the parent chemical may be enhanced (or reduced) by this product, and (2) the degradation product may be erroneously considered as a metabolite formed *in vivo*. If the agent is to be administered in the diet or the drinking water of the animal, the stability in the medium must be ascertained if one wishes to avoid preparing fresh solutions or diets every day. Animal feeds contain plant material including chlorophyll and other components which, taken along with supplemental vitamins and minerals, are highly reactive and can interact with the test substance. Suppliers of animal diets should be consulted concerning the ingredients in their formulations. Many such firms provide analyses of prepared diets.

Consideration should also be given to the availability of reliable methods of analysis of the test substance and biotransformation products in tissues and biological fluids. If suitable methods are not available, the analytical people should be encouraged to develop or modify existing methodology in preparation for this essential requirement. Residue analysis will become an important aspect of your study. The objective of a toxicological study is to develop a relationship between the dose (concentration at target sites) of the test substance and the response (a quantifiable, biological effect). Sensitive and reproducible analytical techniques will be required to quantify the absorption, disposition, biotransformation, and elimination of the administered dosage of the test substance.

III. THE VEHICLE

The physicochemical properties of the test substance will largely dictate how the agent will be administered to the animals. Limited aqueous solubility will force the investigator to consider media such as emulsions or solutions in vegetable oils or organic solvents in order to achieve dosage levels capable of eliciting toxicity. The use of vegetable oils (corn, olive, peanut, sunflower, soya, etc.) poses several problems. First, there may be an enhancement of absorption of the orally administered agent from the intestinal tract, with greater target organ toxicity being observed than that reported in other studies. The converse situation may also be encountered: absorption (and toxicity) being reduced and the agent being retained in the lumen of the gastrointestinal tract with the vehicle (Condie et al., 1986; Kim et al., 1990b). Different vehicles may dramatically affect the pharmacokinetics of organic chemicals absorbed from the intestinal tract (Kim et al., 1990a; Withy et al., 1983). Since both the vehicle and test substance must be metabolized by the animal, interactions can be anticipated. Early studies with DDT, and later with PCBs, revealed that oral administration in corn oil resulted in the appearance of large lipid inclusions in rat hepatocytes, suggesting some difficulty in assimilating this oil into the system. However, if these toxicants were administered in peanut oil, the inclusions were not seen, although comparable levels of toxicant were measured in the tissues (Ecobichon, unpublished). The use of aqueous emulsions, based on Polysorbate®- or Tween®- (polyoxyethylene [20] sorbitan mono-oleate), Triton® (octylphenoxy polyethoxyethanol), or Emulphor® (polyethylene glycol esters of fatty acids) type emulsifiers may pose the same problems as vegetable oils, enhancing or retarding absorption and possibly eliciting differences in pharmacokinetics and tissue responses. The use of alcohols, glycols, dimethyl sulfoxide, etc., as organic vehicles for toxicants administered by the ingestion or intraperitoneal route should be explored with considerable caution since such organic compounds are only relatively "inert".

Suitable vehicles for the dermal application of toxicants pose the same problems as those mentioned above. While solutions of minimally water-soluble chemicals can be prepared in a variety of synthetic or natural organic materials, problems of more efficient penetration of the skin and enhanced systemic toxicity or retarded (delayed) absorption accompanied by reduced toxicity may be encountered. Water-soluble agents do not pass easily through the dermal barrier and emulsification tends to further reduce efficient absorption.

The administration of highly polar test substances, i.e., the salts of synthetic organic chemicals, via the drinking water does not pose a significant problem. However, marginally water-soluble organic compounds (solvents and other industrial chemicals, pesticides, etc.) tend to adhere to glass or plastic surfaces with a substantial fraction of the dose becoming "unavailable" to the animal within minutes or hours of filling the drinking bottle or the aquarium. As the relative water solubility of a chemical decreases, bioavailability becomes a significant problem. Such difficulties are frequently encountered in toxicological studies in laboratory aquatic systems, the toxicant still being present in the aquarium but being unavailable to the target organism as a consequence of adsorption to tank walls, algae, plant material, gravel, etc. It would be essential to carry out analyses to confirm the distribution of the test agent in solution.

The inhalation of aerosolized toxicants, dissolved in suitable organic vehicles, emulsified in aqueous media or in water or physiological saline, pose some major problems. The presence of so-called "inert" emulsifiers and cosolvents may elicit a generalized irritational response of the sensitive pulmonary tissue accompanied by alveolar macrophase mobilization and proliferation, inflammation, interstitial edema, etc., effects totally unrelated to the test agent (Chevalier et al., 1984; Breckenridge et al., 1986). Appropriate control animals must be carried through the study exposed only to the vehicle. An important factor to be considered with aerosols and with suspended solid particles (dusts, fibers) is that the particle size must be in the respirable range of 2.0 to 4.0 µm in diameter in order to ensure efficient uptake of the toxicant by the lungs (Breckenridge et al., 1986).

IV. ROUTES OF ADMINISTRATION

For any toxicological study, the route by which an agent is administered to the test species should mimic, as closely as possible, the route by which that animal would normally acquire the chemical under the circumstances of exposure. In the situation of human occupational exposure, oral ingestion, dermal contact and inhalation may all be important routes of toxicant acquisition. However, industrial hygiene measurements of the "work environment" may identify only one or two hazardous routes of exposure. For the development of toxicity data on drugs, ingestion, inhalation, and topical application may be the proposed routes of treatment, but other routes, including intravenous or subcutaneous or intrathecal injection, may require study. In gathering toxicity data from animal models used as surrogates for the human, the route(s) of administration should be the same as those by which the human would receive the agent. Generally, one has to consider oral gavage, dermal application, and inhalation.

In the area of veterinary medicine, the agent can be given by the most appropriate route in the most appropriate dosage form, using as a test species that animal in which the drug is destined for use. In studies using wildlife species, the potential toxicant can be incorporated into the diet, applied to the skin, or mixed into the medium (soil, water, air) that they inhabit, thereby allowing exposure to occur in the normal manner. As indicated above, dissolution of the test agent in an appropriate medium, the maintenance of concentrations of agent that will be bioavailable to the test animals, and the stability of the agent in the medium are all factors that must receive careful consideration and confirmation by analytical results prior to starting the experiments.

V. SPECIES

Prior to selecting animal species for toxicological studies, consideration should be given to the battery of tests required relative to the end-use of the product (drug, food additive, pesticide, industrial product, home care product, personal care products, cosmetics, etc.). Some of the *in vivo* studies can be replaced by time- and cost-saving, *in vitro*, alternative tests, thereby reducing the numbers of animals required. Regulatory agencies, particularly the European Economic Community (EEC) have shown a strong move toward alternative testing, particularly for certain products, i.e., cosmetics to be banned from sale in the EEC after 1998 if they have been tested in animals (Langley, 1994). There is a greater acceptance of alternative testing protocols by North American regulatory agencies and a move away from the dichotomy of "what would you (government) like to receive vs. what test results would you (industry) like to send for consideration." However, such tests will never entirely replace those carried out in animals and the toxicologist is still faced with pertinent questions in the design of appropriate studies.

In environmental impact studies or the development of veterinary pharmaceuticals, the investigator usually has the luxury of using the species ultimately esposed to the agent. In contrast, the toxicological consequences of chemical exposure of the human requires that animals be used as surrogate models. However, the decision must be made concerning which species will be selected as the test animals. Serious considerations must be given to the biological and physiological differences between the various animals available as is shown in Table 2.1 for eight species. Experience has taught that there is no perfect surrogate for the human, each species coping with the agents — absorption, distribution, biotransformation, and elimination — in a distinctive manner, frequently by rates and routes far different from those used by the human (Williams, 1959, 1974; Parke and Smith, 1977). Remarkable qualitative and quantitative differences in enzymatic activities exist between species. Intraspecies variability is prevalent and is controlled genetically by selecting inbred (homogeneous) or

TABLE 2.1

Biological and Physiological Parameters for Common Laboratory Animals

Parameters	Monkey	Dog	Cat	Rabbit	Rat	Mouse	Guinea pig	Hamster
Adult body weight (kg)	3.5	14.0	3.3	3.7	0.45	0.035	0.43	0.12
Life-span (years)	16	15	14	6	3	1.5	31	30
Water consumption (ml/day)	450	350	320	300	35	6	145	30
Food consumption (adult, g/day)	150	400	100	180	10	5	12	10
Adult metabolism (cal/kg/day)	158	80	80	110	130	600	100	250
Body temperature (°C)	38.8	38.9	38.6	39.4	38.2	37.4	38.6	38.0
Respiratory rate (breaths/min)	50	20	25	53	85	160	90	83
	(40–60)	(10–30)	(20–30)	(40–65)	(65–110)	(80–240)	(70–100)	(35–130)
Heart rate (beats/min)	200	100	120	200	328	600	300	450
Blood pressure (systolic/diastolic, mmHg)	159/127	148/100	155/100	110/80	130/90	120/75	77/50	108/77
Birth weight (g)	500–700	1100–2200	125	100	5–6	1.5	75–100	2.0
Weight at weaning (g)	4400	5800	3000	100–1500	40–50	10–12	250	35
Eyes open (days)	Birth	8–12	8–12	10	10–12	11	Birth	15
Gestation (days)	168	63	63	31	21	20	67	16
Estrus cycle (days)	28	22	15–28	15–16	4–5	4–5	16–19	4
Duration of estrus (days)	1–2	7–13	9–19	30	1	1	1	1
					(1600–2200)	(2200–0100)	(6–15 h)	(4–23 h)
Litter size	1	3–6	1–6	1–13	6–9	1–12	1–5	1–12
Weaning age (weeks)	16–24	6	6–9	8	3–4	3	2	3–4
Breeding age (months)	54	9	10	6–7	2–3	2	3	2
Breeding life (years)	10–15	5–10	4	1–3	1	1	3	1
Breeding season	Anytime	Spring and fall	2–3 mos. (winter)	Anytime	Anytime	Anytime	Anytime	Anytime
Floor space required (ft²)	6	8	3	3	0.4	0.4	0.7	0.34
Environmental temperature range (°F)	68–72	55–65	60–65	60–65	65–75	68–74	65–75	65–75
Blood volume (ml/kg)	75	79	60	53	65	80	75	85
Clotting time (seconds)	90	180	120	300	60	14	60	143
Hematocrit (% red blood cells)	42	45	40	42	46	41	42	50
Hemoglobin (g/100 ml)	12.5	16.0	11.8	13.6	14.8	16.0	12.4	12.0

Data courtesy of ARS/Sprague Dawley, Division of Mogul Corporation, Madison, WI.

TABLE 2.2

Comparison of Features of Inbred and Outbred Strains of Animals

Parameter	Inbred Strains	Outbred Strains
Breeding program	Closed colonies with brother-sister matings over 20 generations	Closed colonies with random or haphazard matings or by a system
Genetic variability	Reduced variability	Reasonably uniform but each animal genetically distinct
Phenotype/Genotype	Greater uniformity	Greater diversity
Genetic stability and characteristics	Stable for prolonged time but eventually will see changes between isolated colonies of the same strain from different sources	Genetic composition will change with time (years) due to selection and genetic drift, particularly when from different sources
Genetic control	Quality control can be measured	Quality control is very difficult to monitor
General health	Susceptible to tumors, degenerative diseases, and shorter lifespan	Hybrid vigor results in lower susceptibility to tumors, diseases, and a longer lifespan
Response characteristics	Uniformity in response to agents	Greater diversity in response due to phenotypic variability

outbred (heterogeneous) strains of the animal. Interspecies variability is the rule rather than the exception, and it is safe to say that no one animal species closely mimics the human in all respects. A living animal model, with definitive capabilities of absorbing, distributing, biotransforming, eliminating, and storing a potential toxicant, provides a closer approximation to another living animal than other "models." While no single species reflects the physiological complexity of any other species, experimental models can produce qualitative/quantitative results that can be extrapolated to other species.

Several authors have addressed the merits of using inbred or outbred strains of rodents (Festing, 1987, 1990, 1995; Gill, 1980; Kalter, 1981; Lovell and Festing, 1982; Yamada et al., 1979). A comparison of significant properties of inbred and outbred strains of animals is shown in Table 2.2 (Festing, 1995). The term "isogenic strain" denotes inbred strains produced by more than 20 generations of brother × sister mating and F_1 hybrids between two such strains (Festing, 1990). An inbred strain may be regarded as "an immortal clone of genetically identical individuals." Being genetically uniform, they should remain genetically constant for many years. The capability of an isogenic strain of animals to biotransform selected groups of drugs can be phenotypically and genotypically profiled, remaining stable for many generations. F_1 hybrids, the first generation cross between two inbred strains, are as isogenic as inbred animals except that they are not homozygous at all genetic loci. They exhibit hybrid vigour in that these animals frequently have a longer life span, appear to be more resistant to common diseases, and show a lower background level of spontaneous tumor formation, many of these being genetically determined. More will be said about this problem when carcinogenicity testing is discussed.

Outbred strains of rodents are closed colonies which are usually propagated through random or haphazard mating or by an established breeding system, avoiding the mating of close relatives (Festing, 1995). While the colony of animals is reasonably uniform in characteristics, each individual is genetically distinct. Outbred strains show genetic variability between colonies from different sources even though they may bear a generic name, i.e., Wistar, Sprague Dawley, Swiss, etc. They will be phenotypically variable and, even within a single colony, the genetic characteristics will change in subtle fashion with time and breeding, distinct phenotypes being identifiable within colonies.

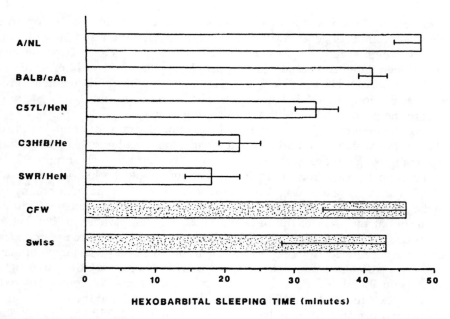

FIGURE 2.1

Differences between inbred (open bars) and randomly bred (closed bars) strains of mice as measured by the mean duration (minutes) of sleeping time induced by an intraperitoneal injection of hexobarbital (125 mg/kg body weight). The small horizontal lines represent the standard deviations of mean values determined from 29 to 63 animals per group (Jay, 1955).

The use of inbred strains allows precise control over the response to the biological parameter being studied, whereas the experiments with outbred strains will be subject to considerable variability between phenotypically and genotypically distinct animals. Frequently, one encounters the use of outbred strains justified by statements that "humans are outbred, so outbred animals represent a better model than inbred animals" or "outbred animals approximate a human population." However, the deliberate use of heterogeneous animals cannot be justified in toxicological research (Festing, 1990). In this age of conservation of animal resources in research, small changes in response(s) can be identified much more easily in fewer animals of inbred strains, thereby reducing the numbers required per treatment group since one can significantly reduce interanimal variability.

Intraspecies (inter- and intrastrain) variability can be measured by examining a simple biological parameter such as the duration of sleeping time induced by the drug hexobarbital in a number of inbred and outbred strains of laboratory mice (Figure 2.1) (Jay, 1955). The duration of sleep — the time interval measured from the loss of the righting reflex to the recovery of the reflex — is largely controlled by the rate of biotransformation of the agent, a factor that is quite different between the five inbred (hybrid) and two outbred mouse strains shown. The results illustrate several important concepts. First, there are obvious differences between the inbred (homogeneous) strains, the mean sleeping time ranging from 18 to 48 min. However, the small standard deviations demonstrate that, with any one inbred strain, the treated animals responded within relatively narrow limits, signifying minimal interanimal variability. In contrast, the results from both outbred (heterogeneous) strains, while showing comparable sleeping times, also show extensive interanimal variations in response, as is indicated by the large standard deviations recorded.

More serious concerns about closed colonies, inbred or outbred, have surfaced with the observations of genetic drift being expressed in more rapid growth, greater mean body weights, reduced 2-year survival rates, and increased incidence and severity of age-related diseases including neoplasia (Roe, 1981; Salmon et al., 1990; Nohynek et al., 1993; Hart et al., 1995a). This subject will be discussed in greater detail under Section VIII since diet, supplied *ad libitum*, appears to be a factor contributing to the problems in addition to breeding practices.

The controversy over the use of inbred vs. outbred strains of animals in toxicological experiments has been addressed at the macromolecular level by DNA fingerprinting, comparing the degree of band sharing between strains (Festing, 1992, 1993, 1995). Theoretically, members of an inbred colony should be like identical twins, with 100% band sharing unless the colonies have been kept separated for many years or genetic contamination has been introduced. Band sharing across 10 different inbred strains of rats was of the order of 34 ± 15%, comparable to that found in humans picked at random (Festing, 1992). Within six stocks of outbred animals (rats), the band sharing ranged from 84 to 95 ± 5%, indicative of a high degree of genetic uniformity far different from that measured between humans. Other investigators have found considerable variations in outbred mouse strains in colonies isolated for many years (Rice and O'Brien, 1980). Festing hypothesized that the reported differences between mice and rats may have been due to the establishment of rat colonies with fewer breeding pairs, accidentally leading to closer inbreeding simply because of the relative greater amount of space required for the housing of rats than for mice (Festing, 1995).

Unfortunately, the choice of animal to be used in a study is frequently based on the objectives of the experiment, previous experience with the species, convenient size, ease of breeding and rearing, and the cost of purchasing, accomodation, and care rather than on the basis of biological similarity to the human. Frequently, national and international regulatory agencies stipulate that toxicity data be obtained from studies conducted in two species, one of which must be a nonrodent. It is too easy to blindly select the rat or mouse as the rodent species and the dog or nonhuman primate as the nonrodent species without serious consideration of the biological similarities and differences between these or other potential surrogate species and the human. While many animal species have been used in the assessment of acute toxicity, the laboratory rat (*Rattus norvegicus*) has become the most commonly used model for predictive acute toxicity testing, partly for reasons of expediency and cost and partly because a vast, comparative data base exists for agents tested in this species, i.e., pesticides and industrial chemicals (Gaines, 1969; Gage, 1970). A similar statement could be made for the laboratory mouse (*Mus musculus*), although far greater strain differences exist than the variability observed between strains of rats. In costly, labor-intensive chronic exposure studies where mechanisms of action are explored concomitant with overt/covert target organ toxicity, the selection of the appropriate test species is far more critical and should reflect, as closely as possible, the species of concern. The rat might well be an appropriate model based upon extensive experience of the background physiology and pathology of the species, as well prior testing of innumerable toxicants and the identification of target organ toxicity. However, valuable toxicity data is just as likely to come from nonrodent species such as the dog, swine, or nonhuman primates. Before initiating any toxicity study, it is crucial to *"know your model"*, to understand something about the pharmaco- or toxicokinetics of the test substance, its biotransformation and elimination from the test organism.

VI. PHARMACOKINETICS/TOXICOKINETICS

Pharmacokinetics is defined as the qualitative and quantitative study of the time course of absorption, distribution, biotransformation, and elimination of an agent in an intact organism (plant or animal). Such information is useful in predicting the duration of toxicant action following exposure, the persistence of the agent and/or transformation products in target organs, and the disposition in storage sites, yielding body burdens of the agent. The time course of the above processes is usually followed by the chemical analysis of serial samples of suitable biological fluids (peripheral blood, urine, milk, amniotic fluid, etc.) or whole organisms, if small, for the content of the parent chemical and/or biotransformation products. Target organ toxicity can usually be correlated with the ability (or inability) of a particular animal species to biotransform and/or eliminate a given dosage of toxicant efficiently from the body, which is frequently reflected in altered pharmacokinetic parameters. Major species differences in toxicity can be anticipated if pharmacokinetic data is obtained from a few animals (rodent, nonrodent) receiving low-to-moderate concentrations of the agent prior to initiating more extensive studies. Such information not only allows the correlation of toxic signs and symptoms with blood/tissue levels of the agent, but also permits the selection of suitable animal species and a regimen including: (1) an acceptable **route of administration**, i.e., in daily diet, by oral gavage, by injection, by dermal application, or by inhalation; (2) **dosage range,** at least some idea of acceptable low, intermediate and high concentrations (mg/kg body wt); and (3), the **frequency of treatment**, particularly important for the oral gavage, injection, or inhalation of single bolus doses once a day or smaller amounts at intervals throughout the day.

To briefly convey some concepts of pharmacokinetic principles, let us examine a theoretical model based upon "buckets" (Figure 2.2). Exposure of mammals, birds, amphibians, fish, etc., to a concentration of agent via any route would result in the initial appearance of the chemical in the bloodstream. Given that each organism has a finite volume of blood, the measurement of chemical residues in serial blood samples would produce the kinetic curve in Figure 2.2A, low levels of agent being detected initially with a gradual increase with time to a plateau level when the agent is completely mixed with the blood volume (dotted line). However, such a model is too simplified. This is not what occurs *in vivo* since agent will be lost from the bloodstream, diffusing out into tissues, the first and foremost group being those in the so-called **central compartment** of the body, the tissues being characterized by having a good blood flow, a high perfusion rate through dense capillary networks, and possessing good "extractive" capabilities, i.e., ability to remove or absorb agent from the blood. Continued analysis of serial blood samples would reveal a decline in blood concentration as the agent is diluted and distributed in this compartment and is removed from the general circulation (Figure 2.2B). The diagram also shows that some excretion can occur from this compartment, with agent being lost through the urine and feces and, in some instances, exhaled via the lungs if the agent is volatile or via gill membranes in aquatic species if the agent is water-soluble. Amphibian species may secrete chemicals through their skin. Further dilution and distribution of the blood-borne agent occurs when the blood reaches the **peripheral compartment**, a much larger fraction of the body mass, composed of the skin, skeletal muscle, adipose tissue, and bone. These tissues have a poorer blood supply, lack dense capillary networks, and have a much lower tissue perfusion rate with less extractive capabilities. Depending upon the physicochemical properties of the agent,

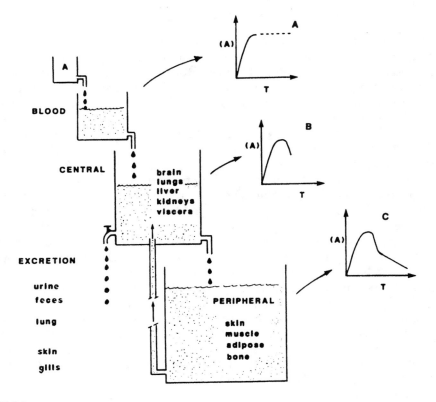

FIGURE 2.2
A schematic diagram demonstrating the dilution and distribution of an agent "A" in the bloodstream and in the central and peripheral tissue compartments of a vertebrate organism. The tissues comprising each compartment are shown as are the routes of excretion, including the skin and gills of aquatic/amphibian species. The results of analyzing serial samples of blood for residues of agent "A" are shown in the theoretical plots of concentration against time indicated as A, B, and C.

extensive deposition can occur in certain of these tissues: lipophilic polychlorinated biphenyls (PCBs) will be localized in the body fat while a toxicant like lead (Pb) will be stored in the long bones. Continued measurement of chemical residues in serial blood samples will reveal the curve (Figure 2.2C), distribution and dilution having been completed and the latter portion of the curve showing a linear relationship between concentration of agent and time. As there are no mechanisms of excretion in the peripheral compartment of most test organisms, the agent and/or biotransformation products must be returned to the central compartment for elimination from the body. However, in other animals, notably aquatic and amphibian species, the skin may be an important route of loss of toxicant and degradation products into the surrounding medium.

While there are any number of complex, computer-derived models for the pharmacokinetics of chemicals *in vivo*, most agents of concern to toxicologists can be accomodated by a classical, simple, two-compartment, open model (Figure 2.3). Administered intravenously to avoid the kinetic complications of absorption into the bloodstream, these theoretical curves demonstrate the disappearance of agent from the blood as the agent is distributed in the **central compartment** (solid line) with the appearance of agent, the attainment of a peak level, and the subsequent disappearance of agent from the **peripheral compartment** (dotted line). Note that

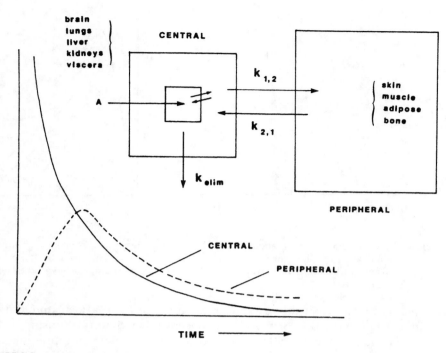

FIGURE 2.3
A diagram of an open, two-compartment kinetic model showing the organs/tissues comprising each compartment and the kinetic constants associated with distribution within compartments and that related to elimination of an agent. The graph of concentration against time portrays the disappearance of an intravenously administered dosage from the bloodstream (solid line) and the theoretical concentrations that might be measured in the peripheral compartment (dotted line) if sampling was done.

the lines are curvilinear since the graph is plotted as concentration against time. The size (volume) of the two compartments can shrink or enlarge depending upon the chemical and its aqueous or lipid solubility and patterns of storage. In addition, nutritional status, general well-being, or disease state can significantly alter adipose and muscle mass or alter the normal hepatic and/or renal function, thereby affecting tissue distribution. Pregnancy, where the developing fetus becomes a component of the central compartment, can increase the size of the volume of this compartment.

Considering the single exposure situation, Figure 2.4 shows the various phases of the time course of a blood level of theoretical chemicals, from absorption through distribution and elimination, with the blood concentration plotted in a logarithmic function. Depending upon the test organism, the route of administration, the vehicle in which the agent is dissolved or suspended, the aqueous and lipid solubility and other physicochemical properties of the test substance and the level of exposure (dosage size), the slope of the absorption phase may be steep or shallow, indicative of a rapid or slow uptake of the agent. However, even low, initial concentrations of circulating agent will be affected by tissue distribution, by biotransformation, by elimination, and by storage. Following the attainment of some peak blood concentration, the full appreciation of tissue distribution becomes apparent, with the initial decline reflecting the dilution of the agent into various tissues governed by a number of physicochemical properties of the agent and physiological properties of the tissues. In addition, the remaining agent circulating in the bloodstream is concomitantly undergoing biotransformation, elimination (agent plus biotrans-formation products), and storage. This portion of the disappearance curve, called the α-phase, is frequently

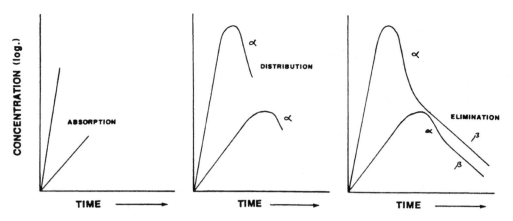

FIGURE 2.4
Theoretical profiles of the blood concentrations of two different dosage forms showing the absorption, distribution and elimination of the agent from the bloodstream with time and denoting the α-phase associated primarily with distribution and the β-phase related to storage, biotransformation, and excretion. See text for discussion.

linear or nearly linear when the residue results are plotted in a logarithmic mode against time. The last portion of the blood concentration–time relationship, called the β-phase, is linear in the logarithmic concentration–time plot and represents only three on-going processes (storage, biotransformation, elimination). With appropriate analytical methods, the latter two functions can be measured in terms of parent compound and/or biotransformation products quantified in exhaled air, blood, urine, and/or fecal samples collected over time. The storage, retention, or body burden of the agent can be estimated indirectly by the difference between the amount to which the animal is exposed and the total of the excretory products quantitated in urine, feces, and exhaled air over a period of time, with samples being obtained from animals housed in metabolic cages.

The β-phase portion of the blood elimination curve is concentration dependent, with the slope of the line reflecting the combination of storage, biotransformation, and elimination and being described by first-order kinetics. A classical example of this concentration dependence is presented in Figure 2.5, showing the disappearance of the herbicide 2,4,5-trichlorophenoxyacetic acid (2,4,5-T) from the bloodstream of rats receiving dosages ranging from 5 to 200 mg/kg body weight. (Piper et al., 1973). These results demonstrated that the slope of the line became concentration dependent above a dosage of 50 mg/kg body weight, the slope decreasing with increasing dosage. The observed linearity can be used to predict the rate of elimination with the development of a kinetic parameter known as the half-life, the elimination half-life, or, more specifically, the β-half-life ($\beta t_{1/2}$ or $\beta t_{0.5}$). This value can be determined, as is shown in Figure 2.6, with the value remaining constant until all of the chemical is eliminated. During each half-life (minutes, hours, days, weeks, or years), 50% of the toxicant in the body at the beginning of that half-life is eliminated. In theory, a toxicant eliminated by first-order kinetics is never completely eliminated from the body but, due to limits of detection of the analytical techniques, the lower end of the line usually becomes asymptotic to the baseline. The half-life of a chemical with first-order elimination characteristics is independent of the dose at low concentrations, as is seen in Figure 2.5 for 2,4,5-T at 5 and 50 mg/kg body weight where the slopes of the β-phase lines are comparable. At higher dosages, the slopes change with the concentration administered. The apparent first-order rate constant, the

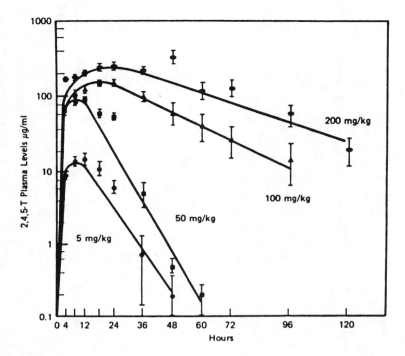

FIGURE 2.5

Concentrations of 2,4,5-trichlorophenoxyacetic acid (2,4,5-T) in the blood plasma of rats as a function of time following a single oral dose of [^{14}C] 2,4,5-T at either 5, 50, 100, or 200 mg/kg body wt. (From Piper et al., *Toxicol. Appl. Pharmacol.* 26: 339–351 [1973]. With permission.)

elimination constant (k_{el}) can be obtained graphically from the slope of the concentration-time relationship, the slope being equal to $-k_{el}/2.303$, with the k_{el} being obtained from the ratio $0.693/t_{1/2}$. Similar semilogarithmic plots of blood levels of agent vs. time after administration can be used to assess strain differences in pharmacodynamic responses, particularly if the agent is extensively biotransformed by hepatic enzymes. This was demonstrated for desmethyl-diazepam in three outbred strains of rats (van der Laan et al., 1993). The short (or long) $\beta t_{1/2}$ values and volumes of distribution (v_d) for desmethyl-diazepam correlated well with the hepatic levels of cytochrome P450 and the activities of 7-ethoxy-resorufin dealkylase (EROD), one strain having an average $\beta t_{1/2}$ of 34 min while the other two strains had $\beta t_{1/2}$ values of the order of 70 min.

The utility of the $\beta t_{1/2}$ and k_{el} is not only in the prediction of the rate of elimination of a single dose of agent from a body fluid in order to attain nontoxic or negligible levels. The same toxicokinetic approach may be used to estimate the disappearance of an acquired body burden of toxicant. One example, shown in Figure 2.7A, demonstrates the progression and regression of neurological signs and symptoms of a patient poisoned by methylmercury dicyandiamide in the 1972 Iraq epidemic, relating these with blood mercury levels (Clarkson, 1987). Replotting the blood mercury concentrations in logarithmic function reveals a linear, first-order relationship between blood level and time, permitting one to predict how long it will take before negligible levels of mercury might be attained (Figure 2.7B).

Frequently, removal of the subject(s) from the source of contaminant results in a linear decline in the body burden of agent that follows the first-order kinetic scenario. An example is shown for the highly lipophilic insecticide DDT and its

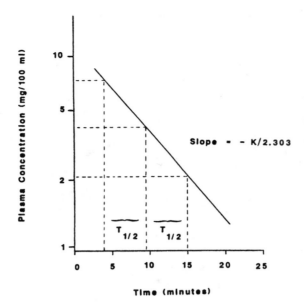

FIGURE 2.6

Plot of the concentration of an agent in blood plasma (as a logarithmic function) against time, with the determination of the plasma, β-phase, and half-life. The slope of the linear relationship = −k/2.303. If C = Co/2, then time "t" = $t_{1/2}$, the half-time. To derive the half-life of the agent: log Co/2 = log Co — k/2.3.$t_{1/2}$; or log 2 = k/2.3.$t_{1/2}$ or 0.693 = k $t_{1/2}$.

metabolites in cattle (Figure 2.8). Another example is that shown by polychlorinated biphenyls (PCBs) such as Aroclor 1254, a highly lipophilic mixture eliminated at extremely slow rates from body burdens in adipose tissue, with median β$t_{1/2}$ values of the order of 2.5 to 6.5 years being measured (Figure 2.9) (Phillips et al., 1989). An important kinetic parameter is illustrated by this data. A concentration-dependent decline in body burden is shown: the lower the tissue concentration, the slower the agent is recycled out of storage from adipose tissue into the bloodstream and the longer is the half-life value for removal from the blood (both biotransformation/excretion and re-storage).

The data shown in Figure 2.9 illustrates another important facet of toxicology: the body burden of a toxicant. Unfortunately, exposure does not occur once but repeatedly or cyclically. Consider wildlife, factory workers, or the general population who experience frequent exposure (daily, weekly, monthly, seasonally, annually) resulting in the acquisition of a body burden of toxicants if the body cannot efficiently biotransform and/or eliminate them. The scientific literature is replete with examples of heavy metal, pesticide, drug, and industrial solvent acquisition, storage, and subsequent toxicity at a later time. Consideration must be given to the toxicokinetics associated with repeated exposure to the agent in the diet, water, and air, or during a therapeutic regimen in treating a disease. The fate of the agent in the organism may be followed by the collection and analysis of residues in suitable biological fluids and/or tissues, and the kinetics for the single exposure scenario can be applied to the repeated exposure situation, making use of the biological half-life value determined in the former.

If the periodic exposure is at an interval such that the test animal can eliminate the agent, there will be little buildup of a body burden, the agent being completely disposed of prior to the next "exposure" (Figure 2.10A). In this situation, the biological

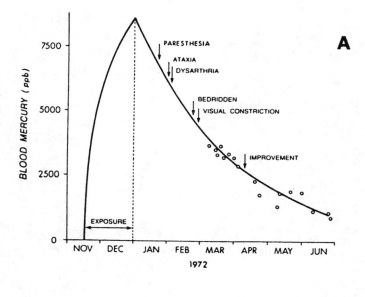

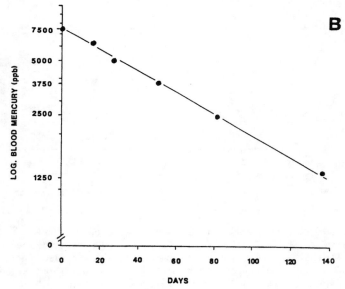

FIGURE 2.7
With no further exposure, the disappearance of an acquired body burden of a toxicant is generally first order. The example shows: (A) the arithmetic plot of theoretical and measured blood mercury concentrations of a victim in the 1971–72 poisoning outbreak in Iraq along with notations of improving clinical signs with time (Clarkson, 1987), and (B) transformation of the data by plotting the mercury concentrations as a semilogarithmic function to yield a linear relationship, thereby permitting the prediction of a rate of disappearance of the toxicant from the bloodstream.

half-life would be small in relation to the exposure interval. However, if the exposure interval was more frequent or the biological half-life was longer as a consequence of the physicochemical properties of the agent (lipid solubility, molecular size, etc.) and/or the unique biochemical/physiological parameters in the test species (selective acquisition by tissues, low rate of biotransformation, etc.), accumulation would

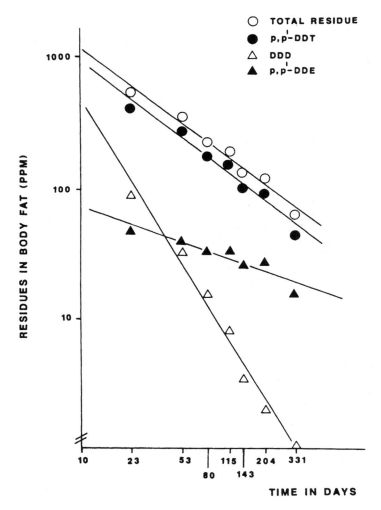

FIGURE 2.8

Regression lines demonstrating the prolonged rate of elimination of body burdens of highly liposoluble organic contaminants such as DDT and two metabolites from bovine body fat. The compound DDD (1,1-dichloro-2,2-*bis*[*p*-chlorophenyl]ethane), an intermediate degradation product, disappeared from adipose tissue within one year of contamination whereas DDE (1,1-dichloro-2,2-bis[p-chlorophenyl]ethylene), a terminal product, persisted in the body fat beyond the period of study. (Redrawn from McCully et al., 1966.)

occur. As is shown in Figure 2.10B, a second exposure to a similar level of agent, occurring before the complete elimination of the previous dose, results in a higher blood level, elevated by that fraction of the previous dose still within the system. A third exposure will increase the blood level even further since, although the agent from the first dosage has completely disappeared, there is a greater fraction of the second dosage still present. If certain assumptions (same level of exposure, same interval between exposures, first order kinetic conditions) are made, this scenario can be repeated, resulting in the pattern of accumulation shown. One important feature should be noted. If the exposure conditions remain relatively unchanged, a maximum concentration or plateau level will be reached within a time period equal to approximately a multiple of four or five times the half-life value. The cumulative

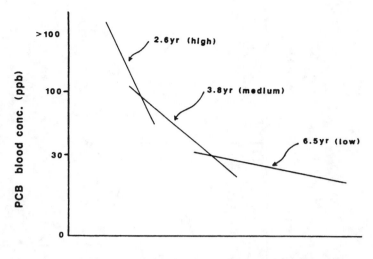

FIGURE 2.9
A schematic diagram of the relationship between the blood plasma half-life of highly lipid-soluble agents such as polychlorinated biphenyls (Aroclor 1254) and the body "burden" reflected in blood levels of agent. The lower the concentration in the blood, the longer the half-life in the bloodstream (Phillips et al., 1989.

concentration in the body fluids (tissues) will fluctuate between the exposure intervals as subsequent blood levels of agent are distributed to body compartments. The time required to attain a plateau is independent of the dosage (Figure 2.11). The **plateau concentration** is dependent upon the concentration or level of exposure, the dosage interval and the half-life (reflecting biotransformation/elimination). The fluctuations in concentration are dependent upon the dosage interval and half-life of the agent, being dramatically altered by enhanced or inhibited absorption of the agent. Within reason, the two-compartment, open model will fulfill the kinetic requirements for repeated exposure to most toxicants (PCBs, trichloroethylene, parathion, 2,4,5-T, cadmium, lead, or fluoride) in most species in defined exposure scenarios. The information necessary to develop such scenarios includes: (1) the level of exposure, (2) the exposure interval, and (3) the biological half-life (in days, months, years) of the agent. A change in either the exposure interval or the concentration of agent will result in an increased or decreased level, with the establishment of a new higher or lower plateau level and possible changes in the biological half-life.

VII. BIOTRANSFORMATION

Selective toxicity may be defined as "the injury of one kind of living matter without harming another kind with which the first is in intimate contact" (Albert, 1973). Major factors contributing to species-specific responses to potential toxicants are the rates and routes by which different animal species biotransform a foreign (xenobiotic) lipophilic agent prior to elimination (Albert, 1987). It is rarely possible to predict the relative rates of formation of particular, individual, toxic (or nontoxic) metabolites in different species, making it essential to obtain some of this information during the study of the toxicokinetic profile of the chemical. Some degree of inter- and intraspecies comparisons can be carried out using *in vitro* preparations of tissues

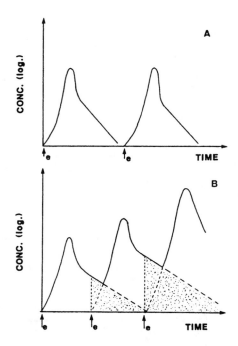

FIGURE 2.10
Schematic diagrams illustrating the toxicokinetic problems associated with repeated exposures or dosages. (A) Treatment (or exposure) was well separated, the residues of agent in the blood having been cleared prior to the second exposure (e). (B) The exposures have occurred at such a frequency that agent from the previous exposure(s) is still present in the blood. The peak blood level of the second exposure is increased by that fraction of the previous exposure still circulating in the blood. The same situation holds for the third exposure, the peak concentration being raised by the amount of agent still present in the bloodstream. Subsequent exposures will result in still higher peak concentrations until an equilibrium (uptake vs. elimination) is reached, reflected in a plateau.

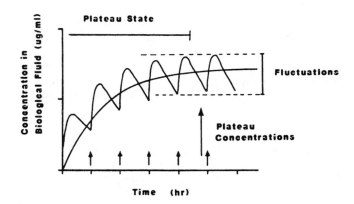

FIGURE 2.11
The effect of repeated treatment (or exposure) on the blood levels of an agent given the assumptions that the concentration of the agent and the intervals between exposure remain constant throughout the duration of the experiment. The time required to attain a plateau level is independent of the dosage (concentration) and will be reached after approximately four times the plasma, β-half-life value of the agent. Plateau concentrations are proportional to the amount of agent administered, the treatment (exposure) interval and the β-half-life. Fluctuations observed at plateau are dependent upon the β-half-life and the treatment interval.

(organ perfusion, subcellular fractions) to identify the spectrum of metabolites that may be found or to examine tissue protein binding which may explain differences in toxicity, thereby avoiding the excessive use of animals (Litterst, 1976). However, it is not possible at the present time to entirely replace *in vivo* rate-controlling processes in *in vitro* preparations. Interspecies differences in biotransformation have long piqued the interest of scientists and is far too broad a topic for this volume. The reader is encouraged to explore the history of this fascinating field by reading Williams (1959, 1974), Parke and Smith (1977), Bachmann and Bickel (1985), Albert (1987), and Hodgson and Levi (1994).

The term **biotransformation** should be used in preference to metabolism or detoxification since, as we shall see, many of the tissue enzyme-induced reactions result in an enhancement rather than in a reduction of toxicity. Given almost any potentially toxic agent, two scenarios present themselves:

1. AGENT → INTERMEDIATE → PRODUCT
   (toxic)   (toxic or nontoxic)   (nontoxic)
2. agent   → INTERMEDIATE → PRODUCT
   (nontoxic)   (toxic)   (nontoxic)

First, the agent may be toxic per se as would be observed with some insecticides (DDT, pyrethroid esters, carbamates), industrial chemicals (halohydrocarbon solvents, etc.), or metals (lead, cadmium, selenium, etc.) which would elicit specific effects on certain tissues of the body. Such agents would be initially biotransformed by tissue enzymes into either toxic or nontoxic intermediates, thereby either enhancing or markedly reducing the toxicity of the parent compound. Some of these intermediates may produce secondary toxicity and tissue damage since they are unstable, highly reactive, and polar in nature. Subsequent biotransformation usually results in the formation of water-soluble, readily excreted, nontoxic products that can be eliminated efficiently. In the second scenario, the agent may have a low order of toxicity per se but is initially biotransformed into a much more toxic intermediate by tissue enzymes. Examples of such chemicals would include insecticides (parathion, malathion, fenitrothion), industrial chemicals (styrene, vinyl chloride), plasticizers (tri-*o*-tolyl phosphate [TOTP], phthalate esters), etc. Additional steps in biotransformation pathways generally result in the destruction of the reactive intermediate and/or conversion into readily excreted, nontoxic products. As an example, the biotransformation of the insecticide malathion is shown in Figure 2.12.

In invertebrate species, the hepatopancreas (lobsters, crabs) and the fat body (insects) are major organs involved in biotransformation. In vertebrates, the liver is principally involved, followed by the kidneys and lungs, with other tissues playing lesser roles. Considering the two-compartment open model discussed earlier (Figure 2.3) and the high extractive capacity of the highly perfused liver, much of an orally acquired toxicant may be removed from the circulation as it passes through the dense capillary bed in the liver. Indeed, there is considerable interest in "first-pass" kinetics in the liver, with the current theories holding that systemic toxicity and biological effects are related to the fraction of agent that "escapes" capture by the liver and is carried on into the systemic circulation. Extrahepatic biotransformation, while not as rapid or efficient, becomes a significant factor in cellular toxicity (Vainio and Hietanen, 1980).

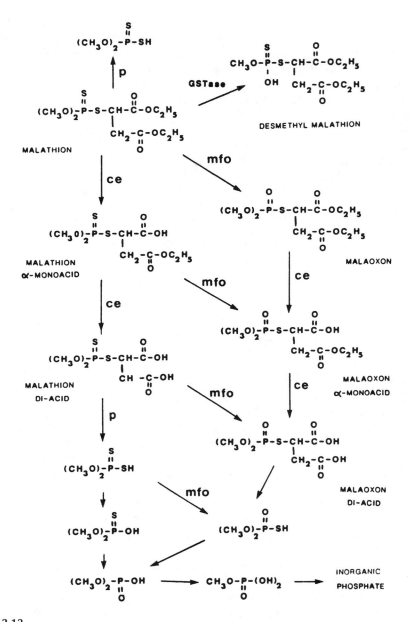

FIGURE 2.12
The biotransformation pathways for malathion (S-1,2-*bis*(ethoxycarbonyl)ethyl, O,O-dimethyl-phosphorodithioate) by cytochrome P-450 monooxygenases (mfo, mixed function oxidases), by nonspecific carboxylesterases (ce), phosphatases (p), and glutathione S-transferases (GSTase) in mammalian tissues. (Modified from Menzie, 1969.)

Whether one is dealing with a toxic agent or an inactive, pro-toxicant, biotransformation usually proceeds in a two-phase process, the aim of the enzymatic reactions being the formation of hydrophilic products that have little or no toxicity and which can be eliminated from the system. The first group of enzymes — **Phase I biotransformation** — promotes the insertion, addition, or exposure of reactive groups on the structure of the lipophilic molecule to create electrophilic substituents

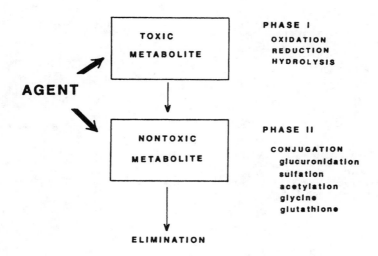

FIGURE 2.13

The biotransformation of foreign (xenobiotic) chemicals by PHASE 1 enzymes capable of adding, changing, or exposing reactive groups to form less liposoluble, polar intermediates and by Phase II enzymes that conjugate normal subcellular chemicals to the intermediates to produce water-soluble (hydrophilic), relatively nontoxic, readily excreted end products.

(Figure 2.13). Phase I enzymes include an impressive array of microsomal monooxygenase functions associated with a group of cellular hemoproteins existing in genetically controlled, multiple forms, the cytochrome P-450 proteins; their role is the oxidation or reduction of existing groups on the molecule or the insertion of molecular oxygen into aromatic rings (Hodgson and Levi, 1994; Leroux et al., 1989; Parke et al., 1991). An additional group of Phase I enzymes includes the hydrolases or esterases, their function being the hydrolysis of peptide and ester bonds of a wide variety of lipophilic endogenous and exogenous substrates to expose polar carboxyl and hydroxyl or amino groups (Ecobichon, 1979). Following the introduction or exposure of reactive groups, a second type of reaction can proceed — **Phase II biotransformation** — in which tissue enzymes conjugate or join normal body constituents (acetyl group, glucuronic acid, ethereal sulfate, glycine, ornithine, glutathione, etc.) to the reactive groups, converting these toxic intermediates into water-soluble, nontoxic products amenable to excretion via the urine and/or feces (Dauterman, 1980). It should be noted that conjugation with glutathione frequently results in the formation of nephrotoxic cysteinyl thioether derivatives (Monks and Lau, 1989). Some xenobiotic molecules may already possess electrophilic groups, thus no longer requiring the need for Phase I biotransformation but permitting Phase II reactions to proceed immediately. An example of the complexity of cellular biotransformation reactions is shown for benzene in Figure 2.14.

One major reason for interspecies, intraspecies, and intrastrain differences in responses to xenobiotic agents is the genetic control of the cytochrome P-450 dependent monooxygenase functions responsible for the biotransformation of the chemical to inactive metabolites as was seen for strains of mice treated with hexobarbital (Figure 2.1). Distinct phenotypic and genotypic animals could be identified between and within colonies. Similar genotypic expression can be observed for the esterases including serum atropinease in the rabbit (Ecobichon and Comeau, 1974), serum pseudocholinesterases (Kalow, 1962; Simpson, 1968), and aryl esterases in man (Carro-Ciampi et al., 1981, 1983), with these genotypic enzymes hydrolyzing drugs

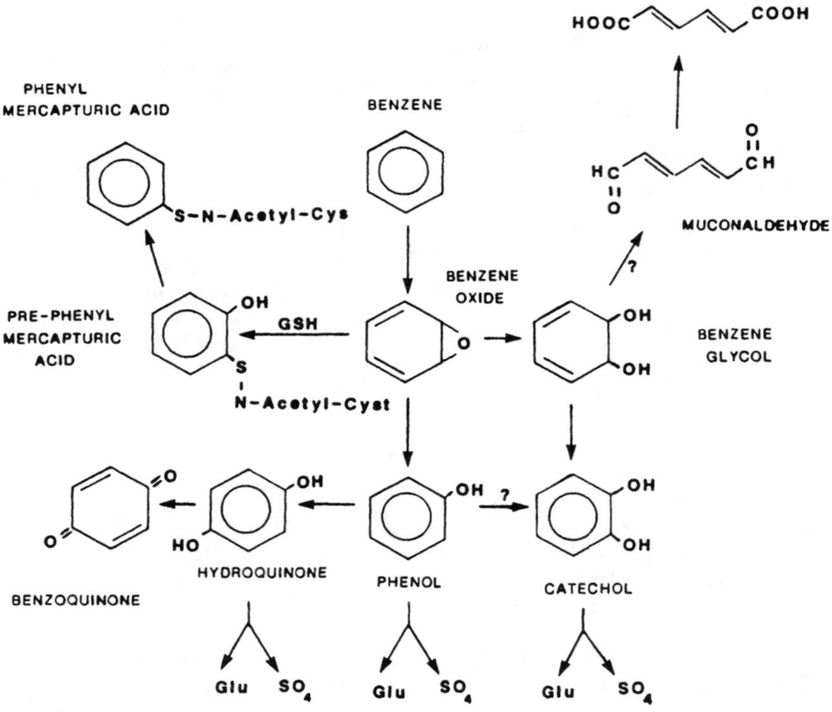

FIGURE 2.14
The biotransformation pathways of benzene. (Modified from Sabourin et al., 1987.)

(atropine, succinylcholine) and insecticides (paraoxon) at distinctly different rates to yield both hypersusceptible and resistant phenotypic individuals. There is considerable interest in the subdisciplines of pharmacogenetics and ethnopharmacology where "ethnogenicity" can be demonstrated in terms of susceptibility to certain drugs. While not explored to as great a depth, the same phenomenon occurs in domestic stock, i.e., succinylcholine in horses and the inbred strains of laboratory rodents. Genetic control of Phase II enzymes also exists, with the bilirubin-glucuronosyltransferase deficiency in the Gunn rat being one of the more famous phenomena (Vainio and Hietanen, 1974). Preliminary *in vitro* and *in vivo* biotransformation studies should be conducted to ascertain what metabolites are formed and which species might serve as acceptable surrogate models for toxicological assessment of test chemicals.

While Phase I and Phase II enzyme systems are found throughout the animal kingdom, vast differences in the ability to biotransform single chemicals have been reported and investigators must pay close attention to inter- and intraspecies variability in chemical biotransformation. Interspecies differences in xenobiotic biotransformation have been extensively studied, particularly those reactions involving the cytochrome P-450 monooxygenase functions. Where selective toxicity toward certain species is desired, e.g., pesticides, it is cogent to explore interspecies biotransformation early in development of the chemical. The range of oxidative/reductive activity from insect species through fish and birds to mammals is frequently as broad as 10- to 100-fold (Bridges et al., 1970; Williams, 1974; Kulkarni et al., 1976; Pan and Fouts, 1978; Kato, 1979; Kulkarni and Hodgson, 1980; Caldwell, 1981; Ronis and Walker, 1989). Extensive studies have even been conducted in various primate species, comparing biotransformation to that in man and demonstrating the phenomenon of unique,

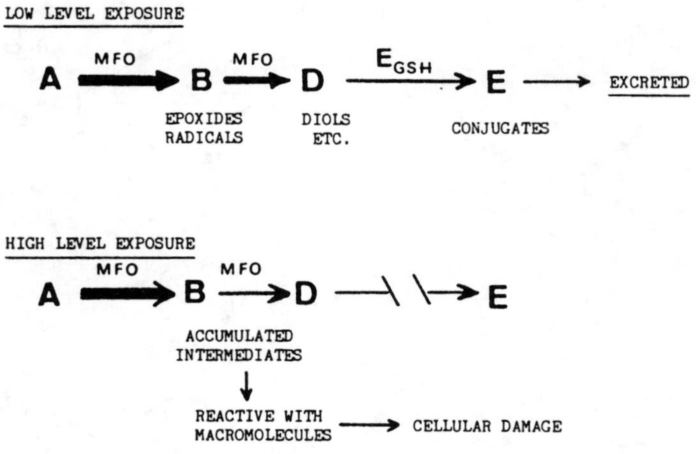

FIGURE 2.15
A comparison of the rate of biotransformation of a xenobiotic agent acquired at a low or a high concentration, demonstrating the rate limiting Phase II reactions at high concentrations due to (1) limited cellular stores and (2) slow resynthesis of "conjugative substrates," with accumulation of highly reactive, unstable, possibly cytotoxic intermediates.

species-specific pathways employed by certain nonhuman primates (Adamson et al., 1970; Williams, 1974). Comparable studies have examined the biotransformation of diverse chemical molecules (substrates) by different strains of animals, using both *in vivo* and *in vitro* techniques. Marked interstrain differences have been reported in mice, rats, and rabbits for both Phase I and II enzyme activities (Cram et al., 1965; Mitoma et al., 1967; Chasseaud, 1973; Williams, 1959, 1974; Hodgson and Levi, 1994).

Clearly related to toxicological effects, one must consider the problems associated with the impact of any concentration of agent administered on the efficiency of biotransformation by tissue enzymes. Since, by design, sufficient chemical must be administered to elicit toxic signs in the test species, it holds that at least one or more dosages will be high enough to pose problems for the tissue enzymes which can be saturated and only function up to a certain maximum rate of reaction. It is imperative to determine the pattern of biotransformation at several different dosages since, at high doses, the pathways of detoxification may be altered significantly. Figure 2.15 shows schematic reactions for a low dose and for a high, potentially toxic dose. The low dose may elicit little toxicity since there is sufficient reserve capacity in the Phase I enzyme pool to deal efficiently with the chemical. Under low-dose kinetics, the rate of reaction is generally first-order, being dependent upon the concentration of the "substrate," the potential toxicant in the case. There would be sufficient reserve capacity of Phase II enzyme activity with, perhaps, one or more routes available to facilitate the efficient formation of water-soluble, excretable products. It is important to emphasize that the kinetics of Phase II reactions is complicated not only by dependency upon the concentration of the reactive intermediate formed but by dependence upon the cellular concentration of the endogenous chemical used by the enzyme in the conjugation. In the high-dose situation, this becomes a significant problem. The schematic reaction for the high dose shows a still-efficient Phase I reaction sequence because of the high catalytic activity of the cytochrome P-450 monooxygenases or esterases. However, toxicity arises because of the accumulation of highly reactive (oxiranes, arene oxides, free radicals) and unstable intermediates that are not efficiently conjugated by Phase II enzymes. Phase II conjugative reactions

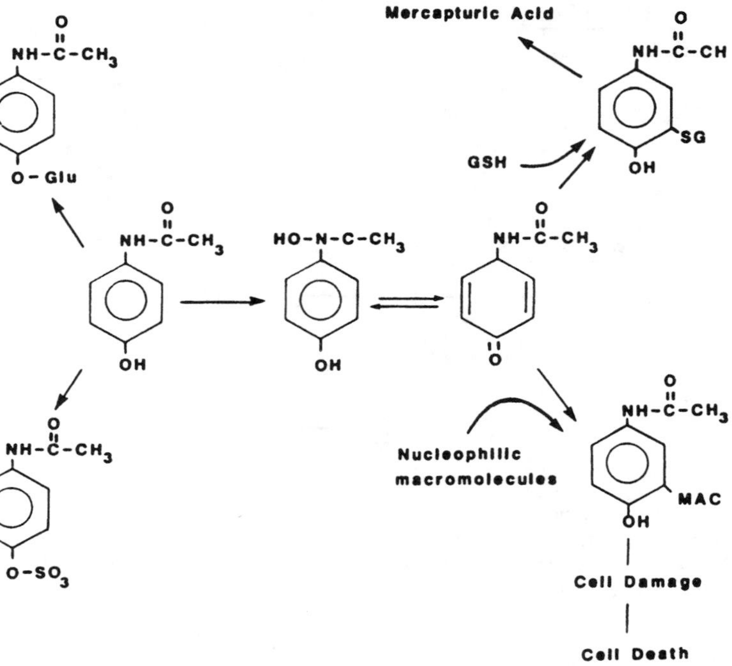

FIGURE 2.16
The pathways of biotransformation of the antiinflammatory agent acetaminophen, showing the dominant Phase II glucuronidation (-Glu), sulfation (-SO$_3$) and glutathione (GSH) conjugation reactions and the fate of an overdose whereby conjugation cannot occur rapidly enough, allowing the accumulating reactive intermediates to elicit cellular damage. (Modified from Hinson et al., 1981.)

proceed at a much slower rate and, therefore, in the high-dose situation, become the rate-limiting steps in the entire sequence of reactions. The individual functions can be saturated more easily and their dependency upon limited cellular stores of endogenous compounds such as glucuronic acid or glutathione is such that, when the levels of these chemicals fall, these enzymatic functions slow down. The recovery of full activity is dependent upon the rate of resynthesis of the required endogenous chemicals. Significantly, many animal species will "activate" a second Phase II system, producing a new conjugated product under high dose exposure conditions that is not detected at low-dose exposures. Phase II reactions tend to be more species specific (Williams, 1974). Guinea pigs make little use of the glutathione-conjugating enzymes since depleted stores of glutathione can be replaced only after 48 h, compared to 12 to 18 h in the rat (Ecobichon, 1984). However, guinea pigs efficiently glucuronidate many agents (Hidvegi and Ecobichon, 1986). The inability to efficiently conjugate reactive, unstable intermediates leaves the cell in jeopardy of having subcellular macromolecules (nucleic acids, proteins, phospholipid membranes) damaged beyond the extent of effective repair, with the subsequent development of necrosis. An excellent example of the interrelationships between biotransformation and drug-induced, hepatic necrosis is seen in Figure 2.16 which describes the toxicity associated with the multifaceted biotransformation of acetaminophen at toxic doses in the mouse and hamster (Hinson et al., 1981).

While attention has been focused on biotransformation in the liver, it should be appreciated that similar pathways may be found in other tissues of the body, although as a rule of thumb, these function at only a small fraction of the rate(s) of those in hepatic tissue. However, at high levels of exposure, where much of the toxicant may escape destruction in the liver, the limited efficiency of extrahepatic biotransformation rates and routes becomes an important factor in the severity and duration of systemic toxicity (Vainio and Hietanen, 1980).

In the preliminary stages of exploring the biotransformation of a new chemical, careful notice should be taken of the rate at which the agent is converted into nontoxic, excretable products. Subchronic or chronic exposure to many chemicals results in a phenomena known as **induction** where a dramatic increase in tissue levels of enzymatic activity is seen. An inducible enzyme is one normally present at very low cellular concentrations but, upon exposure to certain compounds, is newly synthesized in large quantities, with this being reflected in increased activity and in increased cellular protein concentrations. The inducing agent is usually, but now always, a substrate for the enzyme. Invariably, such chemicals are lipophilic in nature, are poorly (and slowly) biotransformed by enzyme systems, and are persistent in the organism. The organ or tissue response appears to be an attempt to cope with the agent, to convert it into water-soluble, readily excreted products. The system most susceptible to inducing agents is the hepatic, microsomal, cytochrome P-450 associated, monooxygenase function(s), although other functions including the Phase II conjugating enzymes may also be induced. While the liver is the most responsive to induction, other tissues may also show moderate increases in enzyme activity. Such inducing agents span a wide range of synthetic, organic chemicals including pesticides (particularly the organochlorine compounds), drugs (phenobarbital, phenytoin), carcinogens (benzo[a]pyrene, chrysene, 3-methylcholanthrene), and industrial and environmental contaminants (polychlorinated benzenes, biphenyls, dibenzo-*p*-dioxins, dibenzofurans). While induction usually results in enhanced biotransformation, the disproportionate increase in Phase I over Phase II enzymes may cause cytotoxicity as a consequence of accumulating reactive intermediates or enhanced biotransformation of endogenous chemicals (neurohormones, steroids, etc.) with serious alterations in normal cellular functions (reproduction, etc.) being observed. Considerable grief can be projected into a study if the problem(s) of bioaccumulation and persistence of a chemical are not anticipated.

Sex-related differences can be observed frequently in responses to treatment, a classical example being that of hexobarbital sleeping time in male and female rats, where, given comparable doses, the interval is markedly prolonged in the female (Kato and Gillette, 1965; El Defrawy El Masry and Mannering, 1974). Closer examination of this phenomenon will reveal that the disposition of the drug is quite different, with the blood plasma half-life being considerably longer in the females and the rate of biotransformation being significantly reduced over that measured in males. This phenomenon is quite prevalent in small rodents but disappears, for the most part, when larger species are studied. Both Phase I and II enzyme systems may be susceptible to the continually fluctuating levels of androgens and estrogens (Kato, 1974). The castration of male rats reduces the activity of hepatic cytochrome P-450 monooxygenases to the levels measured in females while supportive testosterone therapy of these surgically altered males results in maintenance of activity comparable to that found in control male rats (Kato and Gillette, 1965). It is equally important to appreciate that such sex differences in enzyme activity may be specific to only some organs or tissues, e.g., the liver, whereas no sex difference can be detected in the lung or intestinal tract and only some slight sex difference can be seen in the kidney (Chhabra and Fouts, 1974).

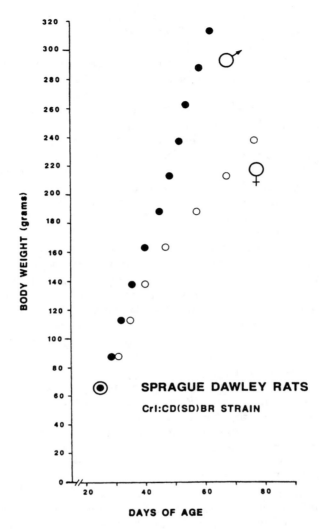

FIGURE 2.17
The growth and development of young Sprague-Dawley rats, illustrating the differences in body weights of males and females of the same age. (Data derived from information provided by Charles River Breeding Laboratories, Wilmington, MA.)

Consideration must be given to the age of the animals in the experiments since age-related variations may introduce significant variations in susceptibility to toxicants. Animals of approximately the same age and sex should be allotted to the treatment groups. Organ functions, including rates and routes of biotransformation and elimination, vary greatly with age, with markedly different levels of Phase I and II enzymes being detected in young and older animals. In particular, activities of Phase I enzyme systems increase significantly during the first 4- to 6-week period after birth and then decline by some 50 to 75% as adulthood is approached (Short et al., 1976). The question of age is further complicated by the fact that males and females of a strain or species frequently develop at different rates, as is seen for one strain of rat in Figure 2.17. Using body weight as an index of age, males and females of the same age will have different body weights.

VIII. DIET

While specifically related to long-term rodent studies, there is a considerable body of evidence that diet plays an important role in the response(s) of animals to potentially toxic agents (Hart et al., 1995a,b). Animals on caloric restriction (approximately 20% less than normal *ad libitum* intake) are leaner, more healthy, live longer, are less susceptible to diseases and age-related changes in organ function, and have a lower incidence of tumors (both sponteneous and chemical-induced) (Tucker, 1979; Turnbull et al., 1985; Rao and Huff, 1990; Roe et al., 1995; Salmon et al., 1990). Total caloric content, rather than any single micro- or macronutrient, appears to have a maximal impact on general health (Hart et al., 1995b). However, results have shown that decreasing the protein (casein) content of the diet by 12 to 15% while increasing the fiber content markedly decreased the severity of age-associated nephropathy seen in older rats (Rao and Huff, 1991). Do we need a sturdier rat (or mouse)? Many say that we do, but we have an enormous body of toxicity (subchronic, chronic, carcinogenic) data built upon the premise that a well-fed rat is a happy, though pudgy one. It will be difficult to wean toxicologists from this viewpoint even given the plentiful, factual evidence that the leaner, meaner animal is very different from the overfed littermate (Hart et al., 1995a,b). Restricted caloric intake opens a virtual Pandora's box and has been the topic of heated discussion at many meetings (Hart et al., 1995a,b). However, such studies are being conducted, with interesting results (Roe et al., 1995).

Caloric restriction, in young animals, has a direct action on sex-specific, growth-hormone-regulated hepatic enzymes, with these enzymes being quickly depressed in both sexes, an action that may be related to the inhibition of pituitary growth hormone (Manjgaladze et al., 1993; Hart et al., 1995a). These same enzymes decline normally in aging rats, and this effect is due to the secretion of abnormal amounts of growth hormone by pituitary adenomas commonly found in old rats (Hart et al., 1995a). Caloric restriction reduces the incidence and delays the onset of pituitary tumors (Turnbull et al., 1985; Thurman et al., 1994). Through the influence on growth hormone, caloric restriction exerts a significant effect on xenobiotic-metabolizing enzymes, reducing the rates of biotransformation/elimination and altering the pharmacokinetics (Hart et al., 1995). The cytochrome P450s, UDP-glucuronosyltransferases, sulfotransferases, and glutathione S-alkyltransferases exist as isoform families, their regulation being controlled by hormonal factors and xenobiotic-inducing agents (Bidlack et al., 1986; Manjgaladze et al., 1993; Hart et al., 1995a). Caloric restriction suppresses enzyme induction. *Ad libitum*-fed rats exhibit hyperinsulinemia which decreases the regulatory expression of these same enzymes, an event that is prevented by caloric restriction (Hart et al., 1995a). Finally, caloric restriction affects the normal nocturnal eating pattern, upsetting the usual circadian rhythm since these animals tend to consume their alloted food rapidly rather than eating it more gradually in the dark portion of the circadian cycle (Hart et al., 1995a,b). Such changes in feeding behavior alter the circadian cycles of serum hormones such as insulin, thyroid hormone, and corticosterone, elevating the levels, although these changes may exert a relatively small effect on xenobiotic-metabolizing enzymes (Hart et al., 1995a). It has been suggested that hypercorticism may be responsible for most, if not all, of the beneficial effects on disease and longevity (Leakey et al., 1994). Overall, caloric restriction suppresses xenobiotic metabolism in young animals and exerts a moderate effect in maintaining these same enzymes in older animals.

Caloric restriction markedly decreases the acute toxicity of several agents whether through elevated glucocorticoids and suppression of the inflammatory response induced by phorbol esters or carrageenan, through reduced rates of metabolism of test chemicals, or by preventing chemicals from inducing their own biotransformation (Hart et al., 1995a). Many studies have shown that caloric restriction reduces the incidence of chemical-induced tumor formation, this phenomenon perhaps being related to suppressed metabolism of the test agents into reactive metabolites (Newberne and Conner, 1986; Hart et al., 1995b). In some cases, previously designated mammalian carcinogens have shown minimal cancer causation in calorie-restricted animals, creating a major risk assessment problem for regulatory agencies.

Under conditions where the test agent is added to the diet, it is the animal that determines how much food it will eat and, by extension, how much test compound. The presence of food at all times predisposes the animals toward obesity and the diseases associated with excess nutrition. While the National Toxicology Program (NTP) protocols continue to offer food *ad libitum* to animals in carcinogenicity studies, the amount of protein has been reduced while increasing the fiber content (Bucher et al., 1995). The U.S. Food and Drug Administration is currently preparing two documents for publication in the *Federal Register* which will identify the problems associated with uncontrolled food consumption and will address which levels of dietary control are appropriate to achieve standardized growth curves (Hart et al., 1995c). Coincident with the problem of diet in toxicological studies is the realization that, with time, there appears to be genetic drift "at work" in rodent strains. In an inbred strain of mice (SPF Swiss, males), mean body weights increased over a 10-year period, with many animals being obese and the incidence of spontaneous neoplasms rising from 10 to 80% (Roe, 1981). Male Fischer 344 rats have shown a 25% increase in body weight, while male Sprague-Dawley rats that once weighed 700 grams now weigh 1000 grams (Rao, 1991). Longevity in strains has been affected. Survival rates of male Fischer 344 rats at 2 years has changed from 80% in 1970, 60% in 1981, and 36% at the current time (Hart et al., 1995b). Comparisons between the CD-COBS strain of Sprague-Dawley rat and a new variant, the CD-COBS-VAF strain, used in the Pfizer laboratories in France, revealed that the latter grew faster, had a decreased 2-year survival time ($41 \pm 3\%$ in males, $44 \pm 7\%$ in females), with increased incidences of pituitary tumors (males), of mammary fibroadenomas (females), of severe glomerulonephritis, and of animals which died without any obvious pathology (Nohynek et al., 1993). Male Sprague-Dawley rats, used in studies at the Merck Research Laboratories, have declined in 2-year survival rates, from 58% in the 1970s, 44% in the 1980s, to a current 24% (Hart et al., 1995b). While some of the problem may arise from genetic drift unwittingly introduced by animal breeders in selecting their stock, *ad libitum* feeding in such stocks may also be playing a role.

IX. ENDPOINTS OF TOXICITY

The consequence of administering a potential toxicant to any animal, by whatever route, is that once the agent is absorbed into the body, the investigator has lost all effective control over the chemical; its disposition, fate, and biological effects are now determined by various biochemical and physiological functions of the "host." Effectively, one is working inside a "black box" (Figure 2.18) where the post-treatment events are controlled by the animal and one has to assume, somewhat on faith, that the agent or some reactive intermediate is attaining a toxic level at some unidentified target site where a subcellular interaction is taking place at a sufficient intensity to be reflected in an altered physiological, biochemical, or morphological state that may be detected or quantitated by some sensitive measuring technique.

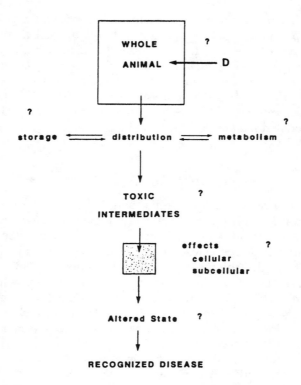

FIGURE 2.18

An overview of the problems encountered in whole animal experiments with a new, toxicologically unknown agent. Essentially, the test agent is being administered to a "box" — the animal, which will proceed to eliminate, biotransform, distribute, and/or store the agent or biotransformation products, and elicit biological effects in target organs thereby causing altered functional states identifiable as definitive target organ toxicity. The question marks (?) indicate where knowledge will be incomplete and must be acquired by additional, specific, *in vivo* or *in vitro* studies to determine the mechanism of action of the potential toxicant.

The question marks remind us of what we do not know concerning the disposition, action, and fate of the agent. Cautious intervention by the investigator may permit monitoring of events. We have already discussed the toxicokinetics/biotransformation/elimination aspects. Innovative technology must be introduced into experiments to quantitate, in terms of dosage administered, tissue levels, binding sites, and mechanisms of action of the toxicant.

As outlined earlier, the objective(s) of any toxicological study is to develop a relationship between one or more biological parameters — measured in the most susceptible species by the most sensitive analytical technique(s) — and the dosage of agent administered. This leads to a consideration of what type of toxicity should be anticipated and what endpoint(s) of toxicity should be quantified. Should an omnibus approach be taken, using a battery of predefined, standardized tests and, essentially, screening the animals throughout treatment for some change in one or more of the tests? Should more specific and perhaps innovative techniques be used, focusing on certain potential target sites? Whatever approach is chosen, one must be able to quantitate the anticipated toxic effects *plus* those serendipidous events that will arise as a consequence of multiple target organ toxicity. With a variety of endpoints of toxicity and dosages, an infinite number of apparent linear and curvilinear relationships may be generated. The dose–effect relationship may be steep, indicating that a small increase in dosage elicits a dramatic increase in the effect, or the slope of the relationship may be shallow, indicative of only a small change in the altered state accompanying a large increase in the dosage of toxicant. Since the potential endpoints of toxicity are as infinite in number as the techniques used in quantitating target organ toxicity, a detailed examination of these aspects is beyond the scope of this text and the reader is referred to more specific volumes such as Galli et al. (1980), Gorrod (1981), Homburger et al. (1983), Arnold et al. (1990), and Hayes (1994) for detailed discussions on the subject.

X. ANIMAL NUMBERS

In testing the potential toxicity of a new agent, the toxicologist cannot afford to miss any significant adverse effects. Invariably, some toxic effects will be observed in all or most of the animals treated. However, other adverse effects may be seen only in a small percentage of the test animals, the observed variability being due to the inhomogeneity of the animal population. To insure that "all" toxic effects are seen, one method is to expand the dosage range to include excessively high doses (overdoses). Confidence in the results of studies is frequently bolstered by the mistaken concept of "safety in numbers," leading to the inclusion of more and more animals in studies. How many animals should be assigned to each treatment group?

An example of this problem is shown in Figure 2.19, with values being derived from data of Zbinden (1973). Assuming an identical incidence of toxicity in humans and animals, if the probability of a toxic effect in the human is 100%, then the number of animals required to demonstrate toxicity at a probability of 0.95 would be very small, i.e., one animal. As the probability of the effect occurring in the human decreases, additional numbers of test animals would be required in order to "guarantee" that at least one subject would show toxic effects, At a 2.0% occurrence rate in humans, 149 animals would be needed. Since the probability of occurrence of many toxic effects in humans is frequently at a level of 0.01% or lower, some 29,956 animals would have to be treated to insure that one of these would show specific toxicity. Understandably, such a study would be impractical, unmanageable, terribly expensive, and very foolish. Few studies have used such large numbers. One of note was the "Megamouse" study of the $ED_{0.1}$ of 2-acetylaminofluorene (2-AAF) in which 24,000 mice were used (Society of Toxicology Task Force, 1981). In usual practice, six to ten animals per treatment group would be used in acute toxicity studies with a minimum of 5 dosages tested. In contrast, subchronic and chronic studies would use no more than 50 animals assigned to each treatment group with a range of 3 selected dosages (low, intermediate, high) plus an appropriate number of control animals, usually two-fold higher than the number in each treatment group. The risk, even with 50 animals in each treatment group, is that not all of the potential adverse health effects will be detected over the dosage range used.

While the above decisions can be readily made for the studies using small laboratory rodent species, the wildlife toxicologist is severely hampered by the availability of suitable numbers of specimens captured in the wild or perhaps reared in captivity. Even the best designed and conducted studies using wildlife will suffer from the problems inherent in using limited numbers of animals: the age and sex differences and the natural genetic inhomogeneity of the population. The degree of variability in responses to the potential toxicant encountered within treatment groups can only be offset by comparison with measurements made in a sufficiently large

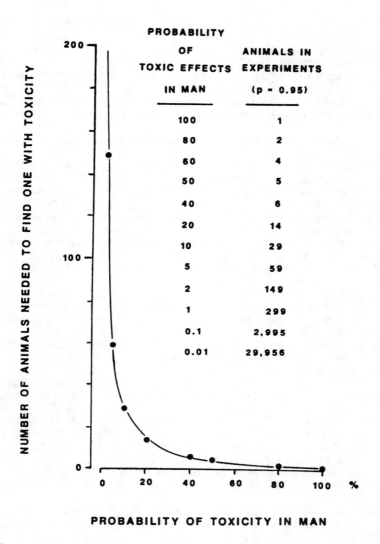

PROBABILITY OF TOXIC EFFECTS IN MAN	ANIMALS IN EXPERIMENTS (p = 0.95)
100	1
80	2
60	4
50	5
40	6
20	14
10	29
5	59
2	149
1	299
0.1	2,995
0.01	29,956

PROBABILITY OF TOXICITY IN MAN

FIGURE 2.19

The interrelationship between the probability (percent) of a given toxic effect in man and the number of animals required in an experiment to insure that the same toxic effect is observed. With a high incidence of occurrence in man, few animals would be needed, but since the incidence frequently is very low in man, i.e., 0.01% or lower, then astronomical numbers of animals would be required to "guarantee" that the same effect would be observed. (Data derived from Zbinden, 1973.)

enough group of control animals. Frequently, one can only wish wildlife toxicologists the best of good fortune in their endeavours.

REFERENCES

Adamson, R.H., Bridges, J.W., Kirby, M.R., Walker, S.R., and Williams, R.T. The fate of sulfadimethoxine in primates compared with other species. *Biochem. J.* 118, 41-45 (1970).

Albert, A. *Selective Toxicity, The Physico-Chemical Basis of Therapy.* Fifth Edition. Chapman and Hall, London, 1973.

Albert, A. *Xenobiosis. Food, Drugs and Poisons in the Human Body.* Chapman and Hall, London (1987).

Arnold, D.L., Grice, H.C., and Krewski, D.R. (Editors). *Handbook of In Vivo Toxicity Testing*. Academic Press, New York, 1990.

Bachman, C. and Bickel, M.H. History of drug metabolism: the first half of the 20th century. *Drug Metab. Rev.* 16, 185-253 (1985).

Bidlack, W.R., Brown, R.C., and Mohan, C. Nutritional parameters that alter hepatic drug metabolism, conjugation and toxicity. *Fed. Proc.* 45, 142-148 (1986).

Breckenridge, C., Lulham, G., Hollomby, B., Bier, C., Losos, G., and Ecobichon, D.J. A subchronic inhalation toxicity study of a Matacil formulation in the albino rat. *Toxicol. Appl. Pharmacol.* 82, 181-190 (1986).

Bridges, J.W., French, M.R., Smith, R.L., and Williams, R.T. The fate of benzoic acid in various species. *Biochem. J.* 118, 47-51 (1970).

Bucher, J.R., Rao, G.N., Abdo, K., Kari, F., and Lucier, G. Letters. *Science* 270, 1421-1422 (1995).

Caldwell, J. The metabolism of amphetamines in mammals. *Drug Metab. Rev.* 5, 219-280 (1976).

Caldwell, J. The current status of attempts to predict species differences in drug metabolism. *Drug Metab. Rev.* 12, 221-237 (1981).

Carro-Ciampi, G., Kadar, D., and Kalow, W. Distribution of serum paraoxon hydrolyzing activities in a Canadian population. *Can. J. Physiol. Pharmacol.* 59, 904-907 (1981).

Carro-Ciampi, G., Gray, S., and Kalow, W. Paraoxonase phenotype distribution in Canadian Indian and Inuit populations. *Can. J. Physiol. Pharmacol.* 61, 336-340 (1983).

Chasseaud, L.F. Nature and distribution of enzymes catalyzing the conjugation of glutathione with foreign compounds. *Drug Metab. Rev.* 2, 185-220 (1973).

Chevalier, G., Henin, J.P., Vannier, N., Canevet, C., Cote, M.G., and Lebouffant, L. Pulmonary toxicity of aerosolized fenitrothion in rats. *Toxicol. Appl. Pharmacol.* 76, 349-355 (1984).

Chhabra, R.S. and Fouts, J.R. Sex differences in the metabolism of xenobiotics by extrahepatic tissue in rats. *Drug Metab. Dispos.* 2, 375-379 (1974).

Condie, L.W., Laurie, R.D., Mills, T., Robinson, M., and Bercz, J.P. Effect of gavage vehicle on hepatotoxicity of carbon tetrachloride in CD-1 mice. Corn Oil vs. Tween-60 aqueous emulsion. *Fundam. Appl. Toxicol.* 7, 199-206 (1986).

Clarkson, T.W. Metal toxicity in the central nervous system. *Environ. Health Perspect.* 75, 59-64.

Cram, R.L., Juchau, M.R., and Fouts, J.R. Differences in hepatic drug metabolism in various rabbit strains before and after pre-treatment with phenobarbital. *Proc. Soc. Exp. Biol. Med.* 118, 872-875 (1965).

Dauterman, W.C. Metabolism of Toxicants. Phase II. Reactions. In *Introduction to Biochemical Toxicology*. Hodgson, E. and Guthrie, F.E. (Editors). Elsevier, New York, 1980, Ch. 5, pp. 92-105.

Ecobichon, D.J. Hydrolytic mechanisms of pesticide degradation. In *Advances in Pesticide Science Part 3. Biochemistry of Pests and Mode of Action of Pesticides, Pesticide Degradation, Pesticide Residues, Formulation Chemistry.* Geissbuhler, H. (Editor). Pergamon Press, London, pp. 516-525.

Ecobichon, D.J. Glutathione depletion and resynthesis in laboratory animals. *Drug Chem. Toxicol.* 7, 345-355 (1984).

Ecobichon, D.J. and Comeau, A.M. Genetic polymorphism of plasma carboxylesterases in the rabbit: correlation with pharmacologic and toxicologic effects. *Toxicol. Appl. Pharmacol.* 27, 28-40 (1974).

El Defrawy El Masry, S., and Mannering, G.J. Qualitative changes produced by castration and the administration of steroid hormones and phenobarbital. *Drug Metab. Dispos.* 2, 279-284 (1974).

Festing, M.F.W. Genetic factors in toxicology: implications for toxicological screening. *CRC Crit. Rev. Toxicol.* 18, 1-26 (1987).

Festing, M.F.W. Use of genetically heterogeneous rats and mice in toxicological research: a personal perspective. *Toxicol. Appl. Pharmacol.* 102, 197-204 (1990).

Festing, M.F.W. Genetic variation in outbred rats estimated by DNA fingerprints: implications for toxicological screening. *Hum. Exp. Toxicol.* 11, 590-591 (1992).

Festing, M.F.W. Genetic variation in outbred rats and mice and its implications for toxicological screening. *J. Exp. Animal Sci.* 35, 210-220 (1993).

Festing, M.F.W. Use of multistrain assay would improve the NTP carcinogenesis bioassay. *Environ. Health Perspec.* 103, 44-52 (1995).

Gage, J.C. The subacute inhalation toxicity of 109 industrial chemicals. *Br. J. Ind. Med.* 27, 1-18 (1970).

Gaines, T.B. Acute toxicity of pesticides. *Toxicol. Appl. Pharmacol.* 14, 515-534 (1969).

Galli, C.L., Murphy, S.D., and Paoletti, R. (Editors). *The Principles and Methods in Modern Toxicology.* Elsevier/North Holland Biomedical Press, New York (1980).

General Medical Council. *British Pharmacopoeia.* The Pharmaceutical Press, London (1953). Appendix XV E, pp. 828-832.

Gill, T.J., III. The use of randomly bred and genetically defined animals in biomedical research. *Am. J. Pathol.* 101, 522-532 (1980).

Gorrod, J.W. (Editor). *Testing for Toxicity.* Taylor and Francis, Ltd., London (1981).

Hart, R.W., Keenan, K., Turtirro, A., Abdo, K.M., Leakey, J., and Lyn-Cook, B. Symposium Overview. Caloric restriction and toxicity. *Fundam. Appl. Toxicol.* 25, 184-195 (1995a).

Hart, R.W., Neumann, D.A., and Robertson, R.T. (Editors). Dietary restriction: *Implications for the Design and Interpretation of Toxicity and Carcinogenicity Studies.* ILSI Press, Washington, D.C. (1995b).

Hart, R.W., Turturro, A., Leakey, J., and Allaben, W.T. Diet and test animals. *Science* 270, 1419-1421 (1995c).

Hayes, A. Wallace (Editor). *Principles and Methods of Toxicology.* Third Edition. Raven Press, New York (1994).

Hidvegi, S. and Ecobichon, D.J. Acetaminophen in the guinea pig: metabolite identification in blood, urine and bile. *Can. J. Physiol. Pharmacol.* 64, 72-76 (1986).

Hinson, J.A., Pohl, L.R., Monks, T.J., and Gillette, J.R. Aceta-minophen-induced hepatotoxicity. *Life Sci.* 29, 106-116 (1981).

Hodgson, E. and Dauterman, W.C. Metabolism of Toxicants. Phase I Reactions. In *Introduction to Biochemical Toxicology.* Hodgson, E. and Guthrie, F.E. (Editors). Elsevier, New York (1980). Ch. 4, pp. 67-91.

Hodgson, E. and Levi, P.E. (Editors). *Introduction to Biochemical Toxicology.* Appleton and Lange, Norwalk CT. (1994).

Homburger, F., Hayes, J.A., and Pelikan, E.W. (Editors). *A Guide to General Toxicology.* S. Karger A.G., Basel (1983).

Jay, G.E. Variations in response of various mouse strains to hexobarbital (Evipal). *Proc. Soc. Exp. Biol. Med.* 90, 378-380 (1955).

Kalow, W. *Pharmacokinetics. Heredity and the Response to Drugs.* W.B. Saunders, Philadelphia (1962).

Kalter, H. Dose-response studies with genetically homogeneous lines of mice as a teratology testing and reassessment procedure. *Teratology* 24, 79-86 (1981).

Kato, R. Sex-related differences in drug metabolism. *Drug Metab. Rev.* 3, 1-32 (1974).

Kato, R. Characteristics and differences in the hepatic mixed function oxidases of different species. *Pharmacol. and Ther.* 6, 41-98 (1979).

Kato, R. and Gillette, J.R. Sex differences in the effects of abnormal physiological states on the metabolism of drugs by rat liver microsomes. *J. Pharm. Exp. Ther.* 150, 285-291 (1965).

Kim, H.J., Bruckner, J.V., Dallas, C.E., and Gallo, J.M. Effect of dosing vehicles on the pharmacokinetics of orally administered carbon tetrachloride in rats. *Toxicol. Appl. Pharmacol.* 102, 50-60 (1990a).

Kim, H.J., Odend'hal, S., and Bruckner, J.V. Effect of oral dosing vehicles on the acute hepatotoxicity of carbon tetrachloride in rats. *Toxicol. Appl. Pharmacol.* 102, 34-49 (1990b).

Kulkarni, A.P., Smith, E., and Hodgson, E. Occurrence and characterization of microsomal cytochrome P-450 in several vertebrate and insect species. *Comp. Biochem. Physiol.* 54B, 509-513 (1976).

Kulkarni, A.P. and Hodgson, E. Metabolism of insecticides by mixed function oxidase systems. *Pharmacol. and Ther.* 8, 379-475 (1980).

Lash, L.H., Anders, M.W., and Jones, D. Glutathione homeostasis and glutathione S-conjugate toxicity in the kidney. *Reviews in Biochem. Toxicol.* 9, 29-67 (1988).

Langley, G. Animals and alternatives in regulatory toxicology. *TEN* 1, 107 (1994).

Leakey, J.E.A., Chen, S., Manjgaladze, M., Turturro, A., Duffy, P.H., Pipkin, J.L., and Hart, R.W. Role of glucocorticoids and "caloric stress" in modulating the effects of caloric restriction in rodents. *Ann. N.Y. Acad. Sci.* 719, 171-194 (1994).

Leroux, J.P., Cresteil, T., and Marie, S. Ontogeny and regulation of drug metabolism in humans. Phase I: monooxygenases. *Dev. Pharmacol. Ther.* 13, 63-69 (1989).

Litterst, C.L. A comprehensive study of *in vitro* drug metabolism in several laboratory species. *Drug Metab. Disp.* 4, 203-207 (1976).

Lovell, D.P. and Festing, M.F.W. Relationships among colonies of laboratory rat. *J. Hered.* 73, 81-82 (1982).

Manjgaladze, M., Chen, S., Frame, L.T., Seng, J.E., Duffy, P.H., Feuers, R.J., Hart, R.W., and Leakey, J.E.A. Effects of caloric restriction on rodent drug and carcinogen metabolizing enzymes. Implications for mutagenesis and cancer. *Mutat. Res.* 295, 201-222 (1993).

McCully, K.A., Villeneuve, D.C., McKinley, W.P., Phillips, W.E.J., and Hidiroglou, M. Metabolism and storage of DDT in beef cattle. *J. Assoc. Offic. Anal. Chem.* 49, 966-973 (1966).

Menzie, C.M. Metabolism of Pesticides. U.S. Dept. of Interior, Fish and Wildlife Service. Bureau of Sport Fisheries and Wildlife. Special Scientific Report. Wildlife No. 127, Washington, D.C. (1969), pp. 230-235.

Mitoma, C., Neubauer, S.E., Badger, N.L., and Sorich, T.J. Hepatic microsomal activities in rats with long and short sleeping times after hexobarbital. A comparison. *Proc. Soc. Exp. Biol. Med.* 125, 284-288 (1967).

Monks, T.J. and Lau, S.S. Sulfur conjugate-mediated toxicity. In *Reviews in Biochemical Toxicology.* Vol. 10. Hodgson, E., Bend, J.R., and Philpot, R.M. (Editors). Elsevier, New York (1989), pp. 41-90.

Newberne, P.M. and Conner, M.W. Nutrient influences on toxicity and carcinogenicity. *Fed. Proc.* 45, 149-154 (1986).

Nohynek, G.J., Longeart, L., Geffray, B., Provost, J.P., and Lodola, A. Fat, frail and dying young: survival, body weight and pathology of the Charles River Sprague-Dawley-derived rat prior to and since the introduction of the VAT variant in 1988. *Human Exp. Toxicol.* 12, 87-98 (1993).

Pan, H.P. and Fouts, J.R. Drug metabolism in birds. *Drug Metab. Rev.* 7, 1-253 (1978).

Parke, D.V., Ioannides, C., and Lewis, D.F.V. The role of the cytochromes P450 in the detoxication and activation of drugs and other chemicals. *Can. J. Physiol. Pharmacol.* 69, 537-549 (1991).

Parke, D.V. and Smith, R.L. (Editors). *Drug Metabolism — From Microbe to Man.* Taylor and Francis, London (1977).

Phillips, D.L., Smith, A.B., Burse, V.W., Steele, G.K., Needham, L.L., and Hannon, W.H. Half-life of polychlorinated biphenyls in occupationally exposed workers. *Arch. Environ. Health* 44, 351-354 (1989).

Piper, W.N., Rose, J.Q., Leng, M.L., and Gehring, P.J. The fate of 2,4,5-trichlorophenoxyacetic acid (2,4,5-T) following oral administration to rats and dogs. *Toxicol. Appl. Pharmacol.* 26, 339-351 (1973).

Rao, G.N. In *Biological Effects of Dietary Restriction.* L. Fishbein (Editor), Springer-Verlag, New York (1991), p. 321.

Rao, G.N. and Huff, J. Refinement of long-term toxicity and carcinogenesis studies. *Fundam. Appl. Toxicol.* 15, 33-43 (1990).

Rao, G.N. and Huff, J. Letter to the editor. *Fundam. Appl. Toxicol.* 16, 617-618 (1991).

Rice, M.C. and O'Brien, S.J. Genetic variance of laboratory outbred Swiss mice. *Nature* 283, 157-161 (1980).

Roe, F.J.C. Are nutritionists worried about the epidemics of tumours in laboratory animals? *Proc. Nutrition Soc.* 40, 57-65 (1981).

Roe, F.J.C., Lee, P.N., Conybeare, G., Kelly, D., Matter, B., Prentice, D., and Tobin, G. The Biosure Study: Influence of composition of diet and food consumption on longevity, degenerative diseases and neoplasia in Wistar rats studied for up to 30 months post-weaning. *Food Chem. Toxicol.* 33, Suppl.#1 (1995).

Ronis, M.J.J. and Walker, C.H. The microsomal monooxygenases of birds. In *Reviews of Biochemical Toxicology.* Vol. 10. Hodgson, E., Bend, J.R., and Philpot, R.M. (Editors). Elsevier, New York (1989), pp. 301-384.

Sabourin, P.J., Chen, B.T., Lucier, G., Birnbaum, L.S., Fisher, E., and Henderson, R.F. Effect of dose on the absorption and excretion of [^{14}C]-benzene administered orally or by inhalation in rats and mice. *Toxicol. Appl. Pharmacol.* 87, 325-336 (1987).

Salmon, G.K., Leslie, G., Rowe, F.J.C., and Lee, P.N. Influence of food intake and sexual segregation on longevity, organ weights, and the incidence of non-neoplastic and neoplastic diseases in rats. *Food. Chem. Toxicol.* 28, 39-48 (1990).

Short, C.R., Kinden, D.A., and Stith, R. Fetal and neonatal development of the microsomal monooxygenase system. *Drug Metab. Rev.* 51, 1-42 (1976).

Simpson, N.E. Genetics of esterases in man. *Ann. N.Y. Acad. Scis.* 151: Art. 2, 699-709 (1968).

Society of Toxicology ED$_{0.1}$ Task Force. Re-examination of the ED$_{0.1}$ Study. *Fundam. Appl. Toxicol.* 1, 26-128 (1981).

Thurman, J.D., Bucci, T., Hart, R., and Turturro, A. Survival body weight and spontaneous neoplasms in *ad libitum* fed and dietary restricted Fischer 344 rats. *Toxicol. Pathol.* 22, 1-9 (1994).

Tucker, M. The effect of long-term food restriction on tumours in rodents. *Int. J. Cancer* 23, 803-807 (1979).

Turnbull, G.J., Lee, P.N., and Roe, F.J.C. Relationship of body-weight gain to longevity and to risk of development of nephropathy and neoplasia in Sprague-Dawley rats. *Food Chem. Toxicol.* 23, 355-361 (1985).

Vainio, H. and Hietanen, E. Drug metabolism in Gunn rats: inability to increase bilirubin glucuronidation by phenobarbital treatment. *Biochem. Pharmacol.* 23, 3405-3412 (1974).

Vainio, H. and Hietanen, E. Role of extrahepatic metabolism. In *Concepts in Drug Metabolism.* Part A. Jenners, P. and Testa, B. (Editors). Marcel Dekker Inc., New York (1980). Ch. 5, pp. 251-284.

van der Laan, J.W., de Groot, G., Wortelboer, H., and Noordhoek, J. Pharmacokinetic differences of desmethyldiazepam in three outbred Wistar strains related to differences in liver enzyme activities. *Pharmacol. and Toxicol.* 73, 229-232 (1993).

Williams, R.T. *Detoxification Mechanisms.* Second Edition. Chapman and Hall, London (1959).

Williams, R.T. Interspecies variations in the metabolism of xenobiotics. *Biochem. Soc. Trans.* 2, 359-377 (1974).

Withy, J.R., Collins, B.T., and Collins, P.G. Effect of vehicle on the pharmacokinetics and uptake of four halogenated hydrocarbons from the gastrointestinal tract of the rat. *J. Appl. Toxicol.* 3, 249-253 (1983).

Yamada, J., Nikaido, H., and Matsumoto, S. Genetic variability within and between outbred Wistar strains of rats. *Exp. Animal* 28, 259-269 (1979).

Zbinden, G. *Progress in Toxicology. Special Topics.* Vol. 1. Springer-Verlag, New York (1973).

Chapter 3

ACUTE TOXICITY STUDIES

I. PURPOSE AND OBJECTIVES

Acute toxicity studies are conducted in animals to ascertain the total adverse biological effects caused during a finite period of time following the administration of single, frequently large, doses of an agent (or several doses repeated over a short interval of time). The effects observed in the animals are usually directly related to the amount of the poisonous substance administered orally, dermally, or via inhalation. The effects are often spectacular since high doses of the agent are administered and death, sudden or otherwise, is frequently the most important endpoint measured. There is a widespread belief that acute toxicity studies are synonymous with mortality of the treated animals. This is untrue as will be seen in a subsequent section where a wealth of information should be obtained from a properly conducted acute toxicity study. The objectives of any acute toxicity test are to discover and report any adverse health effect which could be attributed to the chemical under study.

Acute toxicity studies are frequently designed to express the potency of the toxicant in terms of the median lethal dose (LD_{50}), a value representing the estimated dose causing death of 50% of the universal population of the species exposed under the defined conditions of the test. In situations where the agent is not administered directly to the animals, as in inhalation studies or aquatic studies, toxicant potency is presented as the median lethal concentration (LC_{50}), the estimated concentration, in the environment to which the animals are exposed, that will result in 50% mortality of the population of animals under the conditions defined for the study. It should be appreciated that the LD_{50} value represents only lethality and does not reflect the overall acute toxic properties of a compound. The LD_{50} gives a comparative indication of the immediate toxicity of an agent in a strain, age group, and sex of a particular species of animal, permitting only a comparison of the toxicity of one agent relative to other agents tested in the same manner in the same species (strain, age, and sex). While such comparisons can be made, this ranking does not take into account the obvious, different mechanisms of action by which the agents elicit toxicity, i.e., the oral LD_{50} values for botulinus toxin, nicotine, DDT, and acetylsalicylic acid being 0.00001, 1.0, 100, and 1000 mg/kg body weight, respectively. Significant, interagent comparisons can be made when the agents are homologs of the same class, with the same mechanism of action, e.g., organophosphorus esters such as parathion, diazinon, malathion, and temephos with oral LD_{50} values of 12.0, 250, 750, and 8600 mg/kg body weight, respectively.

The concept of the LD_{50} developed in the early years of the 20th century when many medicinal agents were available as impure, nonuniform, and frequently toxic mixtures, extracts, or tinctures of biologically derived materials rather than pure chemicals. To standardize the potency of the biologically derived medicinal agents, the effective dosages were expressed as **units of activity** rather than units of weight. It was believed that, if one could calculate the lethal potency of the material with precision, one could indirectly assess the therapeutic potency of the same preparation. In this manner, precise, quantitative methods were devised to develop dose-response or dose-effect relationships to standardize the therapeutic potency of the many biological preparations available in terms of their lethal potency. A perusal of the early pharmacology texts such as *Biological Standardization* by Burn, Finney, and Goodman (1950) will illustrate how the LD_{50} was found to be the most accurate means of quantifying the lethal potency of the drug preparations of those days. The utility of this technique will be considered below when the handling of data arising from such experiments is discussed.

The assessment of the lethal properties of chemicals is an integral part of the acute toxicity phase of the safety evaluation process for any agent whether it is a drug, a pesticide, an industrial chemical, a home product, or an environmental contaminant. There are valid reasons for determining the LD_{50} for chemicals. If humans can come in contact with a particular chemical (voluntarily or involuntarily, accidentally or by design), it is essential to know where the lethal range exists if these individuals are to be protected: The safe handling of chemicals in an industrial setting depends upon adequate information of lethal dosages and exposure conditions, with the information appearing in material safety data sheets (MSDSs) for the chemical or product. The interstate, -country, and -continental transport of potentially hazardous chemicals requires that the relative toxicity (lethality) be known so that proper protective and security measures may be instituted to safeguard the health of innocent bystanders in case of unforeseen, acute exposure to high concentrations of agents arising from accidents. Knowledge of the lethal potency of chemicals and of their combustion products is essential to firefighters engaged in combating conflagrations. It is important for the clinical toxicologist to understand the pathophysiology of the intoxications associated with chemicals, information that can only be obtained from conducting acute toxicity studies.

Controversy has arisen over the fact that the LD_{50} is only an estimate of the toxic dose of an agent and that the precision of this estimate does not increase substantially when more animals are "thrown" into an experiment. Animal welfare activists claim that too many animals are "wasted" in acute toxicity experiments. Their position is not without merit, and they raise legitimate questions. A major controversy has centered on the precision that one needs when performing the **LD_{50} test** and whether or not a **range-finding test**, using considerably fewer animals, would not be sufficient for all purposes. Currently, many national and international regulatory agencies no longer require the precise LD_{50} value for an agent, readily accepting an estimate of the potency. It would seem reasonable to propose that the type of test chosen depends largely on the anticipated use that will be made of the results. The controversy has been eloquently discussed by Zbinden (1981, 1986). However, it is important to point out that there are no known, validated alternatives to the use of animals for the assessment of lethal potency, and such alternatives are unlikely to appear in the near future.

II. STUDY DESIGN

Prior to initiating an acute toxicity study, it is imperative to sit down and design a protocol that will cover any unpredictable, as well as possible unexpected eventualities arising from animals' responses to the agent. A sufficient number of animals must be "built" into the front end of the experiment to allow not only an adequate assessment of the predicted toxicity associated with the chemical but, in addition, to monitor the serendipidous or unpredicted observations that might be made. An early decision must include whether or not *in vivo* animal studies are essential or if one or more of the battery of new *in vitro* alternative tests might achieve the same ends, thereby replacing and/or reducing the number of animals involved. Flexibility is of paramount importance. Considering the current moral issues about the use of animals in safety evaluation studies, it is imperative that the protocols used will obtain the maximum amount of scientifically valid information from as economical a use of animals as possible. There is little point in conducting a test with inadequate numbers of animals if it will have to be repeated with larger numbers. Such a practice is wasteful of animal resources, time, and money.

A. Route(s) of Administration

The toxicant should be administered by the route by which the species is expected to be exposed. In mammals, including the human, the toxicant may be acquired predominantly via the oral route and oral LD_{50} determinations would suffice to allow safety evaluation. However, in the industrial scene, workers may be exposed to toxicants via inhalation and/or dermal contact, necessitating the assessment of hazard via these routes as well. Drugs, administered parenterally (intramuscular, subcutaneous, or intravenous) would be assessed using these routes. More than one route of acquisition might exist for environmental contaminants, i.e., trihalomethanes in potable water supplies, where exposure might be a combination of oral (drinking water, cooking of food), dermal (bathing), and inhalation (vapors and/or aerosols from hot water in a bathroom or water boiling in a kettle or pot). In considering the routes of exposure for veterinary drugs, environmental contaminants in domestic animals and wildlife species, the toxicant should be administered via the "medium" whereby the species would acquire it, i.e., in the food, water, or air.

In acute oral toxicity studies, designed to assess the potency of the toxicant, an important question arises as to how the toxicant should be administered. It is unlikely that an animal could be coaxed to eat a sufficient quantity of most chemicals to cause death. Mixing the agent in the food only increases the volume of material that would have to be ingested, and it also results in imprecise dosing and reduces the toxicity of the chemical. It is customary to give the toxicant by gavage, administering the agent dissolved in a suitable, inert, nontoxic vehicle via a "feeding" needle and syringe. In this manner, precise dosages can be given. The volume of solution administered must be kept constant (calculated on a milliliter per kilogram of body weight basis) since absorption rates and subsequent biological effects may vary considerably if different volumes are used. For the rodent species, volumes of solutions of the order of 2.0 to 5.0 ml/kg can be administered without undue stress to the animals. The administration of large volumes should be avoided as this practice tends to retard efficient absorption of the toxicant.

The application of toxicants to the skin to assess the hazards of dermal exposure is a science in itself and the reader is referred to Marzulli and Maibach (1987) for a complete description of the various techniques and approaches used. At this point, it is sufficient to state that the toxicant, in solution or in powder form, is applied uniformly to a closely shaved area of skin on the back or abdomen, representative of a suitable fraction (10 to 20%) of the total body surface. The toxicant and vehicle may readily penetrate the epidermis or it may be necessary to cover the treated area with a wrapping to prevent the animal from licking the unabsorbed material. In the case of powdered material, applied dry or as a moist paste, it will be essential to cover the treated area to keep the toxicant in contact with the site of absorption. With liquids, pastes, and powders, the material is left in place for 24 h at which time any remaining material is washed off with warm water and tissues.

Whether or not the toxicant is acquired via the inhalation of contaminated air by the lungs or via absorption of a water-borne toxicant through the gills, only the medium is different. With inhalation, one is usually dealing with a gas, a vapor, particulate matter, or an aerosolized form of the toxicant. In aquatic studies, the toxicant may be in solution, in a particulate form, or adhering to soil and detritus particles. Studies generally involve placing adequate numbers of the animals in the medium containing a range of concentrations of the toxicant for a suitable length of time (inhalation, 4 h; water, 96 h), transferring the survivors to uncontaminated medium at the termination of the exposure period for further observation. As was indicated above, the potency of the toxicant is usually expressed in terms of an LC_{50}, an estimated concentration in the medium, with exposure having taken place for a finite time period.

B. Animals

Various strains of the laboratory mouse or rat are used routinely in determining the LD_{50}. Preference for these rodent species lies with the economics (relatively inexpensive), the minimal variation between animals, the ready availability of these animals nationwide, and the ease of handling them, rather than the fact that they bear any similarity to the human. In addition, the economics of housing and caring for them frequently outweighs the scientific evidence that might argue for the use of another species. However, one must consider the fact that there is a tremendous amount of acute, toxicological data on these two species, this database being useful when making comparisons between chemicals, as will be discussed below. The studies are usually done in males and females, as well as in young and adult animals, because of known differences in susceptibility to chemicals.

It is desirable to have LD_{50} data from a nonrodent species. This is of particular importance when the mouse and rat LD_{50} values are very different, suggesting clear species differences in the absorption, distribution, and biotransformation and/or elimination of the toxicant. If experience with similar agents suggests that possible biotransformation by the human would be significantly different from that of the rodent, nonrodent species such as the dog or a primate (monkey, baboon, etc.) should be used. Once again, males and females of each species should be treated. However, the costs involved are considerably higher and the use of large numbers cannot be justified. Frequently, the LD_{50} values obtained in the rodent studies will be confirmed by a range-finding study in the nonrodent species (see below). In the fields of veterinary, entomological, and environmental sciences, it is usually possible to use the species of interest, a luxury not available to investigators involved in assessing safety for the human.

Since the animals will be receiving relatively high doses of the test agent, it is imperative that the animals be purchased from a reputable dealer, be placed in a quarantine area of the animal care facility for at least 10 to 14 d prior to being used and be examined to insure that they are healthy (Figure 3.1). Examination may include the euthanasia of a randomly-selected subpopulation of the animals for gross

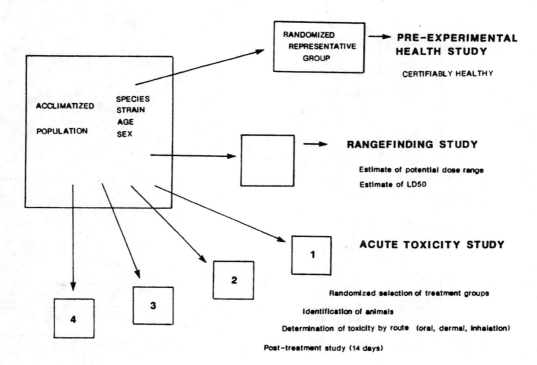

FIGURE 3.1
A schematic flow diagram depicting the acquisition of animals (specified strain, sex, and age) for an acute toxicity study, their acclimatization in an animal care facility for 1 or 2 weeks during which time a representative subgroup undergoes a thorough health study (including hematology, serum biochemistry, urinalysis, and necropsy with gross and microscopic examination of tissues) prior to certifying the health status of the animals. A second, representative subgroup might be selected for a rangefinding estimation of the toxic dose of an unknown agent prior to the determination of acute toxic effects and the LD_{50} value. Many regulatory agencies no longer require the LD_{50} value as an endpoint for acute toxicity, an estimation of this value being sufficient. See text for some protocols for obtaining this value.

and histopathological examination of organs, as well as blood chemistry by experienced personnel. Extra animals should be purchased since the investigators must retain the option to choose and/or reject animals on the basis of the health screening results. All too frequently, transportation from the breeder to the laboratory facility — with the trauma and stress associated with this — in addition to the environment of new quarters (temperature, light, humidity, caging, handling, food, water, etc.), will be sufficient to unmask quiescent infections that can jeopardize the study. Stress associated with exposure to the agent may also promote seemingly dormant health problems. Having some guarantee that the animals are in prime, healthy condition, the investigator can proceed to the actual experiment.

It is imperative that the species, strain, age, and sex of the animal be clearly defined. White laboratory mice or rats are not identical and there are many interstrain genetic differences that can alter the results of studies in significant ways. The age of rodents can be established by referring to growth curves available from most breeders as is shown in the examples in Figure 3.2. Age- and sex-related differences in responses to chemicals are well known. Note that some strains and sexes of rats and mice develop at quite different rates. If other investigators wish to repeat a study, it is essential that they know exactly what animals were used.

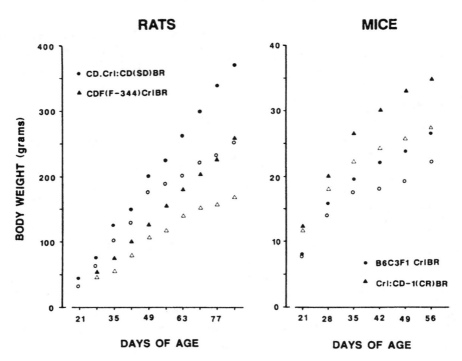

FIGURE 3.2
The interstrain differences in the growth and development of young male and female rats (CD and F-344 strains) and mice (B6C3F1 and CD-1 strains). Over the time period studied, it can be seen that, while male animals are always larger than females of the same strain, there are significant differences between strains. Data from Charles River Breeding Laboratories, Inc., Wilmington MS.

C. Range-Finding Tests

Given the recent controversy about the use of vast numbers of animals to determine the LD_{50} values for chemicals when such precision is not really essential, it is surprising to find that experiments designed to conserve the number of animals used in acute toxicity studies were reported as early as 45 years ago. In the simplest technique to determine the approximate lethal dose, six animals were used, each animal being treated with a single dose of the agent at a concentration 50% higher than the dose administered to the preceding one (Deichman and LeBlanc, 1945). With such a spacing of the doses, one avoids the possibility of killing one animal with a dose but failing to kill the animal with the next higher dose. Such an experiment will allow an investigator to determine the smallest lethal dose which may be close to the LD_{50}. Additional studies using this technique revealed that, for some 87 compounds, 88% of the approximate lethal doses ranged within ±30% of the LD_{50} values determined by the more classical approach using more animals per treatment group (Deichman and Mergard, 1948). This range-finding technique gave reasonably precise lethal concentrations for all but a few of the chemicals tested.

Another technique to determine the approximate lethal dose involved the arbitrary selection of a suitable concentration of toxicant and administration to two animals. After 24 h, having observed what happened to the treated rodents, a second pair receives a dose multiplied by (1) a factor of 3/2 if the dose given to the original pair was tolerated or (2) a factor of 2/3 if the arbitrarily selected dose was fatal. This

TABLE 3.1

Ranking System Used by the
European Economic Community
for Acute Oral Toxicity

Category	LD_{50} (mg/kg)
Very toxic	25
Toxic	25–200
Harmful	200–2000
Unclassified	2000

From European Commission Directive
83/467/EEC., 1983.

procedure can be repeated upward or downward until the maximum nonlethal and the minimum lethal doses have been determined. This type of test was proposed by Smith et al. (1960).

A third technique of ascertaining the approximate lethal dose has been called the **up-and-down** or **staircase method** and was described first by Dixon and Mood (1948) who applied the technique to the sensitivity of explosives to shock, a far cry from animal experiments (Dixon, 1965). However, the technique can be adapted to a biological experiments having different endpoints (Dixon, 1991). The second animal will receive a higher dosage if the first animal survives or a lower dose if the animal dies. By selecting a proper spread of dosages beforehand, most animals would receive dosages of agent close to the true mean lethal dose. Too wide a spread of dosages would require additional animals to fill in the gaps. Renewed interest in this technique has resulted in publications by Bruce (1985, 1987) demonstrating that, while the classical method of LD_{50} determination requires 40 to 50 animals, the up-and-down method requires only 6 to 9 animals per chemical. Studies of estimated LD_{50} values, derived from the up-and-down assay method with 6 to 10 animals, compared favorably with those determined by the conventional assay for 23 of 25 chemicals (Lipnick et al., 1995).

More recently, a newer approach to acute toxicity testing has evolved from the assay suggested by the British Toxicology Society. This **fixed-dose approach** avoids using death of the animals as an endpoint, relying on clear observations of toxicity at one or another of a set of preselected or fixed doses to permit classification or ranking of the chemical according to that system used by the European Economic Community as is shown in Table 3.1 (EEC, 1993). The range of doses was chosen to be in line with this ranking system and was fixed at 5, 50, and 500 mg/kg body weight with an additional test limit dose of 2000 mg/kg. An extensive validation study has been conducted, involving 33 laboratories in 11 countries, measuring the acute oral toxicity of 20 substances or preparations in the rat (van den Heuvel et al., 1990). The results revealed that this fixed-dose method produced: (1) consistent results even given some interlaboratory variations; (2) adequate toxicity data (nature, time of onset, duration, outcome) for risk assessment purposes; (3) a requirement for fewer animals than currently used in the OECD procedure; (4) less pain, distress, and compound-related mortality; and (5) the ability to rank the test agents by the EEC classification system. The procedure has been described in detail, including an interpretive table for the 5, 50, 500, and 2000 mg/kg body weight dose range (van den Heuvel et al., 1990).

One additional method that should be considered is the technique described by Smyth et al. (1962) in which a constant number of animals (two or three) per dosage level is used, the dosage levels are spaced in a geometric progression, and there are a certain minimal number of dosages. This experimental technique, called a **moving average method**, takes the arithmetic mean of three successive values of percent mortality and relates them to the mean of the corresponding doses. The LD_{50} can be computed along with the 95% confidence limit for the value. Earlier studies by Weil (1952) eliminated the need for calculations by developing a series of tables into which one can enter the criteria outlined above to obtain the LD_{50}.

The rangefinding approach to estimating LD_{50} values is particularly suited to situations such as wildlife biology, aquatic toxicology, entomology, etc., where investigators have only a limited number of animals at their disposal. In many cases, this estimate will be sufficiently accurate to use it as a basis for the selection of dosages to be used in longer-term studies.

D. The Classical LD_{50}

Despite the fact that the above-mentioned "quick-and-dirty" methods may be entirely adequate to gain insight into the lethal potency of the toxicant, estimations as accurate as can be made scientifically possible are still being required by regulatory agencies concerned with exposure situations such as industrial and environmental accidents where workers and/or bystander populations may be exposed to high levels of chemical. The Bhopal methyl-isocyanate incident is a case in point where there was little information available on the acute toxicity associated with the inhalation of this chemical. While the criticism may be leveled that these values are just numbers to hang one's hat on, they are valid, particularly if one has decent 95% confidence limits which reflect the reproducibility of the experimental data.

1. The Oral LD_{50}

As is shown in Figure 3.1, some technique of randomization must be developed to maintain an equitable distribution of the test animals into the appropriate number of subgroups having the required number of animals. It is desirable to have a narrow range of body weights within and between subgroups so that all the big animals do not end up in one group and the small ones in another. For rodents, an appropriate number of animals is not less than ten per treatment group. Each animal is then identified in some fashion (ear notches, tattooing, tail markings, ear tags, and corresponding cage tags) and can then be housed individually in a proper cage (wire mesh or stainless steel, with a food and water dispenser) or, if this is not feasible, as a group of four or five animals in a shoe-box cage. In most cases, the animals will be fasted overnight (16 to 18 h) prior to the oral administration of the test agent to insure that there will be no food-related impediment to the absorption of the chemical from the intestinal tract. Water would be provided *ad libidum*. Fasting should also be considered in dermal and/or inhalation studies. The animals should be weighed just prior to dosing.

The range of dosages to be used in the study must be established. Preliminary range-finding studies may reduce the spread of dosages by eliminating the low and high concentrations that elicit no toxicity or lethality, respectively. The precision of the LD_{50} determination can be improved by (1) increasing the number of animals per treatment group (but this is only effective to a certain extent, with ten animals being the maximum) and (2) decreasing the ratio between successive doses. Investigators may use 50 animals per experiment for five different doses having a ratio of 1.5 to 2.0 between successive doses. A more precise LD_{50} can be obtained by using smaller ratios, i.e., 1.2. While such manipulation of the parameters is feasible with an endless supply of rodents, the use of large, nonrodent species or limitations in the absolute numbers of animals available will dictate a careful consideration of the resource(s) before committing it to such a study.

2. The Dermal LD$_{50}$

The acute lethality of a toxicant may be assessed by exposure of a suitable animal species to dermal contact with the agent. Studies are usually conducted because of a possibility of exposure to agents by this route. Lethality is generally assessed in two species, one being a nonrodent, with males and females of the species being treated. The test substance will be applied to the skin in graduated doses to several groups of experimental animals, one dose being used per group. A sufficient number of doses, spaced approximately to elicit a range of toxic effects and mortality rates, should be used. Since total absorption of the test substance through the skin cannot be guaranteed, what is frequently being determined in the study is an LC$_{50}$ — a median lethal concentration — not an LD$_{50}$. If dermal absorption is known to be quantitative, the term LD$_{50}$ may be used.

As described for the oral LD$_{50}$, adequate numbers (n = 10 for rodents and n = 6 for nonrodent species per treatment group) need to be included in the design of the study. The animals will be prepared for the experiment 24 h in advance by clipping or shaving the fur from an area on the back or abdomen equivalent to approximately 10% of the total body surface area, i.e., an area of 3 × 4 cm for rats or 5 × 6 cm for rabbits.

The material, if liquid, should be administered evenly over the shaved area, applying it by syringe and spreading it with a glass rod. If the test agent is a solid, it can be dissolved in 0.9% saline, in a relatively inert organic solvent such as dimethyl sulfoxide or dimethyl formamide, a vegetable oil, propylene glycol, or it can be suspended in 1.0% carboxymethylcellulose. However, the vehicle may have significant effects on absorption. Except in the case of liquid materials, it is recommended that the volume of solution applied remain constant, not exceeding 1.0 to 2.0 ml/kg body weight, and that it be applied uniformly over the exposed skin. Solid, insoluble agents may be applied as dry powders or as water-moistened pastes. The site of application will be occluded by covering it with a suitable gauze pad taped securely to the skin and the entire region will be covered by either a rubber sheet wrapped around the midsection of the body or a form-fitting elastic cloth sleeve. Restraint devices may be necessary to prevent the removal of the coverings and subsequent ingestion of the material during grooming. The test agent is left in place for 24 h, after which the coverings are removed and residual agent is washed off with the aid of a gauze pad and warm soap and water.

Given the variability in physicochemical properties of agents and the physiological properties of the skin, there are a number of problems associated with the acute dermal lethality test. Liquids or solids dissolved in vehicles, having a high degree of lipid solubility as determined by their oil/water (o/w) partition coefficients, will readily penetrate the skin and be absorbed. In contrast, agents that are water soluble will not be absorbed efficiently by this route. Experiments conducted in different laboratories with highly toxic and/or lipid soluble agents generally yield reproducible, accurate estimations of the LD$_{50}$. However, similar interlaboratory experiments conducted with agents of low to moderate toxicity yield highly variable results that are dependent largely upon the conditions under which the experiment was conducted. With chemicals possessing inherent low toxicity, the concentrations required to elicit adverse health effects frequently exceed the dosages that can be applied to the shaved skin. If compound-related toxicity and/or mortality is not observed at a dosage of 2000 mg/kg body weight, further study at higher dosages is unnecessary.

It is imperative that, in dermal lethality studies, an exact description of how the test was conducted be included in any reports since it will facilitate replication of the conditions should the test need to be repeated in other laboratories.

3. The Inhalation LD$_{50}$

The likelihood of exposure to inhalable toxic materials (gases, aerosols, particulates) will necessitate the determination of the acute lethality of the toxicants by this route of exposure. Groups of experimental animals — rodent and nonrodent, males and females of each — will be exposed for a defined period, usually 4 h, to the test substance in graduated concentrations, one concentration being used per group. Essential for such studies is a negative-pressure, dynamic inhalation system having controllable airflow, a suitable system to generate the concentrations of material required, instrumentation to continuously monitor the actual levels attained in the system, and a trapping system to capture the toxicant in the exhausted air (Phalen et al., 1984; Snellings and Dodd, 1990). The animals may be accomodated within the inhalation chamber (whole body exposure) or, alternatively, head-only or oro-nasal exposure to the agent may be used. As was described, a minimum of three doses should be used, spaced appropriately to produce a range of toxic effects and/or mortality rates in order to facilitate the assessment of acute toxicity as well as the concentration-mortality relationship to ascertain the LC$_{50}$ value.

There are a multitude of problems inherent in conducting a well-designed, whole-body exposure inhalation study. Some of the major difficulties that must be considered are outlined below.

1. Exposure data must be presented in terms of (a) the nominal concentration of toxicant (total amount of test substance delivered to the inhalation system divided by the volume of air), (b) actual toxicant concentrations in the animals' breathing zone, (c) airflow rates through the chamber, (d) particle size distribution of aerosols and particulates (median aerodynamic diameter of particles ± standard deviation from the mean), and (e) air temperature and humidity. All of these measurements require sophisticated instrumentation capable of continuously monitoring the experimental conditions for the duration of the study.

2. The physicochemical properties of the toxicant or formulation will dictate the maximum amount of active ingredient that can be suspended in the air in the inhalation device. This may pose few problems with very toxic agents, but frequently insurmountable difficulties with agents having low to moderate toxicity.

3. The particle size of aerosols and particulates must be in the respirable range of less than two μm in diameter for effective inhalation. Larger particles will be trapped in the upper respiratory tract.

4. Invariably, once the animals have been placed in cages in the chamber and have explored the new surroundings, they curl up and go to sleep, thereby reducing their normal respiration rate. If the test agent is noxious, rodents will tuck their heads under a foreleg while sleeping, effectively screening out material and reducing the exposure level. These problems can be minimized to some extent by head-only or oro-nasal exposure.

5. Upon terminating the experiment, the surviving animals will be removed from the chamber and returned to their own cages where they will proceed to groom themselves to remove the toxicant dust or droplets adhering to their fur. The classical whole body inhalation study may actually constitute a mixture of inhalation, dermal, and oral exposure. These complications can be minimized to some degree by head-only or oro-nasal exposure. However, one must anticipate LC_{50} values by these latter routes being several-fold lower (more toxic) than those determined by the classical approach.

6. By inhalation, many substances are highly irritant to the respiratory tract, triggering a mucosecretory response that may severely incapacitate normal respiration and exposure to the toxicant.

7. In the assessment of mixtures or formulations such as pesticide, paints, etc., some of the observed adverse effects may not be associated with the active ingredient but with cosolvents, emulsifiers, and additives, usually considered as "inerts" in the formulation. Localized effects in the respiratory tract are frequently detected. In such studies, at least one group of animals should be included for inhalation exposure to the formulation without the "active" ingredient in order to assess the effects of these other chemicals on the lungs and other organs.

E. Duration of Acute Toxicity Studies

Traditionally, the time interval of 24 h has been used as the deadline in determining the LD_{50}, regardless of the route of exposure. During the first 24-h period after treatment, any moribund, seriously ill animals will be euthanized and examined for clues as to the cause of death. Tissues will be taken for morphological analysis as well as for gross examination. At 24 h posttreatment, the number of dead animals per treatment group is tallied, and the survivors are returned to their regular cages for observation over the subsequent 14 d. Unless otherwise indicated in the reporting of the data, it is assumed that the LD_{50} represents the median lethal dose for deaths occurring in the first 24-h period. By contrast, the LC_{50} values for toxicants in fish or insect toxicity studies are usually based on a 96-h exposure period, the surviving animals being transferred at that time to a toxicant-free environment for subsequent observation.

F. Observations

As was indicated above, mortality is only one parameter to be measured in acute toxicity studies. Close observation of the treated animals through the first 12-h posttreatment period may reveal several clues to the mechanism(s) by which the toxicant is eliciting its effect. The general appearance of the animals should be noted and compared with that of control, untreated, or vehicle-treated animals. In addition to the onset, intensity, and duration of toxicity, it should be possible to monitor obvious changes in behavior, respiration, cutaneous effects, including some associated with the autonomic nervous system, sensory nervous system responses, and gastrointestinal effects. Detailed endpoints of toxicity are listed in Table 3.2 (McNamara, 1976).

Following the acute phase of the study, i.e., the first 24-h period, the moribund and normal appearing survivors should be examined daily over the subsequent 14-d

TABLE 3.2

Observations of Acute Toxicity Pertinent to Ascertaining Target-Organ Involvement

Organ system	Toxic signs
Autonomic	Salivation, nasal discharge, diarrhea, urination, piloerection, exophthalmos, relaxed nictitating membranes, rhinorrhea
Behavioral	Sedation, drooping head, sitting position with head up, panting, staring straight ahead, severe depression
	Restlessness, excessive preening, irritability, aggressive behavior, defensive hostility, fear, bizarre activity, confusion
Sensory	Righting reflex, sensitivity to pain, corneal reflex, placing, hind limb reflex, sensitivity to sound and touch, nystagmus phonation
Neuromuscular	Decreased and increased activity, fasciculations, tremors, weakness, absent or diminished hind limb reflexes, muscle tone, ophisthotonus, ataxia, convulsions, prostration, hind limb weakness
Cardiovascular	Alteration (increase or decrease) of heart rate, cyanosis, vasoconstriction, vasodilatation, hemorrhage
Respiratory	Gasping, dyspnea, apnea, hypopnea
Ocular	Lacrimation, ptosis, nystagmus, mydriasis, miosis, cycloplegia, pupillary light reflex
Gastrointestinal	Salivation, retching, diarrhea, bloody stool, constipation, emesis, defecation
Gastro-urinary	Urinary frequency, blood urine
Cutaneous	Piloerection, alopecia, "wet dog" shakes, erythema, edema, swelling, necrosis

From McNamara, P. B., *New Concepts in Safety Evaluation*, Mehlman, M. A., Shapiro, R. E., and Blumenthal, H., Eds., Hemisphere Publishing, New York (1976), Chap. 4. With permission.

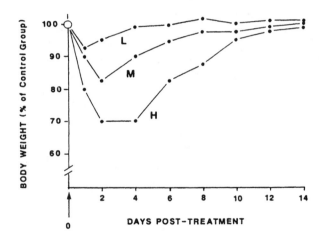

FIGURE 3.3
The influence of low (L), medium (M), and high (H) acute doses of a potential toxicant on the general well-being of surviving animals as reflected in a theoretical plot of body weight changes in the 14-d, posttreatment period. Such results support the adage that, if an animal does not feel well, it does not eat and drink adequately and will lose a significant amount of body weight in a very short period of time. Such an effect is seen particularly in small animals having high basal metabolic rates.

recovery period in order that delayed effects and/or secondary toxicity will not be overlooked. During this time period, the survivors should be weighed daily and the body weight changes should be plotted against time. While this would appear to be a very simple parameter, body weight gain is a good indicator of the general health of the animal and if the animal is not feeling well, it will not eat sufficient food to maintain normal growth and development. In Figure 3.3 is shown a theoretical example of the body weight changes of acute toxicity test survivors in the posttreatment period. Food and/or water consumption may be measured as a confirmation of general well-being.

In both rodent and nonrodent species, blood samples can be obtained from the survivors for hematology and a full range of serum biochemistry without destroying the animals. Urinalysis and fecal analysis can be easily done on samples collected from animals placed overnight in suitable metabolic cages. Neurological assessment can be carried out by noninvasive techniques, i.e., rotarod balancing, activity measurements, nerve conduction velocities with surface electrodes, cognitive deficits, etc. In this manner, one can obtain useful information on target organs affected by the agent.

Gross pathological examination should be performed on all animals during the acute phase of the study. Frequently, this is not very rewarding, particularly when death occurs within a short interval after treatment. Necropsy of all animals dying in the subsequent 14-d recovery period should be done, as well as an examination of all animals, both moribund and healthy, at the termination of the experiment. Selected organs and tissues should be examined histologically to detect morphological changes associated with pathological disease or tissue injury.

III. INTERPRETATION OF DATA

As with any toxicological study, the aim of the acute study is to develop a quantitative relationship between the intensity of a measurable biological response or adverse health effect and the concentration(s) of agent administered. This is best done by preparing a graph with the frequency of the biological response (number of animals responding) on the y-axis of the graph and the corresponding dosage (mg/kg body weight) on the x-axis.

In experiments of this type, one has to be cognizant of biological variation in response to toxicants within the population of animals being tested. However, inbred the strain of animals may be, one has to anticipate that some biological heterogeneity in response will be obtained. Rarely is this assumption ever checked by experimentation. Investigators assume that, if they purchase animals of the same strain, sex, and age from the same supplier, these animals will always possess the same, homogeneous genetic pool and, within reason, will respond in the same manner. Unfortunately, heterogeneity of response will still be observed in inbred animals, as is presented in Figure 3.4, where the normal distribution (Gaussian) curve in the frequency response-dosage diagram is more confined over a narrower dosage range than is that of the heterogeneous strain animals. Investigators using randomly bred strains or captured wildlife should be aware that heterogeneity can cause substantial errors in estimated LD_{50} values, with much broader 95% confidence limits. Significant skewing of the frequency-dosage relationship can be encountered.

Figure 3.5 illustrates another point that investigators must appreciate. The assumption is made that the dosage can be accurately "delivered" to the organism, i.e., weighed out, dissolved or put into a suitable vehicle, the volume to be administered can be accurately measured, and the animal dosed properly without loss of any toxicant. Variation along the x-axis should be minimal and relatively constant. If there is any doubt about the animal's receiving the entire dose, it should be rejected from the study. This still leaves the possibility of variability along the y-axis since each subgroup (n = 6 or 10 animals) should represent the entire population from

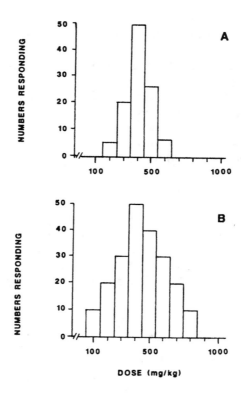

FIGURE 3.4
A diagram showing the relationship between dose and the number of individuals reacting with a specific effect at various doses, i.e., death, the experimental animals being chosen from an inbred, genetically homogeneous strain (A) or from a genetically heterogeneous strain (B). A symmetrical or normal distribution is shown around the median (the dose dividing the frequency distribution into two equal parts) and demonstrates the limited interanimal variability in response in inbred animals while in outbred animals, greater differences are observed, some being very susceptible, while others are quite resistant to the toxic effects. Frequently, plots of a similar nature may be skewed to the left or right, such results denoting some distinct physiological difference(s) within the population of animals.

which they were selected (see Figure 3.1). Each data point represents a mini-Gaussian curve, with variation in response controlled to the best of the investigator's ability in selecting this subgroup to minimize between-animal variability. Greater variation will be seen at the extreme ends of the plotted relationship while variation will be minimal near the center portion.

Given the example shown in Figure 3.6A in which the acute lethality of a hypothetical chemical has been ascertained in three separate experiments, one can see that, over the range of 25 to 250 mg/kg body weight, the agent has been lethal to a large number of animals. However, the reproducibility of the experiments has not been consistent. Initially, a dosage ratio of 2.0 was used in the study, i.e., dosages were 25, 50, 100, and 200 mg/kg body weight. The investigator went back and repeated dosages of 150 and 250 mg/kg body weight because of the observed variability. A "best-fit" line through these points is difficult to achieve by eye. The relationship is sigmoidal or S-shaped. Calculation of the mean percent mortality from the three experiments does improve the relationship between effect (death) and dosage. From this plot, it is obvious that there is a suggestive linear relationship in the middle portion. In this latter region, a given change in dose results in a specific change in effect and the slope of the line can define the magnitude of this relationship.

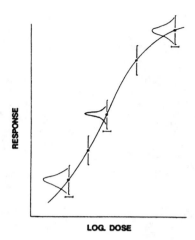

FIGURE 3.5
A theoretical dose-response relationship illustrating the variability in administered dose and the response(s) within the treated subgroup of animals. Variability should be negligible with dosage, competent scientists being able to prepare the amount of drug accurately and to administer the dose to the animal. Variability between animals will be inherent in each subgroup treated at each dosage but should be minimal at the midpoint of the curve, the 50% response point.

Variability, arising from a number of animal- and investigator-related factors, is greatest at the extremes. The fundamental principles illustrated by this example were first defined by Trevan (1927) who pointed out that there was no such thing as a minimal lethal dose, one that would just be sufficient to produce an effect in all animals. He noted that the variability of individuals in a population led to this characteristic S-shaped curve and that there seemed to be less variation at the 50% response value intercept. He proposed the term **median lethal dose**, the LD_{50}, which can be calculated easily from the plotted data (Figure 3.7).

The physical appearance of the experimental results, the ease of drawing a best-fit line through the data points, and the estimation of the slope of the relationship may be improved by transposing the dosage to a logarithmic function as is shown in Figure 3.6B. Linearity of the curve has been improved and a best-fit line is somewhat easier to estimate between approximately 16 and 84% responses. There are several different methods of transposing the data. The conversion of the dosage to the logarithmic function can be done by using a set of logarithm tables or by using semi-logarithmic graph paper (Litchfield and Wilcoxon, 1949). An alternative technique, using probability (probit) semi-logarthmic graph paper, converts the response values to probit units. This derivative plot allows a much wider range of the sigmoidal curve to be "straightened out." The probit unit corresponds to normal equivalent deviations around the mean value, the mean value having a zero deviation. This technique has been described by Miller and Tainter (1944). Variations of these techniques, all designed to improve the accuracy of the LD_{50} estimation, have been described by Bliss (1957) and Finney (1971). A longer treatise on a predictive model for estimating rat oral LD_{50} values has been published recently (Enslein et al., 1983).

Assuming that the variability is at least at the 50% point on the curve, the LD_{50} is obtained by drawing a line horizontally from the 50% mortality point on the y-axis to the point of intersection with the curve (Figure 3.8A). From this point, a vertical line is drawn to the x-axis to derive the LD_{50} value. If one makes the assumption that the population is homogeneous and the results are normally distributed, one can estimate the 95% confidence limits of the LD_{50} by repeating the above

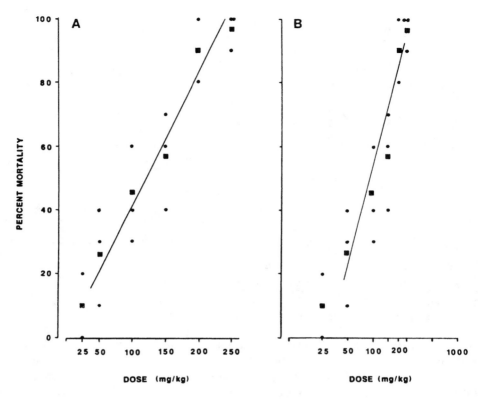

FIGURE 3.6
The acute lethality of a hypothetical chemical, plotting the values obtained from repeated experiments (n = 3) as percent mortality vs. dose on (A) a linear and (B) a logarithmic scale. The conversion of the dose values to the logarithmic values "pulls" the variable points together thereby permitting a better estimation of a "best-fit" line by eye and ruler.

horizontal and vertical lines at the LD_5 and LD_{95} (the $LD_{50} \pm 1.96$ standard deviations) (Figure 3.8A). Should nonlinearity be encountered at these extremes, as it frequently is, the $LD_{50} \pm 1.0$ standard deviations can be obtained by drawing the horizontal and vertical lines at the LD_{16} and LD_{84} (Figure 3.8B), then mathematically determining the 1.96 standard deviation values.

When examining LD_{50} data quoted in the literature, it is imperative to know what the 95% confidence limits are since the narrowness or breadth will signify a very toxic or slightly toxic agent and the relationship of the slope of the line to response. However, one frequently encounters single statements, e.g., the oral LD_{50} for "x" in the rat (or the mouse) is 265 mg/kg body weight, without any identification of the strain, sex, or age of the animals from which this number was generated and without confidence limits. The value has little relevance except in that it can be compared with other single values for homologous or different agents obtained in much the same manner. The vast data base for acute lethality information is of this standard and quality. Without confidence limits, a single value provides no information concerning the dose-response relationship — a steep slope indicating a potent toxicant (a small increase in dosage resulting in a marked response) or a shallow slope suggesting an agent of low potency, requiring a large increase in dosage to cause only a small or moderate change in biological effect. If, in searching the literature, several different LD_{50} values for the same chemical can be obtained from

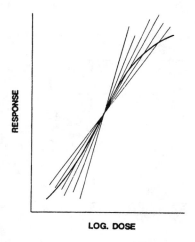

FIGURE 3.7

A diagrammatic representation of the finding of Trevan that, with repeated experiments over the same dosage range, the series of different slopes obtained for the dose-response relationship would intersect at the 50% response point, minimal deviation of the results being observed at this intercept. As one departs from this point, the accuracy of the data declines, greater variability between single values being measured. This observation led to the development of the concept of the LD_{50} being the most accurate estimate of one endpoint of toxicity, the lethality of the agent.

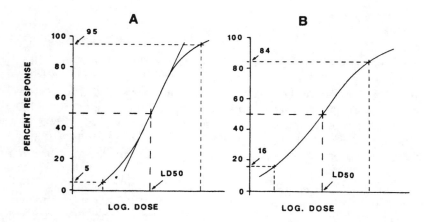

FIGURE 3.8

(A). Estimation of the LD_{50} value and the 95% confidence limits from a plot of percent mortality vs. the logarithmic value of the dose. Note the over-estimation of the confidence limits due to the nonlinearity of the relationship at value points remote from the 50% response value. (B) With nonlinearity frequently being seen in such plots, the variability between the LD_{50} + one standard deviation (LD_{16} and LD_{84}) can be determined, with a subsequent mathematical estimation of the 95% confidence limits by multiplying the standard deviation value by 1.96.

different sources (experiments or laboratories), then an approximate mean value (and a standard deviation) can be determined and a line slope can be generated for the dose-response relationship. The comparison of 95% confidence limits for different isomers or analogs of a class of chemicals, e.g., organophosphorus ester insecticides, may suggest different modes of action, different capabilities of detoxification of the agents, and therefore, different potencies.

TABLE 3.3

Reliability of LD Values Distant from the LD_{50}: Comparison of Calculated LD_{35} to Mortality Observed at That Dose Level

	Calculated		Observed mortality at LD_{35}	
Material	LD_{50}	LD_{35}	Ratio	%
Acetonitrile	5.75	4.24	3/20	15
Aniline	0.48	0.42	2/20	10
Ethanol	6.06	5.40	1/20	5
Ethylene glycol	5.22	4.46	1/18	6
Phenol	0.32	0.28	0/20	0
Propylene glycol	15.9	12.4	1/39	3
Methanol	9.54	8.45	4/20	20
Diethylene glycol monomethyl ether	6.31	5.62	1/20	5

From Weil, C. S., *Toxicol. Appl. Pharmacol.*, 21:454–463 (1972). With permission.

To give some indication of the precarious nature of the dose-relationship used to ascertain the LD_{50} value, an investigator is well advised not to rely on values too distant from the midpoint. Weil (1972), having determined the LD_{50} values for a number of chemicals in rats, treated representative subgroups with dosages equivalent to the LD_{35} (Table 3.3). The results ranged from 0 to 20% mortality, nowhere near the expected 35% mortality. This example illustrates Trevan's hypothesis that, as one moves away from the median lethal dose, the intersubject variability in response increases.

IV. UTILITY OF THE LD_{50} STUDIES

The LD_{50} is a statistical estimate of the acute lethality of an agent administered to a specified sex, age, and strain of a species of animal. It provides a measure of the relative toxicity of an unknown agent compared to other agents administered to the same species, strain, age, and sex of animal. The public conception of the LD_{50} study is limited to the consideration only of the number of animals that died to provide this estimate of toxicity. Nothing could be further from the truth. In fact, if the study has been designed properly, the surviving animals are far more important than those that died.

During the acute phase of the study, the information gleaned from the experiment includes not only a rapid assessment of lethality, but other signs and symptoms of acute toxicity, possible target organs, some minimal information concerning the rate of detoxification and/or elimination, as well as the duration and intensity of the toxic effects. This information is of considerable use to occupational health physicians, the staff of emergency treatment units, and emergency measures organization personnel if and when the agent is misused (accidental poisonings, suicidal overdose) or when an environmental disaster occur. The results will also assist investigators in designing subsequent subchronic and chronic studies, estimating the potential hazard to health and well-being, as well as planning therapeutic trials of drugs in humans.

There is a wealth of information in those animals surviving the doses administered. What can they tell the investigator? The duration of the acute effects can be determined. An indication can be obtained of when the animals begin to recover and whether or not is is dose-related (See Figure 3.3). More importantly, the investigator

TABLE 3.4

Classification of Chemicals
According to Relative Toxicity

Category	LD_{50} (mg/kg)
Extremely toxic	1.0 or less
Highly toxic	1.0–50.0
Moderately toxic	50.0–500.0
Slightly toxic	500.0–5,000.0
Practically nontoxic	5,000.0–15,000.0
Relatively harmless	15,000 or greater

can determine if secondary toxicity develops, possibly involving other signs and symptoms than those observed during the acute phase, indicative of the involvement of other target organs. This information is essential to discovering the mode of action. The information obtained from the survivors is essential in treating poisonings, since it gives the attending physician some idea of how long supportive treatment must be continued and if additional treatment may be required as the toxicant affects other target organs and sites in the body.

The major use of the LD_{50} is a comparative one, allowing the investigator to assess the relative toxicity of an unknown compound in terms of the toxicity associated with other agents tested in the same species (strain, sex, and age). With a massive amount of acute toxicity data tabulated for the white laboratory rat, despite the obvious strain differences, a good indication can be obtained whether the agent is extremely toxic or has a low order of toxicity. One cannot make the quantum leap from rats to the human by saying that, because compound "x" is less toxic than "y" in rats, it should be less toxic in the human. Only if you have comparable acute toxicity data for a group of agents in both rats and humans should such interspecies comparisons be attempted cautiously. Initially, the LD_{50} value of an unknown agent is compared to established classifications of relative toxicity such as that shown in Tables 3.1 or 3.4 in order to categorize the potential potency of the agent. However, the LD_{50} value is misused frequently by industry, government, and the news media in promoting the safety or hazard of the product.

V. DERMAL TOXICITY STUDIES

For the regulation of many products, including household products (detergents, cleaners, waxes, polishes), cosmetics, drugs, pesticides, and all industrial chemicals that may come into direct contact with the skin, studies are carried out on the skin of suitable animal species. Primary dermal irritation studies are routinely conducted as are cutaneous sensitization experiments, but more recently, attention is being directed toward phototoxicity and photosensitization as agents are encountered that elicit these unusual effects in humans. The conduction of these studies has generated much controversy among animal welfare groups who make the valid points that they can cause discomfort and pain, are inhumane, and the results are difficult to extrapolate to man. In defense of these studies which, first of all, are designed to assess the consequences of accidental and/or occupational exposure to high concentrations of agents, it must be pointed out that, to date, none of the *in vitro* alternative tests have proven applicable or acceptable to regulatory agencies.

A. Primary Irritation

A primary irritant is a substance that, as the result of a direct cytotoxic effect, produces inflammatory changes in the skin characterized by the presence of inflammation, vesiculation, and necrosis. The methodology for assessing the potential of a chemical to cause irritation, as measured by edema (the accumulation of excess fluid in the subcutaneous fluid) and erythema (redness of the skin caused by engorgement of the capillaries), was first described by Draize et al. (1944). The **Draize Test** (it should be pointed out that there are two tests, one on the skin and one involving the eye) has been modified and altered as required to test new and unique agents but, essentially, the protocol has remained unchanged. The **Draize Test** was designed as a test of product safety.

Rodents such as rats are generally used in initial studies of dermal irritation but, more frequently, the rabbit or the guinea pig, both of which have relatively sensitive skin, will be used. Larger animals such as the miniature pig or dog may be used. The skin of the rhesus monkey is considered to best mimic the skin of humans (Wester and Maibach, 1975). The choice of species may be dictated by (1) the properties of the chemical, i.e., liquids, solids, low toxicity, etc., which necessitates applying a large amount, (2) solubility of the chemical in aqueous and/or organic media, etc., and (3) known sensitivities of animal skin compared to that of the human. The animals are prepared for the experiment 24 h in advance by removing the hair on the back or abdomen with electric clippers, exposing a bare patch of skin (3.0 to 4.0 cm × 5.0 to 6.0 cm for rats; 6 cm × 10 cm for rabbits) equal to approximately 10 to 15% of the total surface area. Test sites will be approximately 5.0 cm^2 (1.0 inch × 1.0 inch). At one time, it was common to apply a depilatory cream to the exposed skin to remove any "stubble," but concerns were raised about irritation to the skin and subsequent changes in the physiological properties of the test site. This is no longer a common practice. In most studies, some test sites will be abraded with a suitable device (steel comb, hypodermic needle, plastic scarifiers, lancet, etc.) because of the known differences in rate of penetration of chemicals through intact and abraded skin. The abrasions are only minor incisions through the stratum corneum (dead cell layer) and not sufficiently deep to disturb the underlying dermis or to produce bleeding. Adequate numbers of animals, 10 rats or 5 to 6 rabbits per treatment group, should be prepared. With the larger animals, more than one dose may be applied to an animal by marking a grid of squares and treating different and/or adjacent intact and abraded test sites with the same dose. It is important to appreciate that the epidermis is highly variable even within one region and adequate numbers of control, untreated, or vehicle-treated sites should be left for comparison purposes.

The test material, 0.5 ml of liquid or 0.5 g of solid or semisolid, will be applied to one abraded site and one intact site. The material may be applied "neat" if it is a liquid or it may be dissolved in physiological saline or, if insoluble, suspended in 1.0% carboxymethylcellulose. The vehicle should be inert or unreactive. Organic solvents should be avoided unless it is foreseen that the potentially irritant agent will be encountered in such a solvent, i.e., in an industrial process or home product, etc. If different amounts of the agent are to be tested, it is important to keep the volume applied constant (0.5 to 1.0 ml). The liquid should be spread uniformly over the test site with a glass rod. Powders may be applied dry or transformed into a thick paste.

Since the material is to remain in place for 4 h after application, restraining boxes are used to prevent the animals from grooming themselves. The test site will be occluded with a suitable gauze pad secured in place with masking tape. The trunk

TABLE 3.5

Primary Skin Irritation Test: Grading Values for Skin Reactions

Skin responses	Value
Erythema and Eschar Formation	
No erythema	0
Very slight erythema (barely perceptible)	1
Well-defined erythema	2
Moderate-to-severe erythema (beet redness) to slight eschar formation (injury in depth)	4
Edema Formation	
No edema	0
Very slight edema (barely perceptible)	1
Slight edema (edges of area well-defined by definite raising)	2
Moderate edema (raised approximately 1.0 mm)	3
Severe edema raised (more than 1.0 mm and extending beyond the area of exposure)	4

Data from McCreesh and Steinberg (1983).

of the test animal will be wrapped with an impervious plastic sheet to hold the patches in place and to retard evaporation of volatile liquids. At the end of the test period, the plastic sheet and gauze pads are removed, the residual material is wiped off with gauze wetted with warm, soapy water, and the treated areas are evaluated for edema and/or erythema at 1, 24, 48, and 72 h posttreatment. In an attempt to make such a subjective test more quantitative, a number of scoring systems have been developed to measure the degrees of redness and puffiness, that shown in Table 3.5 being the system reported in the *Code of Federal Regulations* (1980) (McCreesh and Steinberg, 1983) and used by the Organization of Economic Cooperation and Development (OECD, 1981). The scoring system involves the assignment of relative numbers ranging from no erythema or edema up to severe reactions. The scores obtained for each effect on each test site (one intact and one abraded site) are averaged for each time period for each animal in each treatment group. A subtotal for erythema is added to the subtotal for edema and the mean for the number of animals being tested is determined to yield a mean primary irritation score for each treatment group, thereby permitting the development of a dose-effect-time relationship. Details of the current regulations of various countries can be found summarized by Rush et al. (1995).

A full discussion of the serious flaws and pitfalls of this test is beyond the scope of this book, but can be found described in various chapters of Marzulli and Maibach's text *Dermatotoxicity* (1987). Species variability in the sensitivity to register irritation is well known but, almost without exception, the albino rabbit was a better predictor for irritation of human skin (McCreesh and Steinberg, 1983). The dermal application of some 40 cosmetic ingredients resulted in a degree of decreasing responsiveness in the order of rabbit, guinea pig, albino rat, human, and swine (Motoyoshi et al., 1979). There are, as one might expect, many exceptions to this order of responsiveness. Indeed, the rabbit frequently appears to demonstrate irritant effects greater than those demonstrated in humans, thereby producing false positive responses. While the Draize technique is effective in identifying strong irritants, it is not as effective in identifying mild or moderate irritants, leading to the misevaluation of some potentially hazardous materials. There has been some controversy over the need to test on abraded skin, and several investigators have demonstrated no correlation between testing on abraded rabbit skin and the potential of eliciting primary irritation of human skin and little if any effect of abrasion on the scores for total irritation values (McCreesh and Steinberg, 1983; Nixon et al., 1975). Differences in the responsiveness of animal and human skin have been associated with the use of the occluded animal model, whereas studies in the human were not conducted under identical conditions.

B. Skin Sensitization

A dermal reaction exists whereby exposure to chemicals (drugs, cosmetics, household products, pesticides, industrial chemicals, etc.) elicit little reaction but following a repeated dermal exposure, an effect is seen that occurs earlier in time, is more severe, and persists for a longer duration. Subsequent exposures, even though weeks or years apart, result in a full-blown "allergy-like," delayed reaction to the chemical(s). Frequently, the reaction can be elicited by much lower concentrations of agent(s) and on areas of the skin other than those involved in the initial contact. The pattern of this dermal condition is suggestive of a developing allergy. Upon penetration of the skin, it is known that such chemicals, called haptens, react covalently with certain carrier proteins, forming "complete antigens" that bind to the membranes of Langerhans cells in the epidermis or to macrophages, thereby initiating the process of antibody formation as well as the immune system "memory." The Langerhans cells express immune recognition (Ia antigen) and have receptors for IgG and C3 on their cell surface. They are capable of absorbing small molecules and can metabolize these to reactive and possibly more haptenic metabolites, which may explain why these cells increase in number in areas showing allergic reactions (Patrick and Maibach, 1994). Subsequent dermal exposure to the same or a closely related chemical, even at lower doses, will trigger an allergic response.

Invariably, the test animal used for skin sensitization studies is the guinea pig. A number of test procedures have been described by various investigators but all are similar in that an attempt is made to build up the immune response by repeated application (dermal or intradermal injection) to shaved regions of the skin over a 14-d period (Marzulli and Maibach, 1987). Treatment with low or moderate concentrations of the chemical in a suitable vehicle may be daily or on a regimen of 4 or 5 days per week. This treatment period is followed by a 10- to 14-day resting period. A challenge dose — usually a lower concentration than used as a sensitizing dose — is applied to a fresh, untreated test site and the reactions to the chemical are scored on the basis of the incidence of animals responding and the severity of the response based on the scheme presented in Table 3.5 at 24, 48, and 72 h after treatment. A greater reaction (edema, erythema) after the challenging dose, when compared to that after the sensitizing dose, is indicative of sensitization.

As was described previously, the sensitization study can be conducted either open and uncovered or occluded. The smaller amounts of liquids, applied topically or injected, pose fewer problems than those used in primary irritation studies, but powders and semisolids are usually tested by the occluded technique. In order to know that the test system is functioning, a positive control group, treated with such known allergens as 2,4-dinitrochlorobenzene (DNCB), p-nitrodimethylaniline (NDMA) or p-phenylenediamine (PPDA), will always be included. A challenge dose of the chemical will be administered after a suitable resting period. A variant of the standard sensitization test is one that includes intradermal injections of Freund's complete adjuvant to enhance the sensitivity by stimulating the general antibody response. Careful selection of the doses of test chemical and of Freund's adjuvant is essential to avoid confusion between the animal's responses to each agent.

TABLE 3.6

Test Methods of Skin Sensitization in Guinea Pigs Arising From OECD Guidelines

Test	Description — Induction/Challenge
Draize Test	Ten daily intradermal injections followed by an intradermal nonirritating challenge dose 25 days after last exposure.
Buehler Test	Three (day 1, 7, 14) topical applications for 6 h duration each time under gauze (absorbent) patch followed by a nonirritating challenge dose on a pad and held in place for 6 h.
Maximization Test (GPMT)	Two intradermal injections (into shoulder) of test agent in vehicle with Freund's complete adjuvant (FCA) followed by a further two injections of FCA alone plus a filter paper saturated with the agent in vehicle and held in place for 48 h. Animals are challenged on a new site (flank) with a nonirritating dose in vehicle on filter paper, held in place for 24 h.
Optimization Test	Ten intradermal injections (two on day 1, one on day 2, 4, and 6, and on every other day in weeks 2 and 3, using FCA). The challenge dose is injected on day 35 after first exposure, with a second, nonirritating, challenge dose on day 45 being applied to the skin and occluded for 24 h.
Freund's Complete Adjuvant Test FCAT	Three intradermal injections (into shoulder) of test agent in vehicle of FCA:water (50:50) on day 1, day 5, and day 9. The challenge doses (minimal irritant concentration, nonirritating concentration and two lower doses are applied to shaved skin (flank) and left uncovered.
Open Epicutaneous Test	Topical application of test agent in vehicle to shaved skin on flank 5 times a week for 4 weeks. Challenge dose is applied 24 h to 72 h after last exposure on previously untreated flank.
Split Adjuvant Test	Dorsal skin is treated for 5 to 10 s with dry ice following close shaving. Test agent is applied to site and covered by gauze throughout study. Agent is reapplied on day 3 and covered again. On day 4, FCA is administered intradermally into edges of test site, and the test material is reapplied and covered. On day 7, the test agent is applied again and is left for 2 days. On day 9, the dressing is removed. Challenge dose is applied topically to a new shaved test site (midback) 22 days after initial treatment, the site being occluded for 24 h.

Data from OECD Test Guideline No. 406, 1981; Patrick and Maibach, 1994; and Seabaugh, 1994.

A variant of the above sensitization test is the closed-patch test developed by Buehler (1964). The test is sensitive enough to detect a moderate-to-strong sensitizer and the probability of false positive results is low. The methodology has been modified and adapted repeatedly, the best description of the protocol being given by Klecak (1983). The flanks and backs of equal numbers of male and female guinea pigs (n = 20 in experimental groups; n = 10 in the control group; n = 4 in the primary irritant group) are clipped to provide test sites of 2 × 2 cm. A 0.4 ml volume of an appropriate concentration of freshly prepared solution, suspension, or emulsion of the test agent or the vehicle is applied to a 20 × 20 mm Webril pad on a 37 × 40 mm bandage or Blenderm tape, this being applied to the test site on the animal held in a special restraining device and the patch being occluded with a rubber dental dam pulled tight and fastened to the bottom of the restrainer with clips. The patches are left in place for 6 h after which they are removed and the residual material is washed off prior to returning the animals to their cages. On days 7 and 14 after the initial exposure, the 6-h, closed-patch (test material or vehicle) is repeated on the experimental and control animals. At 14 d after the last exposure (28 days after the initial exposure), the experimental animals are challenged for 6 h with patches containing nonirritating concentrations of the test material as outlined above. At the end of the treatment period, the patches are removed, the test sites washed free of residual test agent, the areas are depilated, and the test sites are visually evaluated at 24 and 48 h

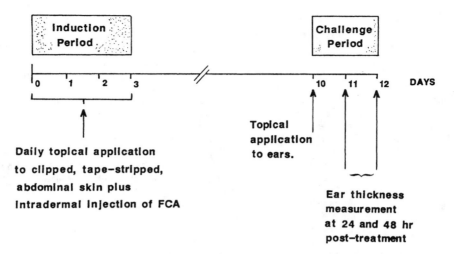

FIGURE 3.9
The mouse-ear-swelling test (MEST) was developed as a rapid assay to detect dermal sensitizing chemicals. The induction phase requires that the test agent be applied topically to the shaved abdominal skin of mice, accompanied by daily intradermal injections of Freund's complete adjuvant (FCA) for 3 consecutive days. Seven days later, in the challenge period, the test agent is applied to one ear, with the vehicle being applied to the other, with the ear thickness being measured by micrometer at 24 and 48 h post-exposure.

posttreatment. The incidence and intensity of erythematous response are calculated, with any response signifying sensitization.

Presently, some seven tests, all using the guinea pig, are accepted by the EEC (Table 3.6), all of these being slight variants of the tests described in detail above (Botham et al., 1991; Patrick and Maibach, 1994). Guinea pigs are used because of their known susceptibility to a wide variety of chemical sensitizers. EEC acceptance is based on validity, requiring test evidence of expected response to standard allergens (2,4-dinitrochlorobenzene or p-phenylenediamine). Agents are applied topically or intradermally, with or without Freund's adjuvant, the skin being left exposed or occluded. Brief details are given in Table 3.6, with complete explanations of the individual techniques being found in Patrick and Maibach (1994). Application sites are examined for erythema and edema at 24, 48, and 72 h posttreatment, the diameter (mm) of the erythematous site and the skinfold thickness (mm) over the site being quantitated by ruler or a caliper. Unfortunately, all of these test methods are empirical in their design and subjective in their means of assessment (Botham et al., 1991). It is essential that more objective, immunologically based test methods be developed to predict delayed contact sensitization, particularly methods that will detect weak as well as strong allergens. However, these methods still require the use of animals since, as yet, there are no adequate *in vitro* systems that mimic the complexity of the immunological reaction involved in contact dermatitis.

The **mouse-ear-swelling test (MEST)** was developed as an accurate, sensitive, and alternative test to evaluate sensitization (Figure 3.9) (Gad et al., 1986). The test includes: (1) **an induction phase**, with the topical application of the test agent in liquid on a suitable, closely-clipped, tape-stripped abdominal site for 3 consecutive days, drying the site quickly with an electric dryer; and (2) **a challenge stage** on day 10, with topical application of the test substance to one ear and vehicle to the other,

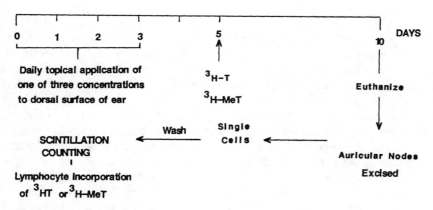

FIGURE 3.10

Dermal sensitization by chemicals can be tested by the mouse local lymph node assay (LLNA). The test agent, in a suitable vehicle, is applied to the dorsal surface of the mouse ear for 3 consecutive days. At 2 days after the last exposure, the mice receive an intravenous injection of tritiated thymidine (^{3}H-T) or methyl thymidine (^{3}H-MeT), the animals being euthanized 5 days later, with the excision of the auricular lymph nodes and the preparation of washed single cell suspensions of lymphocytes. Following incubation overnight, the cells are centrifuged, resuspended in 5.0% trichloroacetic acid and aliquots are taken for β-scintillation counting. Chemical-induced sensitization would be reflected by an increased incorporation of tritium (^{3}H) in the proliferating lymphocytes compared to that found in vehicle-exposed, control cells.

and again, drying the material quickly. The ear thickness is measured by micrometer at 24 and 48 h after exposure. During validation, the **MEST** correctly identified 71 of 72 substances as potential human sensitizers or nonsensitizers. The detection of weak haptens can be enhanced by using abraded skin (Botham et al., 1991).

More recently, a promising sensitization test, **the murine local lymph node assay (LLNA)**, has been developed, being based on an immunological response to agents (Figure 3.10) (Kimber and Basketter, 1992; Basketter et al., 1993). The protocol uses 8- to 12-week old mice treated daily for 3 consecutive days by topical application (25 μL) of the test substance on the dorsum of both ears. Vehicles of choice include acetone-olive oil (4:1), dimethylformamide, methyl ethyl ketone, propylene glycol, and dimethylsulfoxide (Kimber and Basketter, 1992). Five days after the first treatment, the mice received an injection (iv) of 250 μL of phosphate-buffered saline containing 20 uCi of ^{3}H-methyl thymidine or ^{3}H-thymidine. The mice were killed 5 days later and the draining auricular lymph nodes were excised, pooled, and prepared into single cell suspensions of lymph node cells (LNC) by passing through a 200-mesh stainless steel screen. The pooled LNC were centrifuged, the pellet washed twice with buffered saline and was resuspended in 3.0 ml trichloroacetic acid (TCA, 5%). Following incubation overnight, the precipitate recovered on centrifugation was resuspended in 1.0 ml TCA and transferred to 10 ml of scintillation fluid for β-scintillation counting. The proliferative response of the LNC was expressed as mean dpm/node, the ratio of the ^{3}H-incorporation into treated LNC over the value in control LNC (T/C ratio). Chemicals were considered to be sensitizers if the T/C ratio was 3 or greater at one or more of the concentrations of test substance. Several papers have examined the validation of this test, using chemicals that have been assessed in the human maximization test, the results correctly identifying the human sensitizers as well as those that did not cause delayed-contact sensitization (Scholes et al., 1992; Basketter et al., 1994; Basketter et al., 1995).

C. Photoallergic Reactions

A variety of chemicals (halogenated salicylanilides, sulfonamides, thiazides, phenothiazines, chlordiazepoxide, griseofulvin, cyclamates, hexachlorophene, dichlorophene, musk ambrette), when applied dermally or ingested by an individual who is subsequently exposed to sunlight, cause an allergy-like reaction, manifested in the form of an immediate urticaria (rash), a persistent eczema, or a delayed papular eruption (Kornhauser et al. 1983). Frequently, there is an involvement of areas of skin beyond the exposed site, i.e., flare-up of previously exposed sites following ultraviolet (UV) irradiation of another site. The chemicals eliciting this type of reaction all contain ring systems in their structures that are capable of absorbing UV light from sunlight or artificial sources having wavelengths less than 320 nm. While the skin prevents the penetration of short-wavelength (<250 nm) UV light, those having wavelengths in the region of 275 to 325 nm can be absorbed to the depth of the blood capillaries carrying the potentially toxic agent (Kornhauser et al., 1983). The light-induced activation of the chemical results in covalent binding of this reactive intermediate with cellular and plasma proteins to produce antigens which will stimulate antibody formation. The immediate urticarial reactions following exposure to sunlight are considered to be antibody-mediated, whereas the delayed eruptions and eczematous conditions are thought to be related to cell-mediated immune responsiveness.

In conducting photoallergic reactions, the guinea pig or the rabbit are the species of choice. In most cases, small amounts of the test agent will be administered systemically (orally or by intravenous injection) for 10 to 14 d as required in a sensitization study. Dermal application of the agent(s) is also possible. Following a resting period of 14 to 21 d, the animals will be challenged with a dose of the test chemical and exposed to light of an appropriate wavelength on an area of closely-shaved skin. The trick in such studies is to find a light source that will generate the desired wavelengths. Knowledge concerning the absorption of light by the chemical will be crucial to the experiment. It would also be important to carry a positive control group of animals through the procedure, using a known photoallergin. Scoring of the erythema can be done using a scheme similar to that shown in Table 3.5. Details of this type of study are discussed by Harber et al. (1983).

D. Phototoxic Reactions

Phototoxicity is considerably more common than photoallergic reactions and involves a wide variety of chemical agents, the chief characteristics of which include extensive benzene ring systems in the structure. Such chemicals include commonly used drugs (phenothiazines, sulfonamides, sulfonylureas, thiazides, tetracyclines), industrial chemicals (coal tar, phenanthrene, anthracene, pyridine, pyrene), dyes (anthraquinone, aminobenzoic acid derivatives), and other miscellaneous agents (Harber and Bickers, 1981). Current theories suggest that, in the presence of UV light of suitable wavelength (<320 nm), the chemical molecules are converted into reactive intermediates that elicit direct, local (dermal) cellular toxicity manifesting itself in the form of a delayed erythema and hyperpigmentation, followed by desquamation (shedding or scaling) of the skin.

E. Alternative *In Vitro* Dermal Tests

In the spirit of the "3 Rs," considerable effort has been expended by industry in developing *in vitro* test methods to assess the potential dermal toxicity of a vast array

TABLE 3.7

Cell Lines Used in *In Vitro* Cytotoxicity Assays

Origin	Acronym	Cell Type
Human, cervix uteri	HeLa	Continuous
Human, adult lung epithelial	A549	Continuous
Human, trachea	HEP2	Continuous
Human, liver	Chang Liver	Continuous
Human, epidermoid tumor	KB	Continuous
Human, epidermal keratinocytes	XB-2, NHEK, HPKII	Continuous
Human, embryonal lung fibroblasts	HFL1, WI-38, IMR-90, MRC-5	Finite
Swiss mouse, embryo fibroblast	3T3	Continuous
Mouse, lymphoma	L5178	Continuous
Mouse, neuroblastoma	C1300	Continuous
Chinese hamster ovary	CHO	Continuous
Chinese hamster, pulmonary	V79	Continuous
Canine, kidney	MDCK, LLC-PK	Continuous

Modified from Frazier (1992) and Barile (1994).

of chemical mixtures including cosmetics (perfumes, colognes, lotions, powders), personal (soaps, bath gels, shampoos, deodorants), and home (detergents, cleaners, waxes, paints, solvents) care products, pesticides with their emulsifiers and cosolvents, industrial chemicals, etc., all of which will come into contact with the skin through purposeful use or accidental splashing. In the past decade and, more importantly, in the past 5 years, there has been a proliferation of *in vitro* techniques designed to test the above materials. The reader is referred to relevant chapters in a number of recent books presenting overviews on this subject, including those of Frazier (1992), Barile (1994), Gad (1994), and Salem (1995), as well as published proceedings of meetings (Rheinhardt et al., 1985; Purchase and Conning, 1986). As was stated earlier, heightened interest in these *in vitro* alternative methods has been driven largely by the EC directive concerning a ban on the sale, in member countries, of all cosmetics that have been tested in animals after 1998 (EEC, 1995). From the literature, it is quite apparent that the personal and home care products industry has led the way, far in advance of the responses of regulatory agencies.

In vivo tests of dermal toxicity are designed to subjectively assess erythema (redness) and edema (swelling), both indicative of inflammation, as well as eschar (in-depth cellular injury) (Table 3.5). The new test systems being developed range from primary cell cultures, finite and continuous cell lines, through more complex human skin equivalents, to explanted and maintained pieces of mammalian skin (Barile, 1994). There is some overlap between the dermal tests and those used to assess ocular toxicity (Herzinger et al., 1995). What endpoints should be used for *in vitro* systems, with erythema and edema being the only visual aspects of the complex process of inflammation?

The toxicity endpoints encompass cytotoxicity and include: (1) membrane permeation by chemicals; (2) plasma membrane damage with losses of cytoplasmic proteins and changes in electrical conductivity; and (3) effects on subcellular organelles and cell metabolism. All of these tests have been designed to be quantifiable, to provide reproducible "numbers" related to the concentration(s) of test substances, thereby avoiding the somewhat unreliable, qualitative and subjective assessments associated with *in vivo* testing. Other tests, those involving the use of keratinocytes which comprise 95% of the epidermal cell mass, are designed to quantify the signal release of chemotactic factors such as arachidonic acid and eicosanoid-type mediators (prostaglandins, interleukins, leukotrienes, etc.) released during the inflammatory stage (Muller-Decker et al., 1994). In addition to screening for product safety, many of these methods can be used to study mechanisms by which agents elicit dermal toxicity. In this, the selection of techniques is determined by the specific questions to be asked, the flexibility of these methods permitting some of the questions to be answered effectively.

1. Cytotoxicity Tests

Cytotoxicity, usually including more direct measurements of cell penetration or biomarkers of cell leakage, has been a focal endpoint for various *in vitro* techniques. Cytotoxic tests simulate the injury to human epithelium during periods of exposure that are realistic for acute toxicity (Barile, 1994). Cells are exposed to different concentrations of the test agent for predetermined time periods (up to 24 h) followed by the assessment of viability and function. Criteria for these tests include: (1) concentrations of test substance relevant to human toxic or lethal blood concentrations; (2) changes in viability (cell growth, proliferation, morphology); (3) alterations in cellular metabolism; (4) membrane integrity, with leakage of isotope markers or constituent cytosolic enzymes; (5) alterations in function of subcellular organelles (mitochondria, lysosomes, etc.); and (6) histo- and immunochemical staining of proteins, enzymes, carbohydrates, keratin, etc. (Frazier, 1992; Barile, 1994). A list of some of the cell lines used in culture techniques is shown in Table 3.7 and includes both cells capable of growing in suspended culture and those which are anchorage-dependent, requiring attachment to a polyethylene plastic matrix.

A list of the cell culture test systems is shown in Table 3.8, including an indication of the objective endpoint, the technical endpoint, and the mechanism(s) of the test. While many of these assays are conducted with submerged cells in culture flasks, they lend themselves to multi-well frames and automated spectrophotometric analysis of colored dye taken up (or released or excluded) or of colored reaction products formed from substrates and reagents both inside cells and outside in the medium.

2. Nonbiological Test

In contrast to the above systems, the *in vitro* irritation prediction method known as the SKINTEX™ system used nonbiological, nonliving substances. This biochemically based model is a two-compartment cuvette divided horizontally by a keratin/collagen barrier membrane (a biomembrane) with an attached red dye, the lower chamber containing an ordered macromolecular matrix containing lipid components. Test substances, added to the liquid upper layer as liquids, emulsions, or solids, may cause alterations in the barrier membrane, causing the release of the dye in a concentraion-dependent manner into the lower chamber where it can be quantitated. Penetration of toxic agents through the biomembrane may also result in the disruption of the conformation of the macromolecular matrix causing opacity, with a reduction in light transmission to yield "irritational units" described as the potential dermal irritancy index or PDII (Barile, 1994). Considered to be comparable to *in vivo* alterations in the stratum corneum, the *in vitro* results for more than 5300 test substances studied on rabbit skin have yielded reproducibility with standard deviations of 5 to 8% and validation with the *in vivo* rabbit Draize scoring with correlations of 80 to 89% (Gad, 1994). The SKINTEX™ system appears sensitive in ability to predict irritant potential of substances for humans (82% sensitivity, 71% specificity, 82% positive predictive value) (Harvell and Maibach, 1995).

TABLE 3.8

Alternative Test Systems To Assess Dermal Irritation Using Cell Cultures

Test	Assessment	Endpoint of Test	Mechanism
Trypan Blue	Cell viability	Blue stain in dead or damaged cells	Dye is excluded from viable cells only entering those damaged
Neutral Red Uptake	Cell viability	Measure of NR_{50}, the concentration that reduces the dye uptake by 50% compared to control levels	A supravital dye which is sequestered only in viable cells and retained by lysosomal membranes
Kenacid Blue, Coomassie Blue	Cell viability	Quantitates the total intracellular protein concentration. Determine the IC_{50} reduction in protein compared with control levels	Based on the relationship between the measure of total protein, cell number, and binding of the stain
Lowry Method	Cell viability	Protein concentration, determining an IC_{50} for the reduction of protein compared with control levels	Measures total cellular protein, the proline residues, following lysis of intact, undamaged cells after exposure to test agent
Rhodamine or Nile Blue	Cell viability	Increased keratinization of cells	Staining of keratin within viable keratinocytes
Hexosaminidase or	Membrane	Measurement of enzymatic activity in the medium	Measurement of cytosolic enzymes leaking through damaged plasma membranes of cells
Lactate Dehydrogenase		Can determine an IC_{50} for test substance	
^{14}C-Leucine Inclusion	Cell viability metabolism	Reduction in incorporation, into cellular proteins, determining an IC_{50} for the test agent	Incorporation of this amino acid into cellular proteins, a measure of uptake processes and utilization
^{3}H-Uridine or ^{3}H-Thymidine Inclusion	Cell viability metabolism	Reduction in incorporation into nucleic acids	Alterations in cellular metabolism relating to transport and accumulation of nucleotides
MTT Assay (or XTT)	Cell viability	MTT_{50}-representing the concentration of agent that reduces the formation of formazan by 50%	Measures the reduction of yellow MTT (tetrazolium) salt to an insoluble, blue-black formazan
	Mitochondrial function	Measures intact mitochondrial function and intact plasma membrane uptake	XTT is substituted for MTT since it is water soluble, eliminating the need for DMSO
Microtox system	Cellular metabolism	Reduction in the luminescent capabilities of the organism, determining an IC_{50} for the test agent	Uses a luminescent bacterium, *Photobacterium phosphoreum*, which emits light during metabolism

3. Inflammatory Substance(s) Test

Skin irritation consists of more than just cytotoxicity, being a complex process with keratinocytes acting as primary signal receivers and transducers, converting exogenous stimuli into endogenous signals with the release of proinflammatory mediators such as eicosanoids and cytokines (Barker et al., 1991; Furstenberger, 1990). Keratinocytes appear to play a key role in the induction and control of inflammatory

TABLE 3.9

Human Tissue Equivalent Assays for Cutaneous Irritation

Test	Source	Description
SKIN² ZK1200	Advanced Tissue Sciences (La Jolla, CA)	Human neonatal dermis (foreskin)-derived fibroblasts cocultured with layers of neonatal epidermal keratinocytes on a nylon-mesh matrix
SKIN² ZK1300		Comparable to the above but containing a stratum corneum
TESTSKIN™	Organogenesis (Cambridge, MA)	Human neonatal dermal fibroblasts seeded on a bovine collagen-gel matrix cocultured with stratified human neonatal epidermal keratinocytes

responses and signal releases by such cells should provide *in vitro* counterparts of irritancy, i.e., arachidonic acid being transformed into prostaglandins (PGE_2, PGF_2, PGD_2) their metabolic products (hydroxyeicosatetraenoic acids, 5-, 8-, and 15-HETES), and cytokines (interleukin-1 or IL-1) (Furstenberger, 1990). Immortalized human keratinocytes (HPK II cells) have been assessed in submerged culture following incubation with 14 different chemicals ranging from metal salts through solvents, detergents, alkylamides, and phenol, measuring the agent-stimulated release of arachidonic acid, PGE_2, PGF_2, 5-HETE and IL-1 by high pressure liquid chromatography (Muller-Decker et al., 1994). While considerable variability was observed between chemicals, the results showed that human keratinocytes *in vitro* responded to chemicals of graded irritational potency with a graded release of proinflammatory mediators (Muller-Decker et al., 1994). The measuring of multiple mediator endpoints resulted in a better characterization of a test substance than did the evaluation of a single parameter. It would appear that any *in vitro* assay containing keratinocytes or fibroblasts might be coaxed to release chemical mediators, adding other endpoints to the assessment of potential irritants. The release of [³H] arachidonic acid from a prelabeled murine fibroblast cell line (C^3H-$10T_{1/2}$ cells) *in vitro*, in response to treatment with anionic surfactants, suggests one useful approach to dermal irritancy testing (DeLeo et al., 1996).

4. *Human Skin Equivalent Tests*

At least two *in vitro* models, known as human skin equivalents, are available on the market, both of these approaching the complexity of the trilayered, multifunctional living skin (Table 3.9). Cross-sectional, stained photomicrographs of these growing cell systems display an uncanny resemblance to actual mammalian skin, with a layer identical to a stratum corneum lying above layers similar to epidermal cells and basal cells forming a dermis (Osborne and Perkins, 1994; Weideman, 1995). A schematic diagram of the two-chambered, plastic, culture "dish" used in the TESTSKIN™ system is shown in Figure 3.11. Test substances, liquids or solids, can be added to the well in the upper chamber, thereby coming into contact with a "stratum corneum," with penetration into the cell layers and/or through the medium in the lower chamber from which samples of medium can be removed for analysis. Damage to the organized cell layers can be monitored by fluorescent dye uptake/ exclusion techniques or by fixing, staining, and microscopic examination. In a recent comparative study of the Skin™ and TESTSKIN™ models, the set of endpoints measured (cytotoxicity — neutral red uptake, MMT vital dye staining, lactate dehydrogenase and N-acetyl glucosaminidase release, glucose utilization, inflammatory mediator-prostaglandin E_2 release) showed good correlation between the behavior of

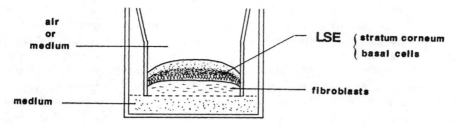

FIGURE 3.11

A schematic diagram of the pre-prepared, two-chambered, plastic culture dish of the TESTSKIN™ system (Organogenesis Inc., Cambridge, MA) containing the living skin equivalent (LSE) complex. A medium containing the test agent(s) can be applied to the LSE surface and penetration into or through the dermis-like layers can be monitored by fluorescein dye uptake or by the removal of aliquots of the lower medium for analysis. The LSE can be fixed, sectioned, and stained for microscopic examination.

test substances in the *in vitro* models and *in vivo* human skin irritation (Osborne and Perkins, 1994). Acids and bases, agents incompatible with submerged culture models, performed well with the TESTSKIN™ model.

5. Isolated Perfused Porcine Skin Flap (IPPSF)

A novel technique of studying percutaneous absorption has been developed using the epigastric region dermis of weanling pigs, suitable because of the presence of direct, cutaneous vasculature — the caudal superficial epigastric artery and its paired venae comitantes (Riviere et al., 1986; Montiero-Riviere et al., 1987; Carver et al., 1989). An isolated, single-pedicle, axial-pattern flap is created surgically *in situ*, producing a tubed flap enclosing the vessels mentioned above, the preparation being isolated 2 to 6 d later with cannulation of the artery and one of the venae comitantes and transfer to an isolated perfusion chamber. In the chamber, the skin flaps remain viable for 10 to 16 h according to the monitoring criteria established (Montiero-Riviere et al., 1986). The system lends itself to a physiological-based, pharmacokinetic (PBPK) approach to the modeling of dermal penetration and toxicity of liquid chemicals or agents in aqueous or nonaqueous solution, with quantitation in the perfusion medium and assessment of agent-related changes in vascular resistance and enzyme release from damaged cells into the perfusion medium (Williams et al., 1990). Light microscopic examination of the tissue layers permits the detection of subtle morphological changes (King and Montiero-Riviere, 1991).

It should be pointed out that this technique is not for the faint-hearted. Both the surgical and the perfusion techniques, the latter a plumber's nightmare, require considerable skills and practice. While not a routine test procedure, the results are comparable to those produced *in vivo* in the same species.

VI. OCULAR TOXICITY STUDIES

Ocular damage as a consequence of accidental contact with splashed industrial chemicals, home products, pesticides, solvents, etc., led to the development of a number of qualitative tests of injury, using animals as surrogate models. Unfortunately, most of these tests were subjective in nature, highly variable, and almost completely devoid of quantitation. In 1944, two papers were published that were purported to be quantitative analyses of the effects of chemicals on the eyes of rabbits.

The first paper, by Friedenwald et al. (1944), examined the effects of acids, bases, and buffered substances of known pH on the eye with the development of "a numerical method of evaluating the severity of the reaction in order to yield data which might be studied statistically and graphically." The second paper, by Draize et al. (1944), was an attempt to transform qualitative observations of physiological effects to quantitative objective measurements by assigning numerical values to physiological phenomena. This became the famous or infamous **Draize Test**, used since 1944 to test the potential of almost every chemical and formulation used by humans to elicit damage to the eye. The basic test used a scoring system related to brief subjective statements of physiological reactions observed in the cornea, conjunctiva, and iris (Table 3.10). The test has been modified by the inclusion of additional, quantifiable parameters such as erythema, thickness of the eyelids, and nictitating membranes to reflect edema, discharge, corneal opacity, capillary damage, and pannus (vascularization) of the cornea (Conquest et al., 1977).

In the past few years, the Draize test has become a target of animal welfare groups, antivivisectionists, and concerned scientists who claim that it is not required, is inhumane, and causes unnecessary pain to the animals and, even with the scoring systems and other measurement, is still subjective and prone to such interlaboratory variation in results that the test is not meaningful. While it is important to point out that there are no alternatives to the Draize test that are acceptable to regulatory agencies, the thought of putting strong acidic or basic solutions in the eyes of animals is repugnant. In fact, if the dermal *in vivo* or *in vitro* irritancy tests are positive, there is little scientific basis for initiating an eye test, since it will almost certainly be positive in this organ. However, between the strong acids and the bases lie a wide variety of near-neutral, slightly acidic or basic soaps, shampoos, cleaners, cosmetic creams and lotions, eyeliners, mascara, disinfectants, mouthwashes, toothpastes, industrial chemicals, pesticides, etc., all of which have considerable potential of accidentally finding their way into the eye. There are chemicals that can produce a severe reaction in the eye, yet cause little or no effect on the skin. Unfortunately, the reverse is also true, some agents being far more irritating to the skin than to the eye. For the sake of occupational, consumer, and bystander safety, these products must be subjected to both irritation tests for lack of a better way to guarantee that they are not harmful. While the ethical concerns about the use of animals in the eye test will not disappear, the 40-odd years of experience with the Draize test has not been supplanted by any satisfactory *in vitro* tests that have been validated. However, as will be discussed below, breakthroughs in this area are imminent given the position taken by the EC concerning cosmetics.

A. Primary Irritation — *In Vivo*

In previous years, groups (n = 6) of rabbits were treated with each dose of the potential toxicant, as with other acute study protocols. Given the number of chemicals that required ocular testing, figures reported for 1983 showed that 509,000 rabbits were used in scientific experiments, many being used in the eye irritation test (U.S. Congress, 1986). Two recent papers have demonstrated that a high level of accuracy can be obtained with fewer rabbits per test. De Sousa et al. (1984) reported that, compared to the standard test, subsample sizes of two, three, four, and five rabbits were 88, 93, 95, and 96% accurate, respectively, at correctly classifying the irritation potential of a series of petrochemical products. Talsma et al. (1988) indicated that five-, four-, three-, and two-rabbit scores were in 98, 96, 94, and 91% agreement,

TABLE 3.10

Eye Irritation Test: Grading Values for Ocular Lesions

Description of lesion	Value
1. Cornea	
A. Opacity, degree of density	
• No opacity	0
• Scattered or diffuse areas of opacity, but details of iris clearly visible	1
• Easily discernible translucent areas, details of the iris slightly obscured	2
• Opalescent areas, no details of iris visible, size of pupil barely discernible	3
• Opaque cornea, iris invisible through opacity	4
B. Area of cornea involved	
• One quarter (or less), but not zero	1
• Greater than one quarter	2
• Greater than one half	3
• Greater than three quarters, up to complete area	4
Score = Part A × Part B × 5 – maximum score = 80	
2. Iris	
A. Normal	0
• Folds above normal, congestion, swelling circumcorneal injection, iris still reacting to light (sluggish reaction, but positive)	1
• No reaction to light, hemorrhage, gross destruction	2
Score = Part A × 5 – maximum score = 10	
3. Conjunctiva	
A. Redness (refers to palpebral conjunctiva)	
• Blood vessels normal	0
• Blood vessels hyperemic (injected)	1
• Diffuse, crimson color, individual vessels not easily discernible	2
• Diffuse vessels, beefy red	3
B. Chemosis (lids and nictitating membranes)	
• No swelling	0
• Any swelling above normal (includes the nictitating membranes)	1
• Obvious swelling with partial eversion of lids	2
• Swelling with lids half closed	3
• Swelling with lids more than half closed	4
C. Discharge	
• No discharge	0
• Any amount different from normal (does not include small amounts observed in inner canthus of normal animals)	1
• Discharge with moistening of lids and hairs adjacent to lids	2
• Discharge with moistening of the lids and hairs of considerable area around eye	3
Score = (Parts A + B + C) × 2 – maximum score = 20	

From Draize, J. H., Woodard, G., and Calvery, H. O., *J. Pharmacol. Exp. Ther.*, 82:377–389 (1944). With permission.

respectively, with the classification assigned to the chemicals tested using the six-rabbit/treatment group protocol.

In the Draize-type test, 0.1 ml of liquid or 100 mg of solid is instilled in the pouched lower conjunctival sac of one eye of each of six rabbits, with the eyelids being held together for 1 s and then released. The treated eye is not washed, allowing the animal's own tear secretions to flush the eye. The untreated eye serves as a control. Both eyes are examined at 1, 24, 48, and 72 h after treatment. In general, the treated eyes are washed with 0.9% physiological saline at the 24 h period. If there is no evidence of irritation at 72 h, the study may be terminated. If residual injury is present, examination of the eyes may be prolonged at the discretion of the investigator. The damage to cornea, conjunctiva and iris is scored numerically as is shown in Table 3.10. Each animal is graded separately, the results being presented as a fraction of the total maximum score of 20. On comparing the scores for each rabbit, if only two or three of the rabbits show a positive effect, the test is considered inconclusive and would be repeated with new animals. If four or more rabbits are positive in response, the test is considered positive.

The large intra- and interlaboratory variations observed in the eye irritancy test has been of great concern to investigators (Weil and Scala, 1971). In an attempt to reduce personal bias and error in scoring the severity of effects, a set of colored photographs showing variable degrees of corneal opacity, iritis and conjunctival effects keyed to a numerical coding system was established by the U.S. government. Copies of this guide used to be available from the Superintendent of Documents, U.S. Government Printing Office, Washington, D.C. Examples of these photographs can be seen in Marzulli and Maibach (1977) or in Dunn (1995). To improve the reproducibility of the scoring of results, magnification, slit-lamp examination, and staining of the eye by fluorescein dye have all been employed. The more simple the endpoint of the test, the better was the reproducibility in that variability was reduced to insignificance if the investigators were asked only to distinguish an irritant from a nonirritant, and if all four criteria (cornea, iris, conjunctival congestion, and conjunctival swelling) were used (Marzulli and Ruggles, 1973).

Concerns have always been raised about the relatively large volume (0.1 ml or 0.1 g) of test material being placed into the conjunctival sac of the rabbit eye. A modification of the standard Draize procedure is the **low-volume eye test (LVET)** in which only 0.01 ml (or 0.01 g) of test substance is applied directly to the cornea instead of into the conjunctival sac, the eyelids not being held shut following treatment (Griffith et al., 1980). Several studies have produced results showing that the LVET more accurately predicts human ocular exposure, good correlations being obtained between LVET results and the human response (Freeberg et al., 1986). The LVET can be successfully conducted with three rabbits rather than the six usually used (Bruner et al., 1992).

As with all animal studies, there are serious limitations in transferring the results to the human with any degree of confidence. While the rabbit is most commonly used in such studies because it is inexpensive, easily handled, and has a large eye, there are serious structural and physiological differences which make the rabbit eye an unsatisfactory model for the human eye (Sharpe, 1985). The rabbit has a nictitating membrane or third eyelid, not found in the human, which could either remove irritants more efficiently or trap material beneath it. The rabbit's tearing mechanism is less efficient than that of the human, thereby altering the degree and/or duration adverse effects. The pH and buffering capacity of the aqueous humor in the eyes of humans and rabbits is quite different; the pH being approximately 7.2 in the human, while in the rabbit it is 8.2. This may explain the susceptibility of the rabbit iris to chemical inflammation. The tissue structure and thickness of the cornea is quite different in the two species; the mean thickness of the rabbit cornea being 0.37 mm, while it is 0.51 mm in the human. Despite these differences, the rabbit is traditionally used to assess eye irritancy and the Draize test would appear to be no better or worse than other *in vivo* or *in vitro* test systems.

B. Alternative *In Vitro* Ocular Tests

The Draize eye irritation test has been criticized for its lack of repeatability, the subjective nature of assessment (Table 3.10) giving rise to variable interpretation, the high dose of test material used, its overprediction of the human response, and, of

TABLE 3.11

In Vitro Ocular Tests

Assessing Cytotoxicity

- Neutral Red Assay ⎫
- Fluorescein Diacetate ⎬ entry only into viable cells
- Propidium Iodide ⎫
- Ethidium Bromide ⎬ entry only into damaged cells
- Trypan Blue ⎭
- MTT — cellular metabolism

Assessing Opacity

- EYETEX™ − nonbiological protein aggregation
- Bovine Corneal Opacity-Permeability (BCO-P)
- Enucleated Eye Test (EET)

Assessing Inflammation

- Bovine Corneal Cup Assay
- Rat Vaginal Tissue Assay — measurement of prostaglandins and thromboxanes released by test agents
- Chorioallantoic Membrane (CAM) or HET-CAM Assays — the scoring of necrosis and vascular changes as well as fluorescein dye penetration 3 days after application in a prepared 10-day-old chick embryo.
- CAM-VA Assay — scoring vascular changes within 30 min of application to a 14-day-old hen's egg.

Immortalized cell lines such as HeLa, CHO, V79, MDCK, etc. are used.

course, the use of animals and the infliction of pain. The normal endpoints of toxicity for the *in vivo* (rabbit eye) test are (1) corneal opacity, (2) inflammation, and (3) cytotoxicity. While no single *in vitro* test can cover all of these parameters, individual tests can address some of these endpoints (Table 3.11). Eventually, it is hoped that a battery of validated tests might suffice to screen the problems associated with ocular toxicity, thereby reducing/replacing the use of animals except for the final and crucial premarket testing of products. The reader is referred to the relevant chapters in Goldberg (1987), Frazier (1992), Barile (1994), Gad (1994), Hayes (1994), and Salem (1995) for specific details on the development and conduction of alternative tests for eye irritation. An excellent review on method development can be found in the published proceedings of a meeting held in 1984 in Switzerland (Reinhardt et al., 1985).

1. Cytotoxicity Tests

The various *in vitro* tests used to assess cellular toxicity are identical to those described in Table 3.8 for dermal cytotoxicity, involving a variety of immortalized cell lines of different origin and examining dye inclusion/exclusion/leakage as indices of membrane integrity (Table 3.11). Dyes include: (1) neutral red or fluorescein diacetate which enter only viable cells, becoming localized there or leaking back out through a damaged plasma membrane; (2) propidium iodide and ethidium bromide, molecules large enough to be excluded from viable cells but entering damaged cells and staining DNA; or (3) Trypan Blue which penetrates only damaged cell membranes, staining proteins in nonviable cells. Some of these cell lines, i.e., MDCK cells, can be grown as confluent monolayers in two-chambered cells supported on a nylon mesh membrane, such systems permitting the study of tight junctions and the penetration of a solution of fluorescein plus test substance from the upper chamber into or even through the cell layer into the lower chamber, with quantitation of the dye and time of incubation.

The problem with these test systems is that, while they produce excellent correlations between cytotoxicity endpoints and *in vivo* irritation within a single class of chemicals, the overall correlations are poor when comparisons are made across different chemical classes (Sina and Gautheron, 1994). This restricts the usefulness of such tests, perhaps limiting them only to a screening role.

2.   *Opacity Tests*

The first test to be considered is the EYETEX™ assay, a completely nonbiological test using a "proprietary reagent" of a soluble protein matrix from the jackbean which turns opaque when an appropriate test substance causes alterations in the hydration/organization of the soluble protein, thereby reducing light transmission through a cuvette placed in a simple spectrophotometer. The change in light transmission is equated with a standard curve provided in the kit relating to *in vivo* eye irritancy scores. The correlations between the arbitrary units and known *in vivo* irritancy were equivocal. With agents strong enough to alter the hydration and organization of the protein, the test showed good correlations (Sina and Gautheron, 1994). However, other investigators showed the correlations to be poor (Brunner et al., 1991).

The **Bovine Corneal Opacity-Permeability (BCO-P) Test** uses eyes (bovine, porcine) obtained from abattoirs, with the cornea dissected free and mounted in a plastic holder fitted into a two-compartment cell having "windows" for light transmission (Figure 3.12). With the epithelial side of the cornea on the top, the corneal cell layers are equilibrated with culture medium in both chambers and then the medium in the upper (anterior) chamber is changed to one containing the test substance. Even suspended materials which settle out onto the cornea can be tested. After an appropriate incubation period, fresh medium is introduced into the upper chamber and the light transmitted through the cornea is measured photometrically in a dual-beam opacitometer, with a comparison being made with a control cornea. A reduction in light transmission indicates damage while an increase in transmission indicates damage, with sloughing off of the epithelial cell layer. The technique has the advantage of permitting an assessment of the reversibility of the lesion by continuing the incubation of the treated cornea in fresh medium following the opacity readings. One modification of this test includes the introduction of a fluorescent dye to the medium (after the opacity readings have been taken) so that the extent of corneal damage may be ascertained by the penetration of the dye into the corneal layers. Diffusion of the dye into the lower (posterior) chamber can be measured by fluorescence spectrophotometry. Correlations between the opacity "index" and *in vivo* Draize test scores have been good for the number of compounds validated to date. The disadvantages of the test appear to be related to hydrophobic agents, weak irritants, and agents that cause minimal *in vivo* irritation initially (24 to 36 h) but which induce increasing irritation at a later stage (Sina and Gautheron, 1994).

The **Enucleated Eye Test (EET)**, using isolated eyes of rabbits, was first introduced by Burton et al. (1981), with the endpoints of the assay being opacity, corneal thickness, and fluorescein dye retention. Other investigators have experimented with the technique using isolated, enucleated eyes of rabbits, cattle, pigs, and chickens held by clamps in suitable chambers containing a suitable medium (Price and Andrews, 1985; Whittle et al., 1992; Prinsen and Koeter, 1993). The test substance is usually applied directly to the corneal surface of a whole enucleated eye held in a frame, the time of contact being a brief (10 s) period, and the excess being washed off with warm saline and an eye dropper. Opacity and corneal thickness are measured by a photoslit-lamp microscope over a post-treatment period of 5 h, with fluorescein

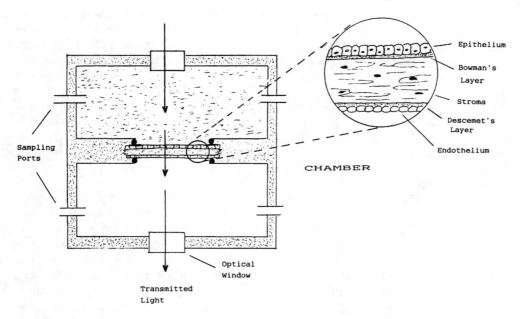

FIGURE 3.12

A schematic diagram of the apparatus used for the bovine corneal opacity-permeability (BCO-P) assay, showing the placement of the isolated cornea, epithelial side upward, into a fitted structure within a two-compartment chamber equipped with "windows." The test agent, suspended or dissolved in medium, can be introduced into the upper chamber, incubated for a specific time period and replaced by fresh medium. Corneal damage (opacity, sloughing of cells) can be assessed by the light intensity transmitted through the windows. Penetration of the test agent into or through the cornea can be assessed by adding fluorescein dye to the medium of the upper compartment and measuring the depth of penetration into the damaged cells or by the analysis of aliquots of medium taken from the lower compartment for fluorescein or the test agent.

dye being applied 4 h after treatment to aid in visualizing damage and to measure the rate and degree of penetration of the corneal stroma. However, this test still uses subjective scoring techniques (Prinsen and Koeter, 1993). This test has been validated with a wide range of compounds, with good correlations being established between *in vitro* effects and *in vivo* irritancy (Price and Andrews, 1985; Whittle et al., 1992). Not surprisingly, the effects of liquid test substances were more successfully predicted *in vitro* than were the effects of solid test agents.

In particular, the **Chicken Enucleated Eye Test (CEET)** correctly classified each of the compounds that must be labeled in the EC as irritant or severely irritant and was able to distinguish slightly irritant chemicals as well (Prinsen and Koeter, 1993). The utility of the **CEET** has been validated for 44 different chemicals/products and has been incorporated into standard contract toxicity testing in the TNO Nutrition and Food Research Institute (Prinsen, 1996). It would appear that the CEET might serve the chemical classification needs of the EC as well as those of other regulatory agencies without the use of laboratory animals, using instead the eyes from slaughterhouse animals which would only be wastage.

3. Inflammatory Tests

Inflammation is a complex event and few *in vitro* cell systems are capable of producing an inflammatory response. Consider just the arachidonic acid cascade phenomenon and the biologically active products produced during metabolism (Campbell, 1990). However, the right type of cells can release chemotactic factors and/or inflammatory mediators such as histamine, serotonin, prostaglandins, thromboxanes, and leukotrienes which can be quantitated indirectly via their chemotactic effects on neutrophils or by direct assay using high-performance, liquid chromatography (HPLC).

In the **Bovine Corneal Cup Assay**, the epithelial surface of the enucleated eye forms the inside of a "well" in a temperature-controlled plastic holder into which is pipetted a volume of physiological medium with or without a test substance. Following an appropriate incubation period, the released chemotactic factors associated with inflammation are removed with the medium for subsequent interaction with isolated neutrophils (Elgebaly et al., 1987). While several different factors may be released from the corneal epithelial cells, the assay does not require the isolation/identification of any specific factors, the chemotactic response of the neutrophils marking the analytical endpoint. Others using the bovine corneal cup assay have quantitated the release of inflammatory mediators from mast cells (histamine, serotonin, leukotrienes), derivatizing the mediators with fluorescamine prior to analysis by HPLC (Benassi et al., 1987). This technique is promising but will require extensive interlaboratory validation with a broad range of known or potential ocular irritants.

In an assay system using rat vaginal tissue *in vitro*, investigators have attempted to quantify and associate the release of eicosanoids with inflammation, measuring the cellular release of prostaglandins (PGE_2, PGF_2, 6-keto PGF_1) and thromboxane B_2 into the medium and using HPLC with fluorescence or radioimmune assay (RIA) techniques (Dubin et al., 1985,1988). This technique is still being developed and validated.

In the **Chorioallantoic Membrane (CAM) Assay** or the **Hen's Egg Test — Chorioallantoic Membrane Test (HET-CAM)**, the vascularized respiratory membrane surrounding the embryonic chicken within an egg is used as the site of irritant activity. The CAM is a comlete tissue but lacks sensory innervation (Leighton et al., 1985; Luepke, 1985). Following the incubation of fertile eggs for 5 d at 37°C, an opening is drilled at the pointed end and 2.0 ml of albumin is withdrawn and the hole is sealed again. A larger rectangular opening is created over the middle of the egg and the CAM is exposed. This opening is resealed with tape and the egg is incubated for a further 14 d, allowing the CAM to develop as the "floor" of the cavity. Removing the tape on the day of experimentation, a 10 mm Teflon ring is placed on the CAM and the test substance is pipetted onto the CAM within the ring. The window is resealed with tape, the egg is incubated for a further 3 d, and then it is examined for the extent of necrosis within the ring application site. A modification of this assay, the **CAM Vascular Assay (CAMVA)**, is carried out in the same manner but vascular changes constitute the lesion, a positive test being indicated by hemorrhage, obstriction, or narrowing of blood vessels 30 min after applying the test substance to the CAM of a 14-day-old fertilized hen's egg (Bagley et al., 1994). While the CAM assays have been validated, the results are mixed. Concerns have been raised about the high number of false-positive results, the subjective nature of scoring, embryotoxicity, no evidence of any inflammatory response, little anatomical similarity to the cornea, the absence of circulating heterophils in the chicken embryo, and an immature immune response in the species (Bruner, 1992). It is improbable that this assay will prove to be very useful since, in addition to the above assay-related defects, the British Animals (Scientific Procedures) Act of 1986 does not recognize developing birds as *in vitro* tests if used beyond the halfway point (10.5 days) in development (Bagley et al., 1994). In Germany, fertile eggs up to 10 days of age are considered as foodstuffs and can be used as nonanimal tests, i.e., the hen's egg test-CAM (HET-CAM) (Bagley et al., 1994). Obviously, some harmonization will have to take place, the focus being on a 9- or 10-day-old fertilized hen's egg for the assay.

In the **Corneal Repair Test**, a defined area of isolated rabbit corneal epithelial cell monolayer is damaged by a 6.0 mm probe frozen in liquid nitrogen and then is covered with medium in the presence or absence of a dissolved test substance. In the absence of an ocular irritant, the neighboring undamaged epithelial cells at the wound periphery migrate over the damaged area, covering the defect with a disappearance of the lesion. The rate of recovery is impeded by potential irritant (cytotoxic) agents, the irritancy potential (IP) being estimated by determining an IP_{50}, the concentration which inhibits wound healing by 50% compared to nontreated controls. This test system requires validation.

More recently, the **Skin™ System (Model ZK1200)**, a coculture of human skin-derived, stratified, squamous epithelial cells and stromal fibroblasts grown on nylon mesh, has been tested to detect potential ocular irritants (Osborne et al., 1995). The culture is air-interfaced to promote epithelial layering to simulate mucosal epithelium such as cornea and conjunctiva. The MTT vital dye metabolism is used as the biomarker of cytotoxicity, measurement being the time (min) of exposure to test agent to reduce MTT metabolism to 50% of control levels (the t50 value). Such values were compared with the rabbit **LVET** assay, a good correlation (r = 0.87) being obtained for a range of solids (granular, powder) and liquids (Osborne et al., 1995).

VII. UTILITY OF ALTERNATIVE STUDIES

Some commentary should be offered concerning the future use of the various *in vitro*, alternative-to-animal testing procedures currently under development. As developed in the early 1940s, the Draize tests, both dermal and ocular, were product safety tests. In the spirit of the "three Rs" and with considerable pressure mounting on regulatory agencies to accept some of these methods as replacements for animal experiments, there has been intensive development, evaluation, and validation of these tests, however, they are still in the mode of product safety assessment. Recent years have seen many papers on evaluation/validation of a wide range of tests to detect and quantify dermal and ocular irritation and damage, with these being applied to a vast array of classes of chemicals (Bruner et al., 1991; Shopsis et al., 1985; Sina et al., 1995). An interesting parallel can be made between the current status of the dermal and ocular testing procedures and the situation that arose with mutagenicity testing a decade or more ago. In both cases, sets of tests, examining a wide range of biological effects, were developed, evaluated, and validated. With mutagenicity testing, regulatory agencies eventually proposed a selected battery of testing procedures, requesting industry to submit results from five or six tests, with some direction being given to guarantee the inclusion of certain tests because of an understanding of the genetics involved and/or the nature of the chemical-induced mutation. Most likely, the same scenario will evolve with the alternative dermal and ocular tests. We are already seeing batteries of representative, validated tests being proposed, with a number of testing procedures being suggested for the screening of the potency of potentially irritant chemicals, the results being submitted as evidence of dermal and/or ocular safety of chemicals and formulations (Shopsis et al., 1985; Bruner et al., 1991; Sina et al., 1995). Testing laboratories will probably develop and maintain a selected group of testing procedures suitable to their needs, e.g., a cosmetic, a personal care product, a household cleaner, etc. (Gettings et al., 1994, 1995). In this fashion, suitable alternative tests will replace the use of animals and reduce the numbers required both at the level of screening as well as at the level of supporting registration. However, it should be emphasized that these alternative tests will never replace animal experimentation completely. In all probability, *in vivo* studies will still be used in the final, premarketing assessment of finished products.

VIII. CONCLUSIONS

From the results obtained in the acute toxicity studies discussed above, a good database of knowledge will have been obtained concerning the potential of a chemical, mixture, or formulation to be hazardous to health in situations of exposure to high concentrations. This information will be incorporated into material safety data sheets which, by law, must be prepared and made available for every chemical and/or product used in North American industries. These results will form the basis for the symptomatic treatment of drug-, pesticide-, home product-, and industrial chemical-induced toxicity by the clinical toxicologist or the family physician. The data obtained from acute toxicity studies will, depending upon the species investigated, be used to gauge the potential and severity of environmental contamination and the impact on the well-being of humans, domestic stock, and crops, as well as wildlife flora and fauna. However, concerns about toxicity go far beyond the situation of acute or short-term exposure to high concentrations. In the workplace, the home, and the outdoors, toxicity may be associated with chronic exposure to relatively low concentrations of toxicants. Acute toxicity data cannot predict the hazards related to long-term exposure. Studies designed to assess these aspects of chemical toxicity will be discussed in the next chapter.

REFERENCES

Anon. Code of Federal Regulations. Title 16. Part 1500.41. (1980).

Bagley, D.M., Waters, D., and Kong, B.M. Development of a 10-day chorioallantoic membrane vascular assay as an alternative to the Draize rabbit eye irritation test. *Food Chem. Toxicol.* 32: 1155-1166 (1994).

Barile, F.A. *Introduction to In Vitro Cytotoxicity. Mechanisms and Methods.* CRC Press, Inc., Boca Raton (1994).

Barker, J.N.W.N., Mitra, R.S., Griffiths, C.E.M., Dixit, V.M., and Nickoloff, B.J. Keratinocytes as initiators of inflammation. *Lancet* 337: 211-214 (1991).

Basketter, D.A., Scholes, E.W., Chamberlain, M., and Barratt, M.D. An alternative strategy to the use of guinea pigs for the identification of skin sensitization hazard. *Food Chem. Toxicol.* 33: 1051-1056 (1995).

Basketter, D.A., Scholes, E.W., and Kimber, I. The performance of the local lymph node assay with chemicals identified as contact allergens in the human maximization test. *Food Chem. Toxicol.* 32: 543-547 (1994).

Basketter, D.A., Selbie, E., Scholes, E.W., Lees, D., Kimber, I., and Botham, P.A. Results with OECD recommended positive control sensitizers in the maximization, Buehler and local lymph node assays. *Food Chem. Toxicol.* 33: 63-67 (1993).

Benassi, A., Angi, M.R., Salvalaio, L., and Bettero, O. Ocular irritancy evaluated *in vivo* by conjunctival lavage technique and *in vitro* by bovine eye cup model. In *Alternative Methods in Toxicology*, Vol. 5, Goldberg, A.M., Ed., Mary Ann Liebert, New York (1987), pp.235-242.

Bliss, C.L. Some principles of bioassay. *Am. Sci.* 45: 449-466, (1957).

Botham, P.A., Basketter, D.A., Maurer, T., Mueller, D., Potokar, M., and Bontinck, W.J. Skin sensitization — a critical review of predictive test methods in animals and man. *Food Chem. Toxicol.* 29: 275-286 (1991).

Bruce, R.D. A confirmatory study of the up-and-down method for acute oral toxicity testing. *Fundam. Appl. Toxicol.* 8: 97-100 (1987).

Bruce, R.D. An up-and-down procedure for acute toxicity testing. *Fundam. Appl. Toxicol.* 5: 151-157 (1985).

Bruner, L.H. Ocular irritation. In *In Vitro Toxicity Testing*, Frazier, J.M., Ed., Marcel Dekker, New York (1944), pp.149-190.

Bruner, L.H., Kain, D.J., Roberts, D.A., and Parker, R.D. Evaluation of seven *in vitro* alternatives for ocular safety testing. *Fundam. Appl. Toxicol.* 17: 136-149 (1991).

Bruner, L.H., Parker, R.D., and Bruce, R.D. Reducing the number of rabbits in the low-volume eye test. *Fundam. Appl. Toxicol.* 19: 330-335 (1992).

Buehler, E.V. A new method for detecting potential sensitizers using the guinea pig. *Toxicol. Appl. Pharmacol.* 6: 341 (1964).

Burn, J.H., Finney, D.J., and Goodwin, L.G. *Biological Standardization.* Oxford University Press, London (1950).

Burton, A.B.G., York, M., and Lawrence, R.S. The *in vitro* assessment of severe eye irritants. *Food Cosmet. Toxicol.* 19: 471-480 (1981).

Campbell, W.B. Lipid-derived autocoids: eicosanoids and platelet-activating factor. In *Goodman and Gilman's The Pharmacological Basis of Therapeutics.* Eighth Edition, Gilman, A.G., Rall, T.W., Nies, A.S., and Taylor, P., Eds., Pergamon Press, New York (1990), Ch.24, pp.600-617.

Carver, M.P., Williams, P.L., and Riviere, J.E. The isolated perfused porcine skin flap. III. Percutaneous absorption, pharmacokinetics of organophosphates, steroids, benzoic acid and caffeine. *Toxicol. Appl. Pharmacol.* 97: 324-337 (1989).

Conquest, P., Durand, G., Laillier, J., and Blazonnet, B. Evaluation of ocular irritation in the rabbit: objective vs. subjective assessment. *Toxicol. Appl. Pharmacol.* 39: 129-139 (1977).

Deichmann, W.B. and Le Blanc, T.J. Determination of the approximate lethal dose with about six animals. *J. Ind. Hyg. Toxicol.* 25: 415-417 (1945).

Deichmann, W.B. and Mergard, E.G. Comparative evaluation of methods employed to express the degree of toxicity of a compound. *J. Ind. Hyg. Toxicol.* 30: 373-378 (1948).

De Sousa, D.J., Rouse, A.A., and Smolon, W.J. Statistical consequences of reducing the number of rabbits utilized in eye irritation testing: data on 67 petrochemicals. *Toxicol. Appl. Pharmacol.* 76: 234-242 (1984).

DeLeo, V.A., Carver, M.P., Hong, J., Fung, K., Kong, B., and DeSalva, S. Arachnidonic acid release: an *in vitro* alternative for dermal irritancy testing. *Food Chem. Toxicol.* 34: 167-176 (1996).

Dixon, W.J. The up-and-down method for small samples. *J. Am. Statist. Assoc.* 60: 967-978 (1965)

Dixon, W.J. and Mood, A.M. A method for obtaining and analyzing sensitivity data. *J. Am. Statist. Assoc.* 43: 109-126 (1948).

Dixon, W.J. Staircase bioassay: the up-and-down method. *Neurosci. Biobehav. Rev.* 15: 47-50 (1991).

Draize, J.H., Woodard, G., and Calvery, H.O. Methods for the study of irritation and toxicity of substances applied topically to the skin and mucous membranes. *J. Pharmacol. Exp. Ther.* 82: 377-389 (1944).

Dubin, N.H. Prostaglandin production as an index of *in vitro* cytotoxicity. In *Alternative Methods in Toxicology* Vol.3, Goldberg, A.M., Ed., Mary Ann Liebert, New York (1985), pp. 45-51.

Dubin, N.H., Ghodgaonkar, R.B., and Parmley, T.H. Differential response of *in vitro* vaginal tissue to various test agents. In *Alternative Methods in Toxicology* Vol. 6, Goldberg, A.M., Ed., Mary Ann Liebert, New York (1988), pp.153-158.

Dunn, B.J. Toxicology of the Eye. In *CRC Handbook of Toxicology*, Derelanko, M.J. and Hollinger, M.A., Eds., CRC Press, Boca Raton, FL. (1995), Ch.4, pp.163-216.

EEC. Sixth amendment of the Cosmetics Directive 76/768 (1995).

Elgebaly, S.A., Forouhar, F., and Kreutzer, D.L. *In vitro* detection of cornea-derived leukocytic chemotactic factors as indicators of corneal inflammation. In *Alternative Methods in Toxicology*. Vol. 5, Mary Ann Liebert, New York (1987), pp. 257-268.

Enslein, K., Lander, T.R., Tomb, M.E., and Craig, P.N. *A Predictive Model for Estimating Rat Oral LD_{50} Values.* Princeton Scientific Publishers Inc., Princeton (1983).

Finney, D.J. *Statistical Methods in Biological Assay.* Charles Griffin, London (1964).

Finney, D.J. *Probit Analysis.* Third Edition. Cambridge University Press, Cambridge, U.K. (1971).

Frazier, J.M. (Ed.). *In Vitro Toxicity Testing. Applications to Safety Evaluation*, Marcel Dekker, Inc., New York (1992).

Freeberg, F.E., Nixon, G.A., Reer, P.J., Weaver, J.E., Bruce, R.D., Griffith, J.F., and Sanders III, L.W. Human and rabbit eye responses to chemical insult. *Fundam. Appl. Toxicol.* 7: 626-634 (1986).

Friedenwald, J.S., Hughes, Jr., W.F., and Herrmann, H. Acid-base tolerance of the cornea. *Arch. Ophthal.* 31: 279-283 (1944).

Furstenberger, G. Role of eicosanoids in mammalian skin epidermis. *Cell Biol. Rev.* 24: 1-111 (1990).

Gad, S.C. (Ed.). *In Vitro Toxicology*, Raven Press, New York (1994).

Gad, S.C., Dunn, B.J., Dobbs, D.W., Reilly, C., and Walsh, R.D. Development and validation of an alternative dermal sensitization test: the mouse ear swelling test (MEST). *Toxicol. Appl. Pharmacol.* 84: 93-114 (1986).

Gettings, S.D., Dipasquale, L.C., Bagley, D.M., Casterton, P.L., Chudkowski, M. et al. The CTFA evaluation of alternatives program: an evaluation of *in vitro* alternatives to the Draize primary eye irritation test. (Phase II) Oil/water emulsions. *Food Chem. Toxicol.* 32: 943-976 (1994).

Gettings, S.D., Lordo, R.A., Hintze, K.L., Bagley, D.M., Casterton, P.L. et al. The CFTA evaluation of alternatives program: an evaluation of *in vitro* alternatives to the Draize primary eye irritation test. (Phase III) Sufactant-based formulations. *Food Chem. Toxicol.* 34: 79-117 (1996).

Goldberg, A.M. (Ed.). *Alternative Methods in Toxicology.* Vol.5, Mary Ann Liebert, New York (1987).

Griffith, J.F., Nixon, G.A., Bruce, R.D., Reer, P.J., and Bannan, E.A. Dose-response studies with chemical irritants in the albino rabbit eye as a basis for selecting optimum test conditions for predicting hazard to the human eye. *Toxicol. Appl. Pharmacol.* 55: 501-513 (1980).

Harber, L.C. and Bickers, D.R. *Photosensitivities: Principles of Diagnosis and Treatment,* Saunders, Philadelphia (1981).

Harber, L.C., Shalita, A.R., and Armstrong, R.B. Immunologically mediated contact photosensitivity in guinea pigs. In *Dermato-toxicology.* Second Edition. Marzulli, F.N. and Maibach, H.I. (Eds.), Ch. 16. Hemisphere Publishing Corp., New York (1983).

Harvell, J.D. and Maibach, H. *In vitro* dermal toxicity assays: validation with human data. In *Animal Test Alternatives. Refinement, Reduction, Replacement,* Salem, H. (Ed.), Marcel Dekker, Inc., New York (1995), pp.145-151.

Hayes, A.W. (Ed.). *Principles and Methods of Toxicology.* Third Edition., Raven Press, New York (1994).

Herzinger, T., Korting, H.C., and Maibach, H.J. Assessment of cutaneous and ocular irritancy: A decade of research on alternatives to animal experimentation. *Fundam. Appl. Toxicol.* 24: 29-41 (1955).

Kimber, I. and Basketter, D.A. The murine local lymph node assay: a commentary on collaborative studies and new directions. *Food Chem. Toxicol.* 30: 165-169 (1992).

King, J.R. and Montiero-Riviere, N.A. Effects of organic solvent vehicles on the viability and morphology of isolated perfused porcine skin. *Toxicology* 69: 11-26 (1991).

Klecak, G. Identification of contact allergens: predictive tests in animals. In *Dermatotoxicology.* Second Edition. Marzulli, F.N and Maibach, H.I. (Eds.), Hemisphere Publishing Corp., New York (1983), pp. 210-213.

Kornhauser, A., Wamer, W., and Giles, Jr., A. Light-induced dermal toxicity: effects on the cellular and molecular level. In *Dermatotoxicology.* Second Edition. Marzulli, F.N. and Maibach, H.I. (Eds.), Hemisphere Publishing Corp., New York (1983).

Leighton, J., Nassauer, J., and Tchao, R. The chick embryo in toxicology: an alternative to the rabbit eye. *Food Chem. Toxicol.* 23: 293-298 (1985).

Lipnick, R.L., Cotruvo, J.A., Hill, R.H., Bruce, R.D., Stitzel, K.A., Walker, A.P., Chu, I., Goddard, M., Segal, L., Springer, J.A., and Myers, R.C. Comparison of the up-and-down, conventional LD_{50} and fixed-dose acute toxicity procedures. *Food Chem. Toxicol.* 33: 223-231 (1995).

Litchfield, Jr., J.T. and Wilcoxon, F. Simplified method of evaluating dose-effect experiments. *J. Pharmacol. Ex. Ther.* 96: 99-113 (1949).

Loomis, T.A. and Hayes, A.W. *Essentials of Toxicology,* Fourth Edition, Academic Press, New York (1996).

Luepke, N.P. Hen's egg chorioallantoic membrane test for irritation potential. *Food Chem. Toxicol.* 23: 287-291 (1985).

Marzulli, F.N. and Maibach, H.I. (Eds.). *Advances in Modern Toxicology.* Vol.4. *Dermatotoxicology and Pharmacology.* Hemisphere Publishing Corp., New York (1977).

Marzulli, F.N. and Maibach, H.I. (Eds.). *Dermatotoxicology.* Second Edition. Hemisphere Publishing Corp., New York (1987).

Marzulli, F.N. and Ruggles, D.I. Rabbit eye irritation test: collaborative study. *J. Am. Assoc. Anal. Chem.* 56: 905-914 (1973).

McCreesh, A.H. and Steinberg, M. Skin irritation testing in animals. In *Dermatotoxicology.* Second Edition. Marzulli, F.N. and Maibach, H.I. (Eds.), Hemisphere Publishing Corp., New York (1983), Ch.6, pp.147-166.

McDonald, T.O., Seabaugh, V., Shadduck, J.A., and Edelhauser, H.F. Eye Irritation. In *Dermatotoxicology.* Second Edition. Marzulli, F.N. and Maibach, H.I. (Eds.), Hemisphere Publishing Corp., New York (1983), pp.555-610.

McNamara, B.P. Concepts in health evaluation of commercial and industrial chemicals. In *New Concepts in Safety Evaluation,* Mehlman, M.A., Shapiro, R.E., and Blumenthal, H. (Eds.), Hemisphere Publishing, New York (1976), Ch.4.

Miller, L.C. and Tainter, M.L. Estimation of the ED_{50} and its error by means of logarithmic-probit graph paper. *Proc. Soc. Exp. Biol. Med.* 57: 261-264 (1944).

Monteiro-Riviere, N.A., Bowman, K.F., Scheidt, V.J., and Riviere, J.E. The isolated perfused porcine skin flap (IPPSF). II. Ultra-structural and histological characterization of epidermal viability. *In Vitro* 1: 241-252 (1987).

Motoyoshi, K., Toyoshima, Y., Sato, M., and Yoshimura, M. Comparative studies on the irritancy of oils and synthetic perfumes to the skin of rabbit, guinea pig, rat, miniature swine and man. *Cosmet. Toiletries* 94: 41-42 (1979).

Muller-Decker, K., Furstenberger, G., and Marks, F. Keratinocyte-derived proinflammatory key mediators and cell viability as *in vitro* parameters of irritancy: A possible alternative to the Draize skin irritation test. *Toxicol. Appl. Pharmacol.* 127: 99-108 (1994).

Naughton, G.K., Jacob, L., and Naughton, B.A. A physiological skin model for *in vitro* toxicity studies. In *Alternative Methods in Toxicology.* Vol.7, Goldberg, A.M. (Ed.), Mary Ann Liebert, New York (1987), pp.183-189.

Nixon, G.A., Tyson, C.A., and Wertz, W.C. Interspecies comparisons of skin irritancy. *Toxicol. Appl. Pharmacol.* 31: 481-490 (1975).

Organization for Economic Cooperation and Development. *OECD Guidelines for Testing of Chemicals.* Paris (1981).

Osborne, R. and Perkins, M.A. An approach for development of alternative test methods based on mechanisms of skin irritation. *Food Chem. Toxicol.* 32: 133-142 (1994).

Osborne, R., Perkins, M.A., and Roberts, D.A. Development and intralaboratory evaluation of an *in vitro* human cell-based test to aid ocular irritancy assessments. *Fundam. Appl. Toxicol.* 28: 139-153 (1995).

Patrick, E. and Maibach, H. Dermatotoxicity. In *Principles and Methods of Toxicology.* Third Edition, Hayes, A.W. (Ed.), Raven Press, New York (1994), Ch.21, pp.767-803.

Phalen, R.F., Mannix, R.C., and Drew, T.R. Inhalation exposure methodology. *Environ. Health Perspect.* 56: 23-34 (1984).

Price, J.B. and Andrews, I.J. The *in vitro* assessment of eye irritancy using isolated eyes. *Food Chem. Toxicol.* 23: 313-315 (1985).

Prinsen, M.K. The chicken enucleated eye test (CEET): a practical (pre)screen for the assessment of eye irritation/corrosion potential of test materials. *Food Chem. Toxicol.* 34: 291-296 (1996).

Prinsen, M.K. and Koeter, H.B.W.M. Justification of the enucleated eye test with eyes of slaughterhouse animals as an alternative to the Draize eye irritation test with rabbits. *Food Chem. Toxicol.* 31: 69-76 (1993).

Purchase, I.F.N. and Conning, D.M. (Proceedings Eds.). International Conference on Practical *in vitro* Toxicology. *Food Chem. Toxicol.* 24: #6/7 (June/July) (1986).

Reinhardt, Ch.A., Bosshard, E., and Schlatter, Ch. Irritation Testing of Skin and Mucous Membranes. *Food Chem. Toxicol.* 23: 135-338 (1985).

Riviere, J.E., Bowman, K.F., Montiero-Riviere, N.A., Dix, L.P., and Carver, M.P. The isolated perfused porcine skin flap (IPPSF). I. A novel *in vitro* model for percutaneous absorption and cutaneous toxicology studies. *Fundam. Appl. Toxicol.* 7: 444-453 (1986).

Rush, R.E., Bonnette, K.L., Douds, D.A., and Merriman, T.N. Dermal Irritation and Sensitivity. In *CRC Handbook of Toxicology,* Derelanko, M.J. and Hollinger, M.A. (Eds.), CRC Press, Boca Raton, FL (1995), Ch.3, pp.105-162.

Salem, H. (Ed.). *Animal Test Alternatives. Refinement, Reduction and Replacement,* Marcel Dekker, New York (1995).

Schlede, E., Mischke, U., Roll, R., and Kayser, D. A national validation study of the acute-toxic-class method, an alternative to the LD_{50} test. *Arch. Toxicol.* 66: 455-470 (1992).

Scholes, E.W., Basketter, D.A., Saril, A.E., Kimber, I., Evans, C.D., Miller, K., Robbins, M.C., Harrison, P.T.C., and Waite, S.J. The local lymph node assay: results of a final interlaboratory validation under field conditions. *J. Appl. Toxicol.* 12: 217-222 (1992).

Seabaugh, V.M. EPA's requirements for dermal irritation and sensitizing tests. *Food Chem. Toxicol.* 32: 93-95 (1994).

Sharpe, R. The Draize test — motivations for change. *Food Chem. Toxicol.* 23: 139-143 (1985).

Shopsis, C., Borenfreund, E., Walberg, J., and Stark, D.M. A battery of potential alternatives to the Draize test: uridine uptake inhibition, morphological cytotoxicity, macrophage chemotaxis and exfoliative cytology. *Food Chem. Toxicol.* 23: 259-266 (1985).

Sina, J.F. and Gautheron, P.D. Ocular toxicity assessment *in vitro.* In *In Vitro Toxicology,* Gad, S.C. (Ed.), Raven Press, New York (1994), Ch.3, pp.21-46.

Sina, J.F., Galer, D.M., Sussman, R.G., Gautheron, P.D., Sargent, E.V., Leong, B., Shah, P.V., Curren, R.D., and Miller, K. A collaborative evaluation of seven alternatives to the Draize eye irritation test using pharmaceutical intermediates. *Fundam. Appl. Toxicol.* 26: 20-31 (1995).

Smith, F.A., Downs, W.L., Hodge, H.C., and Maynard, E.A. Screening of fluorine-containing compounds for acute toxicity. *Toxicol. Appl. Pharmacol.* 2: 54-58 (1960).

Smyth, H.F., Carpenter, C.P., Weil, C.S., Pozzani, U.C., and Striegel, J.A. Range-finding toxicity data. List VI. *Am. Ind. Hyg. Assoc. J.* 23: 95-107 (1962).

Snellings, W.M. and Dodd, D.E. Inhalation studies. In *Handbook of In Vivo Toxicity Testing.* Arnold, D.L., Grice, H.C., and Krewski, D.R. (Eds.), Academic Press, New York (1990), Ch. 10. pp. 189-246.

Talsma, D.M., Leach, C.L., Hatoum, N.S., Gibbons, R.D., Roger, J.-C., and Garvin, P.J. Reducing the number of rabbits in the Draize eye irritancy test: a statistical analysis of 155 studies conducted over 6 years. *Fundam. Appl. Toxicol.* 10: 146-153 (1988).

Trevan, J.W. The error of determination of toxicity. *Proc. Royal Soc.* 101B: 483-514 (1927).

U.S. Congress. *Alternatives to Animal Use in Research Testing and Education.* Office of Technology Assessment. U.S. Govt. Printing Office. OTA-BA-273. Washington (1986).

Van den Heuvel, M.J., Clark, D.G., Fielder, R.J., Koundakjian, P.P., Oliver, G.J.A., Pelling, D., Tomlinson, N.J., and Wlaker, A.P. The international validation of a fixed-dose procedure as an alternative to the classical LD$_{50}$ test. *Food Chem. Toxicol.* 28: 469-482 (1990).

Weideman, M. *In vitro* innovations. *Environ. Health Perspect.* 103: 1014-1016 (1995).

Weil, C.S. Tables for convenient calculations of median effective dose (LD$_{50}$ or ED$_{50}$) and the instructions for their use. *Biometrics* 8: 249-263 (1952).

Weil, C.S. Statistics vs. safety factors and scientific judgment in the evaluation of safety for man. *Toxicol. Appl. Pharmacol.* 21: 454-463 (1972).

Weil, C.S. and Scala, R.A. Study of the intra and interlaboratory variability in the results of the rabbit eye and skin irritancy tests. *Toxicol. Appl. Pharmacol.* 19: 276-360 (1971).

Wester, R.C. and Maibach, H.I. Percutaneous absorption in the rhesus monkey compared to man. *Toxicol. Appl. Pharmacol.* 32: 394-398 (1975).

Whittle, E., Basketter, D., York, M., Kelly, J., Hall, T., McCall, J., Botham, P., Esdaile, D., and Gardner, J. Findings of an interlaboratory trial of the enucleated eye method as an alternative eye irritation test. *Toxicol. Methods* 2: 30-41 (1992).

Williams, P.L., Carver, M.P., and Riviere, J.E. A physiologically relevant pharmacokinetic model of xenobiotic percutaneous absorption utilizing the isolated perfused porcine skin flap. *J. Pharm. Scis.* 79: 305-311 (1990).

Zbinden, G. and Flury-Roversi, M. Significance of the LD$_{50}$ test for the toxicological evaluation of chemical substances. *Arch. Toxicol.* 47: 77-99 (1981).

Zbinden, G. Invited contribution: acute toxicity testing, public responsibility and scientific challenges. *Cell. Biol. and Toxicol.* 2: 325-335 (1986).

Chapter 4

SUBCHRONIC AND CHRONIC STUDIES

I. INTRODUCTION

As early as 1954, Barnes and Denz commented on the status of long-term studies, stating that "a chronic toxicity test is always a makeshift affair to be replaced as soon as possible by a more permanent structure of knowledge built on the foundations of physiology, biochemistry, and other fundamental sciences" (Barnes and Denz, 1954). In the intervening 42 years, great strides have been made in the development of extensive protocols on the design and conductance of such studies but, looking at the paucity of "foundations" built into some investigations and the still prevalent omnibus approach, one might wonder what their comments would be today.

In acute toxicity studies, particularly the LD_{50} determination, one endpoint, death, is examined and the observation of other types of target organ toxicity are limited by the dosage, the short duration of exposure and the length of survival of the test species. While acute exposure to high concentrations of chemicals can occur in any environment (the outdoors, the home, the workplace), living organisms are more frequently exposed over much longer periods of time to agents at levels lower than those that are fatal. The simulation of such exposure requires the development of two distinct types of studies, the short-term (**subacute, subchronic**) and the long-term (**chronic**) studies. Subacute toxicity studies, usually of 2 to 4 weeks duration, are conducted as range-finding studies in order to choose dosage levels to be used in subchronic (up to 90 d) and chronic (6 months to 2 years) studies (Woutersen et al., 1984). A recent examination of newly introduced OECD Guidelines indicates that the subacute/subchronic terminology is being phased out, with the particular test(s) designating the duration of the study, i.e., OECD Guideline 407-Repeated Dose 28-Day Oral Toxicity Study in Rodents, leaving no doubts in the investigators' minds as to how long the study should be conducted. These studies are carried out in selected animal species deemed, hopefully, to mimic the human response. These studies are designed to:

1. Examine the biological nature of the toxic effects, from low dosages, at the cellular level, measuring parameters that cannot usually be obtained in acute studies because of the high dosages administered and the rapidity of onset of toxic signs and symptoms.

2. Ascertain the variation in species response(s) to repeated exposure to the agent, looking for commonality of response and/or distinct species differences.

3. Assess possible cumulative effects of the repeated exposure as body burdens of agent and/or biotransformation products are acquired with time.

4. Determine the nature of macroscopic and microscopic organ or tissue damage as it develops, hopefully in relation to the level and/or duration of exposure.

5. Identify the approximate dosage at which the altered physiological, biochemical, and morphological changes might occur.

6. Predict the long-range adverse health effects in the species arising from intermittent, repeated, or chronic exposure to the particular agent.

Where the human is concerned, an additional factor in the design of surrogate animal studies is to be able to predict whether or not, and at what level(s), similar adverse health effects might be anticipated in the human. The old adage holds true that "the more species of animals in which the same biological response to an agent can be produced, the greater is the chance that, at some dosage, the same effect might be produced in the human."

II. EXPERIMENTAL DESIGN

It is important to appreciate the significance of the term "chronic" in relation to the duration of a study. Environmentally, a 24- to 48-h exposure period could represent a chronic study for some aquatic insects between hatching and flying or a span of some months for birds, etc. In other species, a critical stage of development during which the animal was susceptible might be of the order of 7 to 14 d. Originally, in regulatory parlance, a chronic mammalian study signified a duration of 2 years, the approximate lifespan of a laboratory rodent. However, laboratory rats certainly live longer than that, the 2-year period being approximately 70 to 80% of the lifespan. This 2-year period is only a small fraction of the lifespan of a rabbit (35%), dog (20%), or a monkey (13%) (Table 4.1). To accomodate for the longer lifespan, usually the dosage regimen is adjusted so that the level received in a lifetime will be acquired in the 2-year interval, with all of the attendant problems that such a maneuver could create (see Chapter 2).

In recent years, there have been dramatic shifts in regulatory philosophy on two counts. The first has been a move toward shorter time periods, i.e., 6 or 12 months, for chronic studies in rodents, adjusting the dosage regimen toward higher levels to accomodate the shortened time frame. However, the duration of chronic studies remains variable, depending upon the regulatory agency and the potential end-use of the test substance (Auletta, 1995). Frequently, chronic toxicity/carcinogenicity studies are conducted in tandem to reduce costs. The second philosophical point, to be discussed in greater detail later, concerns the extended, healthy, and tumor-free lifespan of rodents when given a somewhat restricted diet (70 to 80% of normal, *ad libitum*, daily intake), with such animals living longer than 35 or 40 months and raising the question of what a normal lifespan is.

A. Dosage Levels of Test Agent

How is the range of doses to be used in a subacute, subchronic study chosen? First, it is important to differentiate between a study intended to define the shape and nature of the dose-effect curve for some toxicological endpoint (frequently the goal of a subchronic study) and a study in which the objective is to evaluate the

TABLE 4.1

The Duration of Studies in Experimental
Animals and Time Equivalents in the Human

Species	Duration of Study in Months				
	1	3	6	12	24
Percent of life-span					
Rat	4.1	12.0	25.0	49.0	99.0
Rabbit	1.5	4.5	9.0	18.0	36.0
Dog	0.82	2.5	4.9	9.8	20.0
Pig	0.82	2.5	4.9	9.8	20.0
Monkey	0.55	1.6	3.3	6.6	13.0
Human equivalents (in months)					
Rat	34	101	202	404	808
Rabbit	12	36	72	145	289
Dog	6.5	20	40	81	162
Pig	6.5	20	40	81	162
Monkey	4.5	13	27	61	107

Modified from Paget (1970).

presence or absence of a particular toxicological effect (the endpoint in a chronic/car-cinogenicity study) (Grice, 1984). A suitable number of dose levels spanning effect and no effect levels must be employed in order to elicit the spectrum of toxicological effects necessary for the construction of meaningful dose-effect relationships (Grice, 1984). Current guidelines require three dose levels in the selected range for exposure to the test substance plus a vehicle-treated control group, with the use of three doses being based on the premise that the dose-effect relationship is likely to be nonlinear and that three dose levels allow some determination of the shape of the curve (Auletta, 1995). Acute toxicity studies of the type described in Chapter 3 will provide a starting point for dose selection, particularly with consideration of the observed toxicity in the survivors at the doses below the LD_{50} value. The pharmacokinetics of a range of single doses administered to small groups of animals should provide useful information on the rate of disposition, biotransformation, and elimination of the test agent and will be vital to the development of a dosage regimen for repeated daily treatment (See Chapter 2). Theoretically, if a toxicity study is used for risk assessment of human exposure, the lowest dose level used in the animals should, if at all possible, not be less than the pharmacokinetically equivalent human exposure and should produce no toxicological effects. One can appreciate the fact that this may be difficult to achieve, given the physicochemical properties of the test agent and the manner in which the test species handles it. Higher doses could be selected as multiples of this level, giving due consideration to the results of the single-dose pharmacokinetic experiments. The high dose should elicit toxicity without adversely affecting the nutritional status of the test animals or altering their longevity. At least one intermediate dose should be selected so as to provide some identifiable toxicity and sufficient data for purposes of quantitative risk assessment.

Has the question posed at the beginning of the above paragraph been answered? No! There is no finite rule for dosage selection but, based upon observed toxicity with this and related chemicals, and single-dose pharmacokinetic studies with the test agent, the investigator is in some position to make an educated guess. The investigator may have to carry out a repeated dosage, subacute, range-finding study on limited numbers of animals for 2 to 4 weeks to assess the validity of choosing certain dose levels. Such a preliminary study might involve "testing" only the selected high dose, thereby reducing the number of animals committed to the study. It is preferable to do this prior to starting the full scale study since the "in-study" adjustment of dose levels, the addition of another treatment group, or excessive mortality in the high dose group in the early days of the study always create a messy appearance, suggesting that the investigator does not know what he/she is doing.

For carcinogenic studies, results from either a subchronic 90-d or a chronic 104-week study may provide a dosage level known as the maximum tolerated dose (MTD). This may be defined as:

1. The highest dose of the test agent during the chronic study that can be predicted not to alter the animals' normal longevity from effects other than carcinogenicity (Sontag et al., 1976).

2. A dose which, in a subchronic study, causes no more than a 10% body weight decrement as compared to appropriate control groups and does not produce mortality, clinical signs of toxicity, or pathologic lesions (other than those of neoplastic origin) that would be predicted (in a chronic study) to shorten an animal's life span (Sontag et al., 1976).

B. NUMBERS OF ANIMALS

Prior to any experiment, the investigator must plan how the study is to be conducted. It is imperative that the study be as open-ended as possible to accomodate unforeseen and unpredictable events that almost always appear in longer-term studies. Certain questions must be asked, the most important one being **what if** this or that happens during the treatment period? How many animals are needed? When does the "lesion" begin and how rapidly does the toxicity progress toward overt signs and symptoms? Does the toxicity regress when the exposure is stopped? How can the main "theme" of the study be retained (or regained) in the face of serendipidous observations of new "types" of toxicity, sudden excessive mortality within a single treatment group, etc.? These and other questions must be anticipated and addressed before starting the actual experiment in order to avoid the grief that occurs when things go wrong and one of the variations of "Murphy's Law" infests the study. Schematic diagrams showing a sketch plan for a 90-d subchronic is presented in Figure 4.1.

As was indicated by Zbinden (1973) (Figure 2.18), some 30,000 animals would have to be included in the study to insure the detection of a toxic effect occurring even at an incidence rate of 0.01% in the human (see Figure 2.19). The chance of observing toxicity can be improved somewhat by spreading the range of the three selected dosage levels. However, while too few animals give a poor estimate, numbers in excess of 10 per treatment group per study interval (Figure 4.1) are wasteful and really do not improve the statistical estimation of toxicity. Regardless of the scope and/or duration of the study, the number of animals incorporated into the experimental design will only provide an estimate of the potential toxicity of the agent.

When must an animal be euthanized? Based on the results of acute studies, one can anticipate the likelihood of serious adverse health effects making their appearance at one or more dosage levels in subchronic or chronic studies. Animals may become moribund through agent-related effects, giving rise to (1) general impaired

SUBCHRONIC STUDY

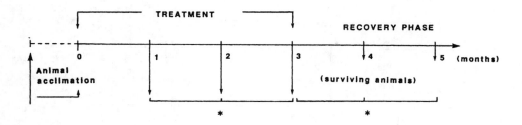

*
Animals (representative subgroups) euthanized periodically for physiological,
biochemical and morphological study.

FIGURE 4.1
The design of a subchronic (3 month, 90 day) and a chronic (12 month, 365 day) study. The planning chart enables the investigator to determine the total number of animals required based on the number of dosage levels, the number of animals required at each study interval when a representative subgroup would be selected for the study of the development of toxicant-related lesions as well as changes in morphological, physiological and/or biochemical tests of organ and tissue function/injury. Included in the designs is a posttreatment recovery phase to assess the permanence or reversibility of the effects of the toxicant.

health; (2) cachexia, with the appearance of bacterial and/or viral infections including chronic respiratory distress (CRD); (3) anorexia and/or adipsia, with accompanying loss of body weight; (4) debility, with the loss of normal organ functions; and (5) pain. Criteria must be developed to govern when a decision will be made to terminate the animal's participation in the experiment by euthanasia. These criteria become an integral part of the study protocol and should appear in the written document. The criteria should follow good laboratory practices and appropriate laboratory, animal care facility, and state and/or federal animal welfare regulations. In general, the decision to euthanize an animal should involve the study director, the attending veterinarian, and the technician responsible for the day-to-day monitoring of the animals following a review of the clinical data base (body weight gain, food consumption, results of diagnostic tests) on the animal and some unfavorable prognosis of the continued health status. Each case for euthanasia should be documented completely in the study records, giving clear evidence why the animal was euthanized and, more specifically, providing the results of a complete autopsy, gross and microscopic examination of organs and tissues. Early identification of specific target organ toxicity in the few more susceptible animals may provide invaluable evidence for predicting what might happen later on when the total dosage on exposure has been much higher.

Given the fact that the ideal design of an experiment should include a control group of animals plus three (low, intermediate, and high dose) treatment groups, one can estimate the total number of animals required (Figure 4.1). Adequate numbers of animals should always be incorporated into a study. The 90-d study schematic describes a scenario in which the animals will be treated or exposed daily for 90 consecutive days, with representative subgroups being euthanized at 30, 60, and 90 d for necropsy, tissue selection, physiological, biochemical, and morphological examination for possible toxic effects, their appearance, and development during the

CHRONIC STUDY

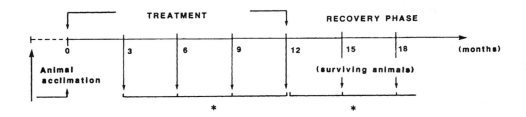

FIGURE 4.2
The design of a chronic (12-month) study. The planning chart enables the investigator to determine the total number of animals required based on the number of dosage levels and the number of animals euthanized at each study interval when representative subgroups would be selected for the study of toxicant-related lesions as well as morphological, physiological and/or biochemical tests of organ and tissue function/injury. Included in this design is a posttreatment recovery phase to assess the permanence or reversibility of the effects of the toxicant.

treatment period. At the termination of treatment, sufficient animals should survive in order that the reversibility of the toxicity can be studied for, perhaps, an additional 30 to 60 d, with suitable, randomized subgroups being euthanized for necropsy and extensive study. If one wanted a minimum of 5 animals randomized into each group selected for euthanasia at a specific time, then 100 animals (five animals multiplied by five 30-d intervals multiplied by 4 treatment groups) would be required. If the study included both males and females, then a minimum total of 200 animals would be required. It would be essential to carry additional animals, e.g., ten, within each treatment group throughout the study period in anticipation of some test agent-related mortality occurring in at least the high dosage group toward the end of the experiment. Such a scenario would require a total of 140 animals per sex for the experiment. Additional animals might be required in order to validate the quality of general health of the group purchases as will be discussed below.

In a similar fashion, the minimum number of animals can be ascertained for a 12-month chronic study, with randomly selected subgroups being euthanized after 3, 6, 9, and 12 months of treatment and with the surviving animals being euthanized at 3 and 6 months posttreatment to ascertain the reversibility of the toxicity (Figure 4.2). Usually, one would consider 5 to 10 animals in each subgroup to be randomly selected, euthanized, and studied for toxic signs and symptoms. Again, additional animals might be carried in each treatment group in anticipation of mortality caused by the agent at higher levels of exposure. Having given due consideration to the above aspects of design and to the various factors discussed in Chapter 2, the investigator is now prepared to begin the study.

It should be remembered that in the labor-intensive, longer-term studies, the animal is the least expensive component in the study. Make certain that there are sufficient numbers. Since these animals are to be kept for a considerable length of time, it is imperative that they be healthy and free of any virus or bacterial infections and other diseases. One cannot anticipate the appearance of latent infections, but

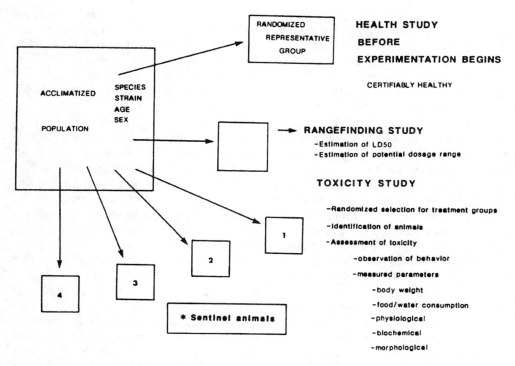

FIGURE 4.3

A diagramatic flow diagram depicting the acquisition of animals (species, strain, sex, age) for longer-term studies and the procedures for determining (1) the health status of the population purchased, (2) the estimation of the dosage range to be used either from the LD_{50} value or a short-term (1- or 2-week) repeated exposure experiment to ascertain toxicity, (3) the randomization of the remaining acclimatized animals into treatment (control, low, intermediate, and high dose) subgroups, and (4) the establishment of a sufficient number of sentinel animals within the facility to monitor the general health of those in experiments.

the stress of transporting the animals from the breeders, the changes in food and water, and the climatic differences in the animal holding facility may unmask such infections. Most assuredly, the stress of treatment and/or the test agent itself can have this effect. The overall, general good health of the experimental animals must be certified.

Adequate numbers of animals, plus "spares", should be purchased or captured prior to initiating a study and should be housed for a suitable time period (1 to 3 weeks) in the animal care facility to allow for acclimatization to the new surroundings (Figure 4.3). During this time period, a subgroup of male and female animals should be selected at random for a thorough health examination, obtaining blood, urine, and fecal samples for appropriate analyses and euthanizing suitable numbers for necropsy and a complete gross and microscopic study of organs and tissues. The results of this preliminary investigation will both determine the health status of the purchased animals and provide a set of baseline values for physiological, biochemical, and morphological endpoints to be studied later, during the treatment and posttreatment period. A second, randomized subgroup of animals will be selected for a rangefinding study to either ascertain what the approximate LD_{50} is (as discussed in Chapter 3) or to select an appropriate range of dosages for the longer studies as discussed above. In the latter situation, some selected animals might be subdivided into small subgroups and receive the test agent by an appropriate route of administration for a period of a week or two to gauge the suitability of the selected dosage range, specific "yardsticks" or endpoints of toxicity being examined in addition to routine hematology, serum biochemistry, urinalysis, and pharmacokinetics/biotransformation studies. This preliminary study also gives the investigator the opportunity to test all of the analytical procedures and modify/correct any methods before the results become crucial.

Having ascertained that the animals are healthy and that they have appeared to tolerate a brief period of repeated exposure to the test agent without serious adverse effects being observed, the experiment can begin (Figure 4.3). Using some predetermined method of randomization (roll of a die, matching rats and groups by selecting a numbered piece of paper from a box, etc.), the animals should be assigned to one or other of the control or treatment groups, assigned to cages (housed singly or in groups of four or five animals to a shoe box cage), and marked in some suitable manner (ear notching, tail marking with a pen, etc.) for the identification of each individual throughout the study period. Since the animals committed to the study will, most likely, be housed together in the same room, attention should be drawn to a potential confounding factor. The position of the cages of the control, low, intermediate, and high dose animals on the racks should be randomized and should be rotated each week in order to minimize between-cage contamination by dusty, test agent-treated powdered food and volatile materials emanating from the food, urine, feces, and/or exhaled air. In contrast, the treatment groups could be subdivided by dosage, each set of cages being housed under laminar-flow hoods. In either situation, **sentinel animals** should be included in the study, these not being a part of the study but residing in the room to monitor the appearance of latent bacterial or viral infections, test agent-related toxicity due to contamination of the facility, etc. Such animals would be subjected to periodic examination, the measurement of hematology and blood chemistry, urinalysis, and bacteriology/virology.

C. Parameters Measured During Studies

An important aspect of any subchronic or chronic study is the daily observation and handling of all animals committed to the study. Subtle between-group differences in appearance (absence of grooming, discolored fur, overall cleanliness), in social behavior (surliness, disinterest, loss of inquisitiveness), in irritability (fighting, barbering, or pulling out fur in patches), and in lack of interest in food, water, and surroundings, etc., may be noted. These signs might not be important if observed independently but, if taken together, may indicate malaise or covert toxicity long before overt signs are seen. In addition to close observation of each animal, investigators rely upon a number of biological indicators of general health. Germane to any extensive study are the parameters or biological endpoints to be measured at each time interval selected for the euthanasia of representative subgroups of the treated animal populations, as well as any moribund animals. The selection of specific biochemical, physiological, and morphological parameters is designed not only to detect target organ toxicity but also to detect pretoxic changes that might predict impending toxicity. A flow diagram, part of the initial planning phase of the experiment, should be prepared (Figure 4.4). The following describes, in general, a spectrum of "biomarkers" used in subchronic and chronic studies.

One measurement, of particular use in extended chronic studies, is the survival time of the control and toxicant-treated animals, presenting the data in a plot of

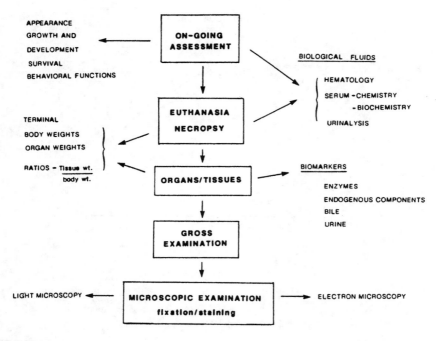

FIGURE 4.4

A flow chart indicating the various physical, physiological/biochemical, behavioral, functional, and morphological "endpoints" of toxicity to be monitored during the ongoing subchronic and chronic toxicity studies, as well as those measured following euthanasia and necropsy. The routine periodic assessment of a chosen selection of such parameters may detect the onset of impending toxicity, proving invaluable for the monitoring of developing lesions and as predictors of target organ toxicity.

percent survival time against time (Borzelleca et al., 1989) (Figure 4.5). From the results of this chronic/carcinogenicity study, one can see that after 104 weeks (2 years), even the control animals begin to die from various causes and it becomes important to ascertain whether or not there is an agent-related, dose-dependent change in the rate(s) of death over that seen in the control animals. As can be seen, little mortality occurs in the first year of a 2-year study, but loss accelerates during the second year presumably due to "natural" causes as well as to agent-related toxicity. The results in this figure demonstrate another frequently observed phenomenon: a slightly better, though perhaps statistically nonsignificant, survival rate in the low-dose treated group than in the control group. It is almost as if a little bit of the toxicant is good for the animal, possibly causing a slight reduction in dietary intake, improving organ function by stimulating the induction of xenobiotic–biotransforming enzymes, and increasing the efficiency of excretory mechanisms. A strategic question must be answered when designing chronic studies, i.e., does one carry on past 104 weeks of treatment, allowing the animals to go "to death" or not? The simple answer to the question is "no" because the entire biochemical, physiological, and morphological picture arising from exposure to the toxicant will be obscured by the normal geriatric changes in the tissues and organs of these aging animals (Grice, 1984). More will be said about this when discussing carcinogenicity.

While it is always a temptation to use highly sophisticated methods of assessing endpoints of toxicity, one of the simplest and perhaps most revealing endpoints is the body weight of the animal, measured every 2 or 3 d (twice weekly) throughout the duration of the study. Regardless of the route of administration, if the toxicant

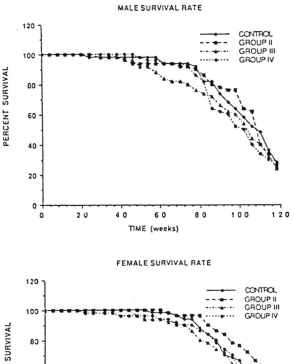

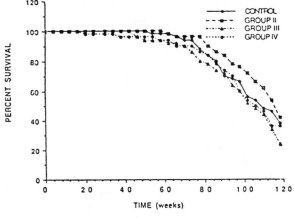

FIGURE 4.5
Treatment-group percent survival rates for male and female Sprague-Dawley rats in a chronic feeding study of F.D. and C red #40 (Allura Red) at dietary levels of 0% (control), 0.37% (group II), 1.39% (group III), or 5.19% (group IV) *in utero* and throughout their lifetimes. Few deaths were observed in the first 52 weeks of treatment, but toxicant-, age-, and other disease-related mortality occurred in the second year, accelerating with age in both sexes. (From Borzelleca et al. *Food Chem. Toxicol.* 27: 701–705 [1989]. With permission.)

is exerting some as yet unidentified biological effect and the animal does not feel well, it will not eat sufficient food and/or drink the usual amount of water (Figure 4.6). A dose-dependent change in body weight will be observed and can be compared with the body weights of the control and the sentinel animals. Such a response is particularly evident in small laboratory or wild animals having high basal metabolic rates dependent upon an adequate daily food intake and may be observed quite early in the study. As is shown in Figure 4.6, a decline in growth and development is observed in the high-dose, treated rats at approximately 20 weeks following the start of the feeding experiment. However, it should be appreciated that such a response may be related either to agent-induced toxicity or an unpleasant taste of the toxicant in the food (or in water if administered via that route) which

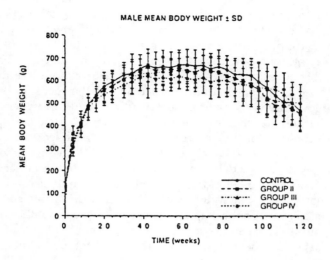

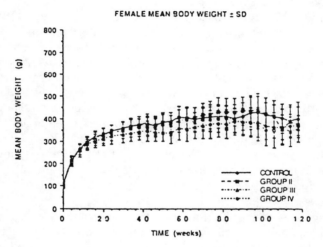

FIGURE 4.6

Treatment-group mean body weights for male and female Sprague-Dawley rats during a chronic feeding study of F.D. & C Red #40 (Allura Red) at dietary levels of 0% (controls), 0.37% (group II), 1.39% (group III), or 5.19% (group IV) from weaning throughout their lifespan. The marked sex differences in growth between males and females can be seen. Maximum body weights in males occurred at about week 60, whereas in females, rapid development reached a plateau at approximately week 40 but continued slowly throughout the remainder of the study. (From Borzelleca et al. *Food Chem. Toxicol.*, 27: 701–705 [1989]. With permission.)

leads the animals to reduce food (or water) intake at one or more dosage levels. Such a response is a particular problem with agents having low toxicity, this necessitating the incorporation of excessively high levels in the diet in order to elicit toxicity. The observed signs and symptoms may be related to nutrient deficiency, not to the test agent. The cause of weight loss may be ascertained by measuring the amount of food (or water) consumed daily by a few animals selected from the control and treated groups.

Such an observation in one group, frequently the high dosage level, introduces an unwelcome confounding factor into the study that must be addressed. Inadequate nutrition will cause significant biochemical, physiological, and morphological changes that might be inadvertently and incorrectly attributed to the toxicant. The investigator may choose to avoid this sort of problem by gavaging the animals each day with the appropriate amounts of toxicant in a suitable, nontoxic vehicle and providing water and food *ad libitum*. Control animals should be gavaged daily with the vehicle. In this situation, body weight loss at one or more treatment levels can usually be attributed to the toxicant, particularly if the measured food intake is reduced. If the loss in body weight is observed in a study in which the toxicant is added to the diet, the investigator may have no other recourse than pair-feeding, a situation in which some of the control animals will be selected as a new control subgroup to receive the same weight of diet (untreated) or food allowance as that consumed daily by the affected, toxicant-exposed group. In this situation, the control animals are always 1 or 2 d behind the treated animals in the experiment, since the investigator must know what weight of food to provide to this control subgroup. This food-restricted control subgroup will be carried throughout the study, providing samples of biological fluids and tissues for comparison with those of the high-dose, affected animals. Such a phenomenon is another good reason to initiate a study with sufficient numbers of control animals.

A third simple measurement, carried out with all moribund animals euthanized *in extremis* and with those euthanized at each study interval, is to weigh the animals and, at necropsy, to weigh the major organs dissected free of adhering tissue and kept moist prior to weighing. Given the fact that body weights of animals will vary within groups, each organ weight should be related to the body weight of the animal from which it was removed and organ weight/body weight ratios should be determined. Frequently, before any overt toxicity is observed, significant shifts in the normal ratios may be seen. As an example, hepatomegaly (enlarged liver) following treatment with polychlorinated or polybrominated biphenyls will be indicated by a higher liver/body weight ratio while atrophy of the thymus gland in the same animals will be reflected in a reduced thymus/body weight ratio. Physiological changes in the organ can be subsequently confirmed by light microscopic examination of the tissues.

The ongoing assessment of animal behavior, neurological function, hepatic and renal function, etc., can be carried out periodically without the destruction of valuable animals. Small blood samples can be obtained periodically, as well as the terminal samples from animals at specified treatment intervals. Animals can be placed overnight in metabolic cages to collect urine and feces for analysis. A variety of noninvasive techniques have been developed to test neuronal conduction velocities, sensory and motor dysfunction, and cognitive and neurobehavioral deficits (Tilson and Mitchell, 1984; Moser et al., 1988). All can be conducted with minimal trauma to the toxicant-exposed animals. Once again, accidents can happen, emphasizing the need to have extra animals in each group.

In both subchronic and chronic studies, routine clinical examinations should be conducted periodically on control animals to provide a baseline of changes with age and on the treated animals to ascertain whether or not exposure to the toxicant can elicit any agent-related and, more importantly, dose-dependent changes in organ function. While groups of animals (n = 5 or 10) may be selected from control and treated populations at 1- or 3-month intervals to detect whether stages are preliminary to overt toxicity, the samples of biological fluids collected are terminal since the animals have been euthanized. One does not want to miss "events" that might occur between these study intervals, and plans for more routine blood sampling of five or ten animals from each group every 7 or 14 d should be incorporated into the study

TABLE 4.2

Clinical Determinations to be Made During Subchronic and Chronic Studies in Animals

Hematology

Erythrocyte count	Mean corpuscular volume (MCV)
Leukocyte count	Mean corpuscular hemoglobin (MCH)
Differential leukocyte count	Neutrophils
Hemoglobin	Lymphocytes
Hematocrit	Eosinophils
Platelet count	Basophils
Reticulocyte count	Monocytes
Packed cell volume	Thrombocytes
	White blood cells

Blood Chemistry

Serum bilirubin	Alkaline phosphatase
Blood glucose	Amylase
Blood urea nitrogen	Alanine aminotransferase (ALAT)
Serum cholesterol	Aspartate aminotransferase (ASAT)
Serum creatinine	Lactate dehydrogenase (LDH)
Serum proteins	Sorbitol dehydrogenase (SOD)
Albumin/globulin	Calcium, sodium, and potassium
Serum triglycerides	Phosphorus, inorganic
Serum fatty acids	Chloride
Serum creatine	
Serum cholinesterase	

Urinalysis

Volume	Bile pigments
Color	Hemoglobin
Specific gravity	Calcium, sodium, and potassium
pH	Phosphorus, inorganic
Protein (total)	Precipitates (cells, urates, crystals, casts, bacteria) examined by microscope
Glucose	
Ketones	
Nitrate	

design. These animals will not be euthanized; small blood samples will be obtained by venapuncture while urine and feces will be collected following confinement in metabolic cages overnight. Routine hematology should be carried out during this ongoing assessment; a standard protocol is shown in Table 4.2. A vast array of blood chemistry tests is available, and care must be taken to select those parameters that may reflect certain types of target organ toxicity rather than using a broad spectrum of analyses on the chance that "something" will be changed. A list of potential clinical tests is given in Table 4.2. It has long been recognized that a correlation exists between such biochemical parameters as AST, ALT, SDH, etc., and morphological changes in hepatic tissue (Buttar et al., 1976; Clampitt, 1978; Tyson et al., 1985). Most of the enzymatic parameters are not tissue-specific but are found at highest levels in the hepatic cytoplasm (SDH) or in the cytoplasm and mitochondrial fractions (AST, ALT) (Mitoma, 1985). Normally, only low levels of such enzymes would be detected in the blood plasma, but with toxicant-induced damage to the integrity of hepatocyte membranes, the cytoplasm leaks into the bloodstream carrying these enzymes with it and resulting in sharp 5- to 10-fold elevations of activity within a few hours of chemical insult. An example where such enzymatic endpoints have been used to monitor the severity of hepatocellular injury can be seen in Borzelleca et al. (1990). While the analysis of blood plasma levels of various enzymes considered to be unique to other organs has been used to identify other target organ toxicity, this has been less successful than for the liver. Invariably, the levels of activity found in these other tissues are low. Second, the liver is frequently affected by the same toxicant, releasing such quantities of enzymes as to mask the contribution by other toxicant-damaged organs. Whatever species is being used in the assessment of target organ toxicity, adequate numbers of control animals must be included in order to determine baseline levels and interanimal variabilities in the biochemical parameters selected as indicators of toxicity.

Detailed analysis of the urine may provide evidence of toxicant-induced changes in intermediary metabolism as well as target organ toxicity. Considerable information can be obtained from measurement of the normal (or abnormal) amounts of endogenous body constituents appearing in the urine as well as the excretion of the toxicant and/or biotransformation products. Enzymes released into the urine as a consequence of toxicant-induced nephrotoxicity may provide essential information concerning the target site(s) involved (Wright and Plummer, 1974; Stroo and Hook, 1977).

Detailed, specific information on target organ toxicity can be obtained from fresh tissues removed at necropsy and from the measurement of various biochemical parameters including nucleic acids, phospholipids, phosphatidyl fatty acids, peroxidation of lipids, protein, glutathione, and a vast array of enzymes localized in such subcellular organelles as the mitochondria, and from the cytoplasm. The number of available parameters is almost unlimited, and it is advisable to carry out an in-depth search of the literature relevant to the particular species being studied in order to select the most appropriate "biomarkers" indicative of cellular and subcellular changes in target organ toxicity.

The key to any adequate subchronic or chronic study rests on the extent, diligence, and accuracy with which tissues and organs of treated and control animals are examined for morphological changes. At necropsy, gross pathological examination of all major organs should take place, weighing each entire organ and commenting on the visible condition. Tissue samples from most body organs will be obtained and fixed in buffered formalin or other preservative solutions for eventual mounting in plastic or paraffin blocks, cutting by microtome with subsequent mounting on glass slides, staining with hematoxylin and eosin (or other more selective staining dyes), and examination under a light microscope. Concomitant with the above, samples may be prepared for examination by electron microscopy. Lists of tissues routinely removed from euthanized animals vary considerably, and one such list is shown in Table 4.3. Other lists can be found in Zbinden (1976) and Kamrin (1989). Because of the almost limitless possibilities of tissues collected from control and three treatment groups (males and females in each) and a possible range of effects from minimal to striking changes, some priorization must occur if the pathologist is ever to complete the assessment of tissue damage. First-priority organs — including liver, kidney, adrenals, heart, spleen, thymus, testis, epididymis, lung, bone marrow, mesenteric lymph node, and all organs showing gross changes in shape, weight, color or structure — will be examined from all animals including controls. Second-priority tissues from the high-dose animals and some of the controls will be examined, those of the medium- and low-dose groups being studied if significant changes are observed in the high-dose group. A third priority — extensive collection of

TABLE 4.3

Organs and Tissues to be Examined Following Necropsy During Subchronic
and Chronic Animal Studies

Aorta	Urinary bladder	Brain
Myocardium	Testis/ovary	Spinal cord
Larynx	Epididymis/uterus	Eye
Trachea	Prostate/vagina	Harderian gland
Lung	Seminal vesicles	Peripheral nerves
Liver	Mammary tissue	Skin
Pancreas	Salivary gland	Striated muscle
Spleen	Tongue	_M. longissimus dorsi_
Kidney	Esophagus	_M. gastrocnemius_
Adrenal	Pituitary	Site of injection (if agent is
Stomach (glandular and nonglandular regions)	Thyroid	administered via this route)
Jejunum	Thymus	
Ileum		
Cecum		
Colon		
Rectum		

tissues — will not be examined routinely unless clinical observations merit this or
there is some motivation by scientific interests (Zbinden, 1976). However, they will
be preserved and retained in fixative for future reference.

A colleague of mine presented an analog in which he said that looking for tissue
lesions in a chronic study was like driving through a snowstorm with your headlights
on and attempting to focus on individual snowflakes while ignoring the remainder.
There are so many changes occurring normally in the animals that it is frequently
difficult to spot the subtle, abnormal, agent-induced changes. The purpose of the
detailed morphological examination of moribund animals and those at preselected
study intervals is simply to detect effects, physiological or pathological, which are
manifested as differences between control and treated groups and between high-
and low-dose groups. Macroscopic findings are extremely important and should be
communicated to the pathologist in order to make any histopathological evaluation
meaningful. This is particularly important if all that the pathologist sees is the fixed
and stained tissue slides. It will save considerable time and effort on his part to be
able to focus on the nature of the target organ toxicity. The pathologist should not
be kept completely "blind" to the results of the experiment! An excellent summary
of the experimental design around the role of the pathologist has been presented by
Roe (1981). The pathologist will likely begin with control and high-dose animal
tissues, scanning quickly to get the "feel of the toxicant-induced situation," and
subsequently return for a more detailed documentation of the observed differences.
The severity or prominence of the changes will lead the pathologist to examine the
slides for the intermediate- and low-dose animals. Given the facts that (1) some 400
animals may be involved, (2) approximately 40 tissues are subjected to microscopic
examination, (3) several different lesions may be identified, and (4) there may be a
gradation in severity of the effect over the dosage range administered; the number
of histopathological data points may be of the order of 200,000. This will necessitate
detailed record keeping amenable to statistical analysis. Roe (1981) has prepared a
data-keeping system that can be computerized for easy access and analysis
(Table 4.4). A more detailed presentation of an interactive-integrated data system for
toxicological studies has been described by Arnold et al. (1990).

TABLE 4.4

System for the Recording of Morphological Information from Subchronic and Chronic Animal
Studies

---

1. Report findings in a series of tables, each line of which represents one animal.
2. Organs and tissues are examined in logical order from a series of sections presented to the pathologist in that same order.
3. For each tissue, each column used for a parameter becomes an obligatory parameter for all animals of the same sex in the study.
4. Unusual findings are recorded separately.
5. Meaningful abbreviations are used as headings for parameter columns and for describing unusual findings.
6. A glossary of all abbreviations used should be provided as well as a list of criteria for the diagnosis of all grades of all lesions.
7. The tables are designed so that the data can be "fed" directly into a computer having the capacity and the ability to prepare summary tables, analyze data statistically, and print out full histopathological reports for all organs of all animals.
8. The unusual findings can be (a) tabulated in the computer data base, to appear in the printed-out histopathological reports under one column, or (b) simply bound into the study report separately.
9. A two-letter code is used to describe tissues.
10. Sizes of lesions are recorded, where appropriate, as mean diameters (in mm).
11. Numbers of lesions are recorded up to an arbitrary maximum. Appropriate severity is recorded using a 6-point scale (0, 1, 2, 3, 4, or 5), the highest being the most severe.

Data from Roe (1981).

D. Duration of Studies

As was stated previously, subchronic studies are generally 21 to 90 d in duration, depending upon the route of administration and toxicological endpoints of interest. However, the duration of chronic studies has been a controversial issue for many years. Originally, chronic studies, regardless of the species used, were of 2 years' duration, this time interval being based on the approximate life span of a rodent (mouse, rat). More recently, several regulatory agencies have reduced the duration of a chronic study to 18 months and, currently, to 6 to 12 months for rodents. Chronic studies in nonrodents are of 1-year duration. No doubt, this controversy will continue in the scientific literature and within and between national regulatory agencies (Frederick, 1985; Lumley and Walker, 1985, 1986; Auletta, 1995).

Scientific arguments have been presented to suggest that there is no need to carry out 2-year studies, because documented toxicity observed in the second year is not different from that produced in the first year with the selection of an appropriate range of doses to simulate a lifetime exposure. Since one usually begins a chronic study with healthy, young, post-weanling rodents of 5 to 6 weeks of age, there should be little "natural" mortality in the first year (Figure 4.5); any incidence occurring should be agent-related and possibly even dose-dependent. However, a 1-year study in mice or rats requires a range of doses that would be equivalent to what the animals might consume or be exposed to over a lifetime, i.e., approximately 2 years. As was discussed in Chapter 2, the amount of toxicant administered may lead to complications with the inability of the animals to efficiently biotransform and eliminate the elevated dosages given to simulate a lifetime exposure in the shortened period of time. In addition, the ability of an animal to "cope" with any given toxicant decreases with age, and the dosages administered to the young, healthy animal may elicit toxicity at a later age. In any animal species, including the human, adverse health effects begin to appear in the older individuals, be they natural geriatric changes or toxicant-related target-organ toxicity. If one is attempting to assess the potential toxicity of "lifetime exposure," surely the effects of the agent during pre-geriatric and geriatric periods of the animals' life should not be ignored. In the case of chronic rodent studies, should the study start with 6-week-old animals and terminate at 52 weeks, or should it begin with animals of 6 months of age and end at 18 months of age? The conduction of lifetime exposure studies in dogs or primates would not be practical due to the time period involved and the associated astronomical costs of the order of several millions of dollars. The few such studies that have been attempted have been unsatisfactory, with adverse health effects and mortality occurring generally from infections and diseases seemingly unrelated to the toxicant. Currently, studies in nonrodent species of 1 or 2 years' duration are considered acceptable. This controversy will continue in the literature, and it is sufficient to draw the reader's attention to the pitfalls and to what constitutes a normal life-span for the particular species being used as an animal model. "Lifetime" may be as little as a few hours or days, a few weeks or months or, in the case of the human, three score plus ten years (and a little bit more).

What has been the experience of investigators making comparisons between the results of short- and long-term studies for the same chemicals? Using the NOEL and the minimum effect level (MEL) as indices in subacute (2 to 4 wk) and subchronic (13 to 18 wk) studies in rats, a comparison of 82 chemicals tested revealed that the NOEL values in each test were comparable for 56% of the compounds while, for 44%, the NOEL for the subchronic test was lower than that for the subacute test (Woutersen et al., 1984). These results indicate clearly that the subacute test cannot simply replace a subchronic test. However, the shorter term studies, relatively low in cost, might be sufficient for the initial registration and estimation of human exposure, particularly when such nonregulated agents might be the subject of investigation for several years. Reliable information can be obtained from the subacute studies if selected hematological and biochemical parameters are included along with body weight, food intake, and histopathology of the livers and kidneys (Wautersen et al., 1984).

Can subchronic studies replace chronic studies? A retrospective evaluation of the toxicity results for 117 pharmaceutical compounds in subchronic (90 d) and chronic (24 month) studies in dogs revealed that little new qualitative toxicity data was obtained which was not seen in the shorter study or in short- and long-term studies in rats (Parkinson et al., 1995). Animal toxicity studies of longer than 6 months duration are not required except those investigating carcinogenesis. This finding confirmed that of an earlier study (Lumley and Walker, 1985). A similar finding was reported in a Japanese study of 90 pharmaceutical products (Igarashi, 1993). However, a Canadian study supported the current national guidelines' requirement for the duration of final long-term toxicological tests of drugs being at least 18 months (Frederick, 1986). This position created considerable controversy (Emmerson, 1987; Frederick, 1987). Newer guidelines in Europe and Japan recommend 6-month studies in rodents and dogs in conjunction with applications for marketing authorization for new drugs. The U.S. FDA still requires 12-month studies in nonrodent species for drugs to be used chronically in the human. Such requirements may be changed in the future, given the impetus to harmonize national regulatory guidelines, both within and between countries. Canada's position on chronic studies has changed to a 12-month duration.

E. Reversibility of Toxicity

In the original design of the longer-term studies (Figure 4.2), adequate numbers of animals were included so that, at the termination of the treatment period, sufficient subjects would remain to study the reversibility of lesions and recovery from the toxicity elicited by the various doses of the test agent. Questions to be answered include whether or not the toxicant-induced lesions are permanent and continue to progress, with deterioration of the animals' health, or if, with time, the effects disappear and less impaired or even normal function is regained. Over a posttreatment period of 1 to 3 months, representative subgroups of these "survivors" would be selected at random for ongoing hematological and clinical chemistry evaluation and for eventual euthanasia and necropsy at selected intervals with subsequent complete biochemical, physiological, and morphological examination. The answers on the ability of the animals to recover from the insult of the toxicant are well worth the time and effort of extending the study by 3 months.

III. EVALUATION OF RESULTS

The aims of the subchronic and chronic studies are (1) to ascertain the biological effects of repeated administration of the test agent on potential target organs of the body at dosages that do not elicit acute toxicity, (2) to establish a dose-effect relationship between biochemical, physiological, and morphological effects over the dosage range and the duration of administration (or exposure) of the agent, (3) to ascertain the maximum dosage level that produces no discernible ill effects following repeated exposure, and (4) to explore the possible mechanism(s) by which the toxicant elicits its effect(s). A series of dose-relationships may be generated, as is shown in the theoretical plots in Figure 4.7, for a number of different endpoints of toxicity at each chosen study interval. A series of sigmoidal curves or linear plots may be generated, each having a different slope. In this manner, given specific endpoints and estimating the total dosage (mg/kg/day) multiplied by the number of days of treatment, the appearance and early detection of functional and morphological changes in organs may be documented and the appearance of lesions may be observed. However, it must be emphasized that these relationships are based on different groups of animals being used at each study interval. Hopefully, these subgroups are representative of the larger group(s) being treated. Having carried out such a detailed stage-by-stage analysis of the experimental results, what values can be measured in terms of the dosages administered?

If an appropriate range of low, intermediate, and high doses has been arbitrarily chosen, several values may be determined although it is impossible that every parameter will be available (Figure 4.8). Since, by experimental design, the highest dosage should elicit toxicity, at least one treatment level should produce frank (overt) effects, the **Frank Effect Level** (FEL) (Dourson, 1986). One somewhat lower dosage should produce some evidence of mild adverse health effects, this dosage being labeled the **lowest observed adverse effect level** (LOAEL). A still lower dosage may cause some minor biological changes but no effects associated with the target-organ toxicity observed at higher levels of treatment; this dosage is defined as the **lowest observed effect level** (LOEL). It is entirely possible that the measured biological effect(s) drop off too rapidly as one reaches the lower dosage levels and that either **no observable adverse effects** will be seen — this level of treatment being the NOAEL value — or no observable effects will be seen at all, providing the **no**

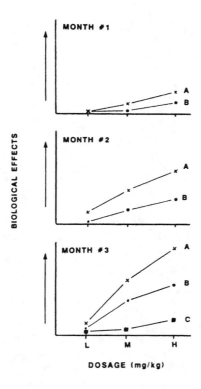

FIGURE 4.7

A theoretical graphic representation of the time- and dose-related development of three toxicologically significant effects (A, B, C) at treatment levels of low (L), medium (M), and high (H) over a 3-month period of a subchronic study. For parameters A and B, the effects were detected early in the study and the severity increased with "total dose" (dosage level × time), whereas with parameter C, no effect was detected until 3 months into the study and then only at the highest level.

observable effect level (NOEL). As will be seen in a later chapter, it is very important to either obtain this latter value from the actual study or to be able to derive a good estimate of it from study results.

What is the difference between the NOEL and NOAEL? The NOEL is defined as "... that level of a substance administered to a group of experimental animals at which those effects observed at higher levels are absent and no other significant differences between the exposed animals and the unexposed control group are observed. The effects observed need not be severely toxic or even adverse." (Study Group, 1979). Other definitions of the NOEL state that it is "... the *maximum* dosage level that has not induced any sign(s) of toxicity in the *most susceptible species* of animal tested using the *most sensitive indicator(s)* of toxicity" (Lu, 1985). In contrast, the NOAEL is the level of substance administered at which those effects observed at higher levels are absent, but some toxicant-related biological effects are still detectable. The utility of these values will be explored in Chapter 7.

IV. CARCINOGENICITY STUDIES

A simple definition of cancer is that it is a disease characterized by the proliferation of abnormal body cells and by the spread of these cells to other tissues by invasion or metastasis (Roe, 1993). Cancer is one of the most feared words in any

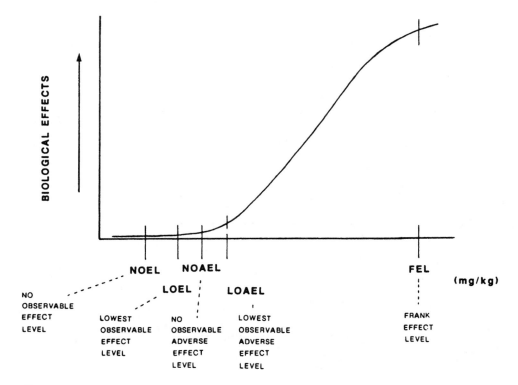

FIGURE 4.8

A dose-effect relationship and the development of dosage-related indices based on the detection or absence of toxicant-related adverse health effects or other nontoxic changes. Generally based on the results of chronic or lifetime exposure to the agent, the values constitute a single, constant daily intake rate that is low enough to produce no observable adverse effects (NOAEL), lowest observable effects (LOEL), i.e., decrement in body weight and no observable effects (NOEL). Such values are used in risk assessment practices.

language and a major concern of the public is that chemicals (natural or synthetic) to which they are exposed daily in the workplace, in the home, and as components in their lifestyles can cause cancer. Despite certain lines of evidence pointing out that, with the exception of lung cancer, cancer incidence at other sites in the body has remained the same or is in decline, the controversy rages on with other reports seemingly at odds with this evidence (Davis et al., 1990; Marshall, 1990; Cahow, 1995). The situation has made it mandatory that manufacturers of industrial chemicals, pharmaceuticals, agrichemicals including pesticides, etc., must demonstrate that their chemicals are noncarcinogenic. While some rapid *in vitro* and short-term *in vivo* bioassays (Chapter 6) can provide evidence that the agents are not carcinogenic, sooner or later the chemical must either be abandoned on the basis of this evidence or undergo a full-scale assessment on at least two suitable animal models. The mouse and the rat are the species of choice because of ready availability, cost, size, ease of handling and housing, short lifespan, and the presence of a solid base of background information on both the "natural" incidence of type- and site-specific carcinogenesis in the two species and various strains and their responses to other carcinogens. Only rarely are other, larger species (i.e., dog, monkey) used, the cost, size, numbers needed, and the required long duration of exposure (7 to 10 years) all being factors against their use in standard protocols.

TABLE 4.5

Operational Definition of a Carcinogen

An agent having the ability to induce tumors as evidenced by:

1. An increased *incidence* of tumor types found in controls
2. The occurrence of tumors *earlier* than in controls
3. The development of tumor types *not seen* in controls
4. An increased *multiplicity* of tumors in individual animals

Note: See Interdisciplinary Panel on Carcinogenicity (1984).

The operational definition of a carcinogen is given in Table 4.5. A carcinogen is any agent that increases the frequency of tumors, causes an earlier appearance of tumors, introduces new types of tumors not seen in controls, or causes a multiplicity of neoplasms at different body sites, all these being compared with the same parameters measured in untreated animals maintained under identical conditions except for exposure to the test agent (Interdisciplinary Panel on Carcinogenicity, 1984). Carcinogenicity may be defined as the "enhancement of age-standardized incidence of malignant neoplasia" (Roe, 1993). Enhancement of benign tumor (proliferating cells but neither invasive nor capable of metastasizing) incidence does not constitute carcinogenicity although it may — and often does — provide grounds for "suspicion of possible or probable carcinogenicity" (Roe, 1993). In many studies, a combination of benign and malignant neoplasms will be considered as constituting sufficient evidence of carcinogenic potential.

In past years, a major endpoint in chronic toxicity studies concerned the incidence of tumors found in the treated animals. However, with the duration of chronic toxicity studies being reduced to 12 months or less, there is little likelihood of seeing any extensive tumorigenicity associated with the chemical except in cases where particularly potent agents are tested. Therefore, carcinogenicity studies must be carried out over a longer time period — traditionally to 18 months in mice and 24 months in rats -in order to be certain that the time interval of exposure is of a length such that the chemical would be certain to induce carcinogenicity if it was capable of doing so. Figure 4.9 depicts a schematic diagram of a standard 24-month mammalian carcinogenicity bioassay.

Originally, these long-term bioassays were designed for the qualitative identification of potential human carcinogens to identify which agents required more extensive study for quantitative risk assessment (Fung et al., 1995). However, the qualitative data are usually used for quantitative risk assessments, and additional in-depth studies are never carried out because of time, cost, and the urgency to test too many new agents. Thus, quite by accident, this qualitative bioassay has become a quantitative one and has given rise to the criticism that this assay identified too many "rodent carcinogens" (Ames and Gold, 1990). The concordance of target organs between the animal surrogates and humans, for those agents identified as carcinogenic in the latter, is discussed by Fung et al. (1995). However, the statement above about the qualitative nature of the carcinogenicity assay must be kept in mind considering the viewpoint of the International Agency for Research on Cancer (IARC) that "in the absence of adequate data in humans, it is biologically plausible and prudent to regard agents and mixtures for which there is sufficient evidence of carcinogenicity in experimental animals as if they presented a carcinogenic risk to humans."

A signal feature of the animal carcinogenicity assay is the singular endpoint of toxicity — cancer, whatever the type and site of origin. Therefore, in contrast to the

CARCINOGENICITY STUDY

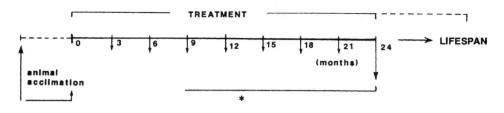

FIGURE 4.9
The planning strategy for a carcinogenicity study (24-month) showing the duration of treatment and the intervals when representative subgroups of the toxicant-exposed populations of animals would be euthanized and studied morphologically for the appearance and progression of tumors (frequency, site, and type). Animals surviving to 24 months may be euthanized at that time or may be allowed to live out their lifespan either with or without continued exposure to the test substance.

detailed biochemical, physiological, and morphological assessment that accompanies a chronic toxicity test, the efforts of the carcinogenicity test are somewhat limited, with more attention being focused on the morphological examination of body tissues to determine the number of various types of tumors (both benign and malignant), the number of tumor-bearing animals, the number of tumors in each animal, and the onset of tumors whenever determined. Throughout the study, the survival, the body weight as an indicator of growth and development, weekly examination for "lumps and bumps," and signs of toxicity will be recorded, but in the interest of carrying animals in the study as long as possible, few routine blood chemistry tests, urinalysis, etc., will be done, except for periodic hematological assessment. All dead, and moribund animals will be subjected to a gross autopsy with all major organs, lymph nodes, etc., being examined carefully. Evidence of abnormalities will result in tissue samples of the region being taken for preparation and microscopic examination. The study may be designed to include a randomized selection of representative animals from each treatment group for euthanasia and extensive biochemical, physiological, and morphological study. Those surviving to the end of the treatment period will be euthanized for extensive study. As described under the design for chronic studies, animals in a carcinogenicity study should not be allowed to go "until death" after the 104-week period. Tumorigenicity increases sharply in older animals and the agent- and dose-related carcinogenicity will become confused with natural tumor formation.

An example of an interesting variant of the usual carcinogenicity study is shown in Figure 4.10 (Lijinsky et al., 1982). Two important environmental carcinogens — nitroso-1,2,3,6-tetrahydropyridine (NTHP) and dinitrosohomopiperazine (DNHP) — were administered in the drinking water of female F344 rats for different periods of time at different levels and were then followed either to death or to when they became moribund. The plots are Kaplan-Meier survival curves (Kaplan and Meier, 1958). Note that, at high concentrations, both agents were highly toxic, an almost complete loss of these groups occurring before the end of 1 year. The survivability of the untreated control group and of at least four NTHP low-dose groups were comparable out to 130 weeks. However, the survivability of the various DNHP-treated groups was spread throughout the study period. It is important to note the manner in which the exposure was estimated, i.e., as the total dose (in milligrams) of agent acquired during the study period. This format of dosage presentation is found in other studies (Morgan et al., 1989).

Numbers of animals, the dosage range, and the duration of the study are important considerations in carcinogenicity testing. Generally, regulatory agencies require a minimum of 50 animals of each sex per treatment group. The upper dose should be the maximum tolerated dose (MTD, the maximum amount of agent that can be administered without adversely affecting the animal due to toxicity other than carcinogenicity), with two arbitrarily chosen lower doses, say 25% and 5% of the MTD. Controversy has arisen over the MTD, the problem being that for compounds of low toxicity, very large doses having little relevance to human exposure may be required, the results being clouded when the agent acts by some nongenotoxic mechanism. The duration of carcinogenic studies vary with regulatory agencies. European (EEC) guidelines specify a minimal duration of 18 months for mice and 24 months for rats, while those of the U.S. and the OECD require study for at least 18 to 24 months in mice and 24 to 30 months in rats, or for the lifespan of the species if there is a high survival rate.

It is worth examining one of the more famous large-scale studies of carcinogenicity which set out to answer the question: "Given a known carcinogen selected by well-defined criteria, can the ED_{001} be accurately described for that agent?" Prior to starting the study, it was scaled back to the ED_{01} since the required 80,000 animals could not be accomodated and the cost was prohibitive. I refer to the study of the ED_{01} of 2-acetylaminofluorene (2-AAF), a known hepatocarcinogen, in female BALB/cStCrfl C3H/Nctr mice, more commonly but incorrectly referred to as the "megamouse" study (Staffa and Mehlman, 1980). This strain of mouse has a low background tumor incidence and lives for a long time. The study took 18 months to plan and 9 months to produce and allocate the 24,192 mice to treatment groups (0, 30, 35, 60, 75, 100, and 150 ppm 2-AAF in the diet for 15 months). Animals were euthanized for study at 9, 12, 14, 15, 16, 17, 18, 24, and 33 months. It took close to 4 years to conduct and evaluate at a cost of approximately 7×10^6. The test substance induced hepatocellular carcinomas in an almost linear, dose-dependent manner, their late appearance occurring only after 18 months, with no tendency for a threshold level. The conclusions and predictions for this study in relation to other, more limited (both animal numbers, dose levels, and cost) carcinogenicity studies are worth reading (Gaylor, 1980). The bottom line is that it will be impossible, with animal bioassays, to study dose-response curves with precision at low levels of tumor incidence!

The present-day exorbitant costs associated with carrying out independent chronic toxicity and carcinogenicity studies has led to a blending of these studies together. In addition to the range of doses used in the chronic study, at least three additional doses, the highest being the MTD or a close approximation of it and two lower concentrations will be administered to groups of animals throughout the chronic study and for the subsequent time period of the carcinogenicity study. Sufficient control animals will be incorporated into the design for the second stage assessment of natural tumor incidence in older animals. One positive aspect of the combined study is that the investigator will have surviving animals, from higher doses, in the recovery phase of the chronic study that can be used for tumor assessment when they are euthanized at appropriate intervals. In addition, there will be a better data base on other toxicity endpoints and parameters measured, from a larger group of animals — all from the same population housed and treated alike — than if the carcinogenicity study was completely independent and conducted at a different time.

NTHP

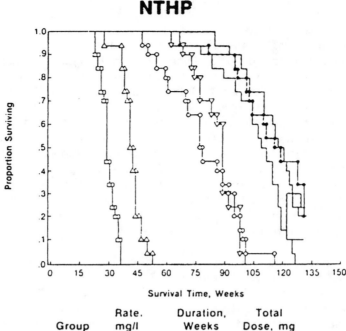

Group		Rate, mg/l	Duration, Weeks	Total Dose, mg
0	●	0	0	0
1	▢	100	25	250
2	△	40	25	100
3	○	16	25	40
4		6.4	25	16
5	▽	6.4	70	45
6		2.6	25	6.5
7		2.6	100	26
8		1.0	25	2.5
9		1.0	100	10

FIGURE 4.10
An interesting variant of a chronic toxicity study in which Kaplan-Meier survival curves are shown for deaths (from all causes) in female F344 rats receiving various concentrations of two carcinogenic nitrosamines, nitroso-1,2,3,6-tetrahydropyridine (NTHP) and dinitrosohomopiperazine (DNHP) in drinking water for various time intervals. Twenty 8-week old animals were assigned to each treatment group, receiving the test agent in drinking water for five consecutive days each week for the prescribed number of weeks after which the animals were kept until natural death or killed when moribund. This technique of plotting adjusts for "censored" observations, those made on relatively few animals in lower dose groups and controls surviving to the end of the study. For NTHP, the data for groups 4 and 6 to 9 lie within the shaded region. NTHP is a hepatic carcinogen while DNHP is a potent esophageal carcinogen. From Lijinsky et al. (1982) with permission.

The complexity and the long duration of carcinogenicity studies presents ample opportunity for confounding factors to influence tumor prevalence within and between experiments, thereby introducing variability in the interpretation of the studies. Haseman et al. (1989) have addressed this issue, stating that the major sources of variability include the animal room environment, strain (genetic) differences, food consumption/weight gain, survival/age of the animals, the identification of gross lesions, pathology sampling procedures, the preparation of the histology slides, and the histopathological diagnosis. Investigators should be aware of these potentially confounding factors and attempt, in the study design, to reduce or eliminate

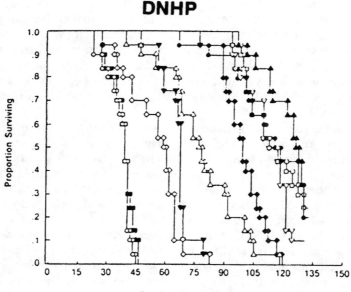

Group		Rate, mg/l	Duration, Weeks	Total Dose, mg
0	●	0	0	0
1	■	110	30	330
2	○	44	30	132
3	◇	18	30	54
4	△	7	30	21
5	▼	7	60	42
6	▽	2.8	30	8.4
7	◆	2.8	120	34
8	□	1.1	30	3.3
9	▲	1.1	120	13

FIGURE 4.10 (continued)

their impact on the interpretation of the results. In keeping with this, the ultimate interpretation of the data should be based on biological judgment and not on the rigid application of statistical decision rules (Haseman, 1990). While analysis of the data may be statistical, the interpretation of the results should not be limited to this method. The investigator should consider such key biological factors as (1) a dose-related effect, (2) if the increased tumor incidence was supported by an increase in related preneoplastic lesions, (3) whether the effect was observed in other sex-species groups, (4) the historical (spontaneous) control rate of the tumor type, (5) the effect being seen in a suspected target organ, (6) the relative survival of dosed and control animals, and (7) the appropriateness of combining tumors from varying sites and histogenesis for evaluation. While statistical decision rules should be applied to experimental evidence, they should not be employed as a substitute for sound scientific judgment in the evaluation.

It would be remiss to finish this chapter and ignore the problems of (1) trends toward more rapid growth and development in various established strains of mice and rats, attaining adult body weights far greater than those measured a decade or more ago; (2) the decreased longevity and increased incidence rates of tumors in untreated animals over the same time period; and (3) the extended longevity and improved health status (reduced neoplasia and degenerative diseases) of animals given a diet restricted to approximately 80% of the normal *ad libitum* daily intake. While these observations are not new, they have raised new concerns about the design and conduction of chronic/carcinogenicity studies, have opened several new avenues of research, and have called into question the interpretation of earlier and current carcinogenicity assays carried out in these strains of rodents. Particularly, I refer the reader to the recently published "Biosure Study" which addresses many of these problems (Roe et al., 1995).

There is solid evidence of "genetic drift" in many inbred strains of mice and rats, the animals having much larger adult body weights than those of a couple of decades ago, being more obese, showing dramatic changes in survival rates and in the pathology of degenerative diseases, as well as marked increases in the incidence rates of various tumors (Haseman et al., 1994; Roe, 1981; Roe et al., 1991; Selikop, 1995; Turnbull et al., 1985). That such changes do not require decades of time is shown in Figure 4.11, comparing body weights for a well-established strain of Spra-gue-Dawley rats (CD-COBS = Caesarian Obtained Banier Sustained) with those of a specific, pathogen-free, variant (CD-COBS-VAF = Virus Antibody Free) introduced only in 1988 (Nohynek et al., 1993). The new variant, particularly the male, is larger throughout the entire growth and development period compared to the older strain. For animals fed *ad libitum*, both individual and group mean body weights in early adult life were predictive for individual and group live expectancy. The VAF-variant showed increased incidences of pituitary tumors (males) and mammary fibroade-nomas (females), increased incidence and severity of glomerulonephritis, and a greater incidence of animals which died without any obvious pathology. The decreased longevity was due to disease and degenerative processes associated with the rapid growth and development (Nohynek et al., 1993). Relationships between body weight gain, reduced longevity, increased nephropathy, and increased neopla-sia have been reported in numerous other studies (Roe et al., 1991,1995; Turnbull et al., 1985; Weindruch, 1989).

Despite the renewed interest in the multiple biological effects of dietary restric-tion in rodent studies in the mid-1980s, such effects were reported in mice as early as 1914 by Peyton Rous (Rous, 1914). Another flurry of reports, linking dietary or caloric restriction with increased survival time and decreased tumor incidence, appeared in the 1930s and 1940s, these studies being summarized and discussed by Pariza (1986). It seems incredible that such important observations could be ignored since caloric restriction appears to be the most effective inhibitor of cancer formation in both mice and rats. However, it has been suggested that, if the freely fed animals had been described as obese instead of the restricted ones being described as small, the phenomenon might have had more impact on modern cancer research (Doll and Peto, 1981).

As much as anything, *ad libitum* feeding arose from the concept that it was "normal" and also that it fitted in with the 5-day work week of investigators, the animals not starving over the weekend if unattended (Roe, 1981). Rodents fed *ad libitum* eat almost continuously since they have nothing more interesting to do, whereas those on restricted diet are usually presented with their daily, reduced ration at one time of the day and are hungry enough to eat it quickly. The effects caused by dietary restriction seem to depend on a complex interaction between energy (calories) utilization (intake/retention) rather than on fat restriction. Studies have shown that animals on a high fat, restricted diet were significantly healthier in all respects than were other groups (Albanes, 1987; Pariza, 1986,1987; Roe, 1981). Various possible mechanisms of the effects of caloric restriction have been presented, including

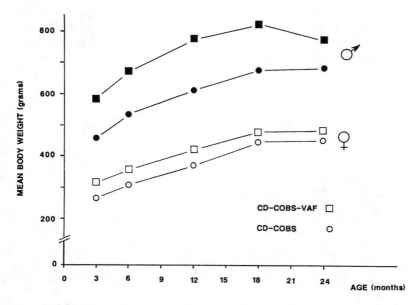

FIGURE 4.11
The growth and development differences observed between an established strain of Sprague-Dawley rat (CD-COBS) and those of a derived variant, the specific virus antibody free strain (CD-COBS-VAF) introduced in 1988. The newer variant is larger throughout development, has a shorter lifespan, an increased incidence and severity of glomerulonephritis, as well as increased incidences of site-specific tumors (Nohynek et al., 1993).

less damage by free radical-reactive, oxygen species; retarded immunosenescence; neuroendocrine changes; altered gene expression; increased protein turnover; or a combination of such cellular activities (Weindruch, 1989). It brings to mind the effect often observed in older, chronic studies where the growth, development, general health, and longevity of the low-dose, treatment group was better than that of the *ad libitum* fed, control animals. A little bit of toxicant appeared to perk up the animals' systems. It has been observed that increased body weight enhanced tumor risk (Haseman et al., 1954; Rao et al., 1987; Roe et al., 1991; Seilkop, 1995). Dietary restriction or caloric reduction (approximately 20%) caused significant decreases in the incidences of tumors at different sites including endocrine tissues (pituitary, pancreatic islets, adrenal cortex and medulla, thyroid follicular, thyroid c-cell) and of hormone-controlled tissues (mammary gland) (Rao et al., 1987; Roe, 1981; Roe et al., 1995; Salmon et al., 1990; Seilkop, 1995). Other parameters causing a reduction in body weights, i.e., exposure to thyroid hormones, low environmental temperature, or high level of physical activity, also caused a reduction in tumor incidences (Albanes, 1987). Housing animals individually or in groups also influenced the outcome of carcinogenicity studies, body weights of the former being higher concomitant with an associated increase in liver tumor incidence (Haseman et al., 1994). Other than animal segregation, other factors such as isolation (single-sex rooms vs. housing in a mixed-sex room), virginal status, or periodic access to virgin females (5 days each alternate week) had only marginal influence on tumor outcomes (Salmon et al., 1990).

Within the past 2 years, large studies have been conducted or initiated to revisit the problems of dietary or caloric restriction and the overall effects on general health, tumor incidence, and longevity (Roe et al., 1995). Hopefully, this time around, the obvious message will not be lost on those involved in the design and conduction of carcinogenicity studies. In contrast to the uncontrolled nature of *ad libitum* feeding, moderate dietary restriction does not adversely affect the animals' health and improves the carcinogenicity bioassay as a model for the evaluation of human safety (Keenan, 1995).

REFERENCES

Albanes, D. Total calories, body weight and tumor incidence in mice. *Cancer Res.* 47: 1987-1992 (1987).

Ames, B.N. and Gold, L.S. Too many rodent carcinogens: mitogenesis increases mutagenesis. *Science* 249: 970-971 (1990).

Arnold, D.L., McGuire, P.F., and Nera, E.A. The conduct of a chronic bioassay and the use of an interactive-integrated toxicology data system. In *Handbook of In Vivo Toxicity Testing.* D.L. Arnold, H.C. Grice, and D.R. Krewski (Eds.). Academic Press, New York (1990), pp. 589-607.

Auletta, C.S. Acute, subchronic and chronic toxicology. In *CRC Handbook of Toxicology,* Derelanko, M.J. and Hollinger, M.A. (Eds.), CRC Press, Boca Raton, FL. (1995), Ch.2, pp. 51-104.

Barnes, J.M. and Denz, F.A. Experimental methods used in determining chronic toxicity. *Pharmacol. Rev.* 6: 191-242 (1954).

Borzelleca, J.F., O'Hara, T.M., Gennings, C., Granger, R.H., Sheppard, M.A., and Condie, L.W. Interaction of water contaminants. I. Plasma enzyme activity and response surface methodology following gavage administration of CCl_4 and $CHCl_3$ or TCE singly and in combination in the rat. *Fundam. Appl. Toxicol.* 14: 477-490 (1990).

Borzelleca, J.F., Olson, J.W., and Reno, F.F. Lifetime toxicity/carcinogenicity study of FD and C Red No. 40 (Allura Red) in Sprague-Dawley rats. *Food Chem. Toxicol.* 27: 701-705 (1989).

Buttar, H.S., Nera, E.A., and Downie, R.H. Serum enzyme activities and hepatic triglyceride levels in acute and subacute acetaminophen-treated rats. *Toxicology* 6: 9-20 (1976).

Cahow, K. The cancer conundrum. *Environ. Health Perspect.* 103: 998-1004 (1995)

Clampitt, R.B. The tissue activities of some diagnostic enzymes in ten mammalian species. *J. Comp. Pathol.* 88: 607-621 (1978).

Davis, D.L., Hoel, D., Fox, J., and Lopez, A. International trends in cancer mortality in France, West Germany, Italy, Japan, England and Wales and the U.S.A. *Lancet* 336: 474-481 (1990).

Doll, R. and Peto, R. The causes of cancer: Quantitative estimates of avoidable risks in the United States today. *J. Natl. Cancer Inst.* 66: 1191-1308 (1981)

Dourson, M.L. New approaches in the derivation of acceptable daily intake (ADI). *Comments on Toxicol.* 1: 35-48 (1986).

Emmerson, J.L. Letter to Editor. *Fundam. Appl. Toxicol.* 8: 134 (1987).

Frederick, G.L. Letter to Editor: Reply. *Fundam. Appl. Toxicol.* 8: 135-138 (1987).

Frederick, G.L. The necessary minimal duration of final long-term toxicologic tests of drugs. *Fundam. Appl. Toxicol.* 6: 385-394 (1985).

Fung, V.A., Barrett, J.C., and Huff, J. The carcinogenesis bioassay in perspective: application in identifying human cancer hazards. *Environ. Health Perspect.* 103: 680-683 (1995).

Gaylor, D.W. The ED_{01} study: summary and conclusions. *J. Environ. Pathol. Toxicol.* 3: 179-183 (1980).

Grice, H.C. *Current Issues in Toxicology. The Selection of Doses in Chronic Toxicity/Carcinogenicity Studies.* Springer-Verlag, New York (1984a), pp. 9-49.

Grice, H.C. *Current Issues in Toxicology. Age-Associated (Geriatric) Pathology: Its Impact on Long-Term Toxicity Studies.* Springer-Verlag, New York (1984b), pp. 57-107.

Haseman, J.K. Issues in carcinogenicity testing: Dose selection. *Fundam. Appl. Toxicol.* 5: 66-78 (1985).

Haseman, J.K. Use of statistical decision rules for evaluating laboratory animal carcinogenicity studies. *Fundam. Appl. Toxicol.* 14: 637-648 (1990).

Haseman, J.K., Bourbina, J., and Eustis, S.L. Effect of individual housing and other experimental design factors on tumor incidence in B6C3F1 mice. *Fundam. Appl. Toxicol.* 23: 44-52 (1994).

Haseman, J.K., Huff, J.E., Rao, G.N., and Eustis, S.L. Sources of variability in rodent carcinogenicity studies. *Fundam. Appl. Toxicol.* 12: 793-804 (1989).

Igarashi, T. A review of the Japanese Pharmaceutical Manufacturers' Association database currently established to examine retrospectively the value of long-term animal toxicity studies. *Adverse Drug Reaction Toxicol. Rev.* 12: 35-52 (1993).

Interdisciplinary Panel on Carcinogenicity. Criteria for evidence of chemical carcinogenicity. *Science* 225: 682-687 (1984).

Kamrin, M.A. *Toxicology, A Primer on Toxicology Principles and Applications.* Lewis Publishers, Chelsea, MI. (1989).

Kaplan, E.L. and Meier, P. Non-parametric estimation from incomplete observations. *J. Am. Stat. Assoc.* 53: 457-481 (1958).

Keenan, K.P. Comments on findings in the Biosure Study. *Food Chem. Toxicol.* 33: Suppl.#1, 98S-100S (1995).

Lijinsky, W., Reuber, M.D., Davies, T.C., and Riggs, C.W. Dose-response studies with nitroso-1,2,3,6-tetrahydropyridine and dinitrosohomopiperazine in F344 rats. *Ecotox. Environ. Safety* 6: 513-527 (1982).

Lu, F.C. *Basic Toxicology. Fundamentals, Target Organs and Risk Assessment.* Hemisphere Publishing Corp., New York (1985).

Lumley, C.E. and Walker, S.R. The value of chronic animal toxicity studies of pharmaceutical compounds: A retrospective analysis. *Fundam. Appl. Toxicol.* 5: 1007-1024 (1985).

Lumley, C.E. and Walker, S.R. A critical appraisal of the duration of chronic animal toxicity studies. *Regul. Toxicol. Pharmacol.* 6: 66-72 (1986).

Marshall, E. Experts clash over cancer data. *Science* 250: 900-902 (1990).

Mitoma, C. Test for hepatobiliary function. In *Organ Function Tests in Toxicity Evaluation.* C.A. Tyson and D.S. Sawhney (Eds.), Noyes, New Jersey (1985), pp. 90-108.

Morgan, D.L., Jameson, C.W., Mennear, J.H., and Prejean, J.D. 14-Day and 90-day toxicity studies of C.I. Pigment Red 3 in Fischer 344 rats and B6C3F$_1$ mice. *Food Chem. Toxicol.* 27: 793-800 (1989).

Moser, V.C., McCormick, J., Creason, J., and McPhail, R.C. Com-parison of chlordimeform and carbaryl using a functional observational battery. *Fundam. Appl. Toxicol.* 11: 189-206 (1988).

Nohynek, G.J., Longeart, L., Geffray, B., Provost, J.P., and Lodola, A. Fat, frail and dying young: Survival, body weight and pathology of the Charles River Sprague-Dawley-derived rat prior to and since the introduction of the VAF variant in 1988. *Human Exper. Toxicol.* 12: 87-98 (1993).

Paget, G.E. (Ed.). *Methods in Toxicology.* Blackwell Scientific Publ., Oxford (1970), p. 49.

Pariza, M.W. Caloric restriction, *ad libitum* feeding and cancer. *Proc. Soc. Exp. Biol. Med.* 183: 293-298 (1986).

Pariza, M.W. Fat, calories and mammary carcinogenesis: net energy effects. *Am. J. Clin. Nutr.* 45: 261-263 (1987).

Parkinson, C., Lumley, C.E., and Walker, S.R. The value of information generated by long-term toxicity studies in the dog for the nonclinical safety assessment of pharmaceutical compounds. *Fundam. Appl. Toxicol.* 25: 115-123 (1995).

Rao, G.N., Piegorsch, W.W., and Haseman, J.K. Influence of body weight on the incidence of spontaneous tumors in rats and mice of long-term studies. *Am. J. Clin. Nutr.* 45: 252-260 (1987).

Roe, F.J.C. Testing *in vivo* for general chronic toxicity and carcinogenicity. In *Testing for Toxicity.* J.W. Gorrod (Ed.). Taylor and Francis Ltd., London (1981), Ch. 4, pp. 29-43.

Roe, F.J.C. Are nutritionists worried about the epidemic of tumours in laboratory animals? *Proc. Nutr. Soc.* 40: 57-65 (1981).

Roe, F.J.C. What does carcinogenicity mean and how should we test for it? *Food Chem. Toxicol.* 31: 225-231 (1993).

Roe, F.J.C., Lee, P.N., Conybeare, G., Tobin, G., Kelly, D., Prentice, D., and Matter, B. Risks of premature death and cancer predicted by body weight in early adult life. *Human Exper. Toxicol.* 10: 285-288 (1991).

Roe, F.J.C., Lee, P.N., Conybeare, G., Kelly, D., Matter, B., Prentice, D., and Tobin, G. The Biosure Study: Influence of Composition of Diet and Food Consumption on Longevity, Degenerative Diseases and Neoplasia in Wistar Rats Studied for up to 30 Months Post Weaning. *Food Chem. Toxicol.* 33: Suppl.#1 (1995).

Rous, P. The influence of diet on transplanted and spontaneous mouse tumors. *J. Exp. Med.* 20: 433-451 (1914).

Salmon, G.K., Leslie, G., Roe, F.J.C., and Lee, P.N. Influence of food intake and sexual segregation on longevity, organ weights and the incidence of non-neoplastic and neoplastic diseases in rats. *Food Chem. Toxicol.* 28: 39-48 (1990).

Selikop, S.K. The effect of body weight on tumor incidence and carcinogenicity testing in B6c3F$_1$ mice and F344 rats. *Fundam. Appl. Toxicol.* 24: 247-259 (1995).

Sontag, J.M., Page, N.P., and Safiotti, U. *Guidelines for carcinogen bioassays in small rodents.* DHHS Publ. (NIH/76-801). National Cancer Institute, Bethesda, MD. (1976).

Staffa, J.A. and Mehlman, M.A. (Eds.). Innovations in Cancer Risk Assessment (ED$_{01}$ Study). *J. Environ. Pathol. Toxicol.* 3: #3, 1-246 (1980).

Stroo, W.E. and Hook, J.B. Enzymes of renal origin in urine as indicators of nephrotoxicity. *Toxicol. Appl. Pharmacol.* 39: 423-434 (1977).

Study Group on Pesticide Tolerances. Review of EPA's Tolerance Setting System (Draft Report). U.S. EPA, Washington (1979).

Tilson, H.A. and Mitchell, C.L. Neurobehavioral techniques to assess the effects of chemicals on the nervous system. *Ann. Rev. Pharmacol. Toxicol.* 24: 425-450 (1984).

Turnbull, G.J., Lee,P.N., and Roe, F.J.C. Relationship of body-weight gain to longevity and to the risk of development of nephropathology and neoplasia in Sprague-Dawley rats. *Food Chem. Toxicol.* 23: 355-361 (1985).

Tyson, C.A., Story, D.L., Green, C.E., and Meier-Henry, E.F. Traditionally used indicators in relation to pathologic lesions. In *Organ Function Tests in Toxicity Evaluation.* C.A. Tyson and D.S. Sawhney (Eds.), Noyes, NJ. (1985), pp. 23-89.

Weindruch, R. Dietary restriction, tumors and aging in rodents. *J. Gerontology* 44: #6, 67-71 (1989).

Woutersen, R.A., Til, H.P., and Feron, V.J. Sub-acute vs. sub-chronic oral toxicity study in rats: comparative study of 82 compounds. *J. Appl. Toxicol.* 4: 277-280 (1984).

Wright, P.J. and Plummer, D.T. The use of urinary enzyme measurements to detect renal damage caused by nephrotoxic compounds. *Biochem. Pharmacol.* 23: 65-73 (1974).

Zbinden, G. *Progress in Toxicology. Special Topics.* Vol. 1. Springer-Verlag, New York (1973).

Zbinden, G. *Progress in Toxicology. Special Topics.* Vol. 2. Springer-Verlag, New York (1976).

Chapter 5

REPRODUCTIVE TOXICOLOGY

I. INTRODUCTION

Reproductive toxicology is the study of the occurrence, causes, manifestations, and sequelae of adverse effects of exogenous agents on reproduction (Johnson, 1986). Reproductive "hazards" encompass adverse health effects to the prospective mother, father, and the unborn and the newborn child and includes loss of libido, sterility, mutagenesis, teratogenesis, abortion, fetal death, perinatal death, and delayed toxicity (Smith and Costlow, 1985). Public concern has been focused on the susceptiblity of human reproduction to xenobiotics such as drugs, substances of abuse, industrial chemicals, pesticides, airborne contaminants, trace metals, and food additives as well as foods and lifestyles. Such concern is justified by reports demonstrating that, between 1965 and 1982, there was a threefold increase in infertility among couples in the 15- to 24-year-old age group, the group in which fertility is considered to be the highest (Mosher and Pratt, 1985; Mattison et al., 1990). For the most part, the causes of infertility — derived approximately one third from the male, one third from the female, and one third between the couple — remain unknown. Not surprisingly, considerable attention is paid to the development of definitive tests to assess reproductive toxicology.

The mandate to study the toxicity of an agent encompasses the entire breadth of the life cycle. In the studies described to this point, there has been no assessment of toxicant-related effects on the conceptus, the fetus, or the early postnatal animal. This is a most challenging facet of toxicology, not only because agents may elicit cellular damage in either the male or female, but also because such damage may be inflicted on the unseen conceptus, with pre- and post-implantation pregnancy loss reflected only as "infertility." It is not simply that the target organ(s) could be identified as the testes or the ovary, but also the myriad of direct and indirect effects on the normal functions of the reproductive cycle (Table 5.1). Each of the items listed consists of multiple components. In addition, one must be cognizant of the fact that there are sensitive time frames or "windows" in gamete production/function and embryo development when the cells (or organisms) are highly susceptible to either frank, overt, frequently lethal effects or to subtle, covert, cytogenetic damage from exposure to exceptionally low levels of toxicants. These hypersensitive cell systems respond to concentrations of toxicant(s) far lower than are required to elicit any toxicity in an older animal. Add to this the factors of species differences in response(s) dependent on anatomy, pharmacokinetics and metabolism, and mechanisms of hormonal control plus gender differences in reproductive vulnerability, and the complexity is complete. The challenge in reproductive toxicology is to design tests capable of

117

TABLE 5.1

The Human Reproductive/
Development Cycle

Fecundity	Embryo formation
Libido	Differentiation
Gametogenesis	Organogenesis
Gamete	Fetal maturation
Transport	Parturition
Function	Neonatal
Mating	Viability
Fertilization	Development
Zygote transport	Lactation
Implantation	Nutrition
Placental	Postnatal maturation
Formation	Sexual maturation
Function	Gametogenesis

detecting any possible adverse effects caused by the chemical in any segment of the reproductive cycles of male and/or female animals vulnerable to toxic insult.

Since it is impossible to investigate the entire array of reproductive toxicity endpoints with one set of experiments, techniques are used to examine particular sets of endpoints that are manageable (Figure 5.1). **Segment I** testing provides the most comprehensive overview of reproductive toxicity, with protocols varying from the treatment of both sexes of rodents throughout gametogenesis (60 and 15 d for males and females, respectively), mating the treated animals, and exposure of the maternal animal throughout pregnancy until weaning. The evaluations will assess the reproductive process from gonadal function through mating behavior, pregnancy loss, frequency and type of teratogenicity, difficulty with delivery, postnatal viability, survival, growth, and development. Many different **Segment I** protocols are seen, some in which only the female is treated while in others only the male is exposed to the potential reproductive toxicant. **Segment II** testing pertains specifically to the screening of the capability of agents to elicit toxicity during the period of primary organogenesis, the experiments beginning with normal conceptuses (untreated females bred with untreated males) and examining the influence exerted by given levels of the agent on cellular development during organogenesis. Since organogenesis continues throughout *in vitro* development and even into the postnatal period, **Segment III** testing relates to the ongoing assessment during fetal and neonatal life, particular endpoints assessing the effects of the agent on delivery, lactation, neonatal survival, and vitality of the offspring. Additional segments of the reproductive cycle, i.e., gametogenesis, can be examined independently, linked closely to *in vivo* reproduction and *in vitro* culturing of normal pre- and post-implantation embryos exposed to potential cytotoxic agents in the incubation medium at concentrations approximating those encountered *in vivo*.

In reproductive toxicology, the investigator is continually extrapolating toxicity data across species in the hope that a prediction of the likelihood of hazard and an estimation of risk to humans can be attained. If one examines the data found in Table 2.1 of Chapter 2 and tables in this chapter for the species listed, the most striking feature is the interspecies variability in the reproductive endpoints. Several decisions must be made prior to initiating any study. Which species should be used? Within any one species, which strain(s) should be selected as test animals? Is there adequate knowledge about the experimental animal response to the test agent itself or to similar chemicals? What dosage range of the test chemical should be tested?

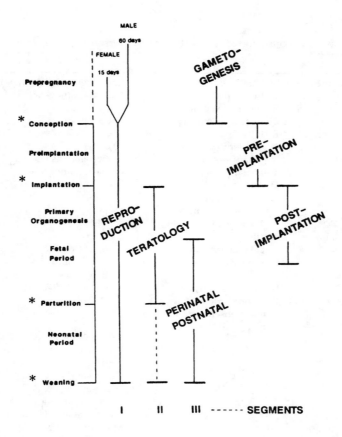

FIGURE 5.1
Various formats of testing reproductive toxicology in mammalian (rodent) species on distinct endpoints (*) in the reproductive cycle. In **Segment 1** reproduction studies, either the male or female animals (or both) are exposed to the test agent for 60 and 15 d, respectively, prior to mating with comparably treated or control, untreated animals. The pregnant animals will be treated at the same dosage throughout gestation and parturition to the point of weaning the offspring. In **Segment II** teratology studies, healthy, untreated pregnant animals are exposed to the test agent from day 6 through day 15 (mouse, rat) or from day 6 through day 18 (rabbit) with either: (1) euthanasia on the day before parturition and examination for anomalies, or (2) allowed to give birth and examination both at birth and at weaning for anomalies. In **Segment III** perinatal/postnatal studies, the healthy, pregnant animals are treated with the test agent through at least 15 d of gestation and 21 d of lactation, with effects on the newborn and postnatal offspring being quantitated by a number of indices throughout development. **Gametogenesis** may be studied by treating either male or female animals throughout one gametogenic cycle followed by an extended breeding program with unexposed animals of the opposite sex. The *in vitro* culturing of unexposed animals pre- or postimplantation embryos in the presence of suitable concentrations of test agent(s) in the incubation medium can be used as screening techniques to assess mechanisms of cytotoxicity up to approximately day 14 of *in utero* development. In all the above studies, at least three exposure groups plus controls, with adequate numbers (n = 10 or 20) of animals in each treatment group, should be used.

Is the entire reproductive cycle to be examined in one sex or both? Is it necessary to examine only certain portions of the reproductive cycle in one sex or the other? How long should a study be conducted?

Reproductive toxicology requires detailed knowledge of the species differences in reproductive biology and development. No animal species used routinely in reproductive toxicity studies exactly mimics the human in reproductive physiology. Certain species lend themselves to the study of agent-induced actions on certain facets of reproduction (Table 5.2). For decades, rodents (mice, rats) and rabbits have

TABLE 5.2

Species Recommended for Evaluation of Reproductive Endpoints

Species	Male	Female
Mouse	Spermatogenesis	Embryogenesis (cleavage)
	Testicular pathogenesis	Ovarian pathogenesis
	Epididymal sperm	Estrus cycle
	Cellular biochemistry	Endometrium
	Fertility	
	In vitro fertilization	
Rat	Spermatogenesis	Embryogenesis (cleavage)
	Testicular pathogenesis	Ovarian pathogenesis
	Hormone profiles	Estrus cycle
	Hormone challenge	Endometrium
	Epididymal sperm	Fertility
	Cellular biochemistry	
Rabbit	Motility	Oviduct
	Ejaculation function	Hormone profiles
	Sperm function	*In vitro* fertilization
	Fertility	Embryogenesis (cleavage)
	Secondary sex organs	Hormone challenge
	Hormone profiles	
	Artificial insemination	
	In vitro fertilization	
Pig		Ovarian morphology
		Estrus cycle
		Fertility
		Hormone profiles
		Hormone challenge
		In vitro fertilization
		Embryogenesis (cleavage)
Monkey		Menstrual cycle
		Oviduct
		Uterus
		Endometrium
		Fertility
		Hormone challenge
		Follicle development

From Mattison et al., *The Effect of Pesticides on Human Health*, Baker, S. R. and Wilkinson, C. F., Eds., Princeton Scientific, Princeton, NJ (1990), Chap. 6. With permission.

provided the bulk of reproductive toxicity data since the species and strains are relatively standardized — they are of small size and they have high fertility (large litters), thereby providing adequate numbers of progeny for meaningful statistical analysis of the results. However, while they are frequently used for all of the wrong reasons, there is a massive data base on chemical-induced reproductive toxicity in these species that cannot be ignored (Schardein, 1985). They remain the species of choice to test a variety of reproductive endpoints. With other species, our knowledge of the reproductive cycle of the female may be far more complete than that for the male, and only studies of endpoints in the female can be conducted with any assurity.

The dosage range of the test agent to be used will evolve following close scrutiny of the pharmacokinetic profile of the agent in males and females of the species plus the results obtained from appropriate subchronic (90-d) studies. Particularly for the female, dosages that induce maternal toxicity should be avoided since subsequent effects on the developing fetuses may have little to do with the agent than with nutritional deficiency if the pregnant animal is ill and not eating properly. A similar case can be made for extended breeding studies in which the dosages given elicit adverse health effects thereby interfering with estrus, copulation frequency, etc.

It is crucial in reproductive toxicology that the investigator comprehends that the developing female mammalian fetus possesses the entire complement of oocytes within the ovaries that will be used in a breeding lifetime. Theoretically, this means that exposure of a pregnant animal to sufficient reproductive toxicant could affect the oocytes of the daughter's ovaries, such damage not becoming detectable until the reproductive life of the daughter begins. Of course, morphological damage and dysfunction can also occur in the adult individual during folliculogenesis and the estrus cycle, with effects on either or both the ovum and the corpora lutea. In contrast, spermatozoa are not formed in the male until puberty, the primordial germ cells and supporting precursor cells remaining dormant until then. Spermatozoa in the post-pubertal adult are constantly being replenished by a nucleus of stem cells (gonocytes or early spermatogonia) which appear to replicate at a slow mitotic rate that minimizes cellular damage from all but an extremely prolonged exposure.

While a complete discussion of reproductive physiology/function is beyond the scope of this text, some appreciation of mammalian reproductive cycles is necessary in order to design adequate protocols for toxicity assessment as well as for interpretation of the results obtained. The reader is referred to appropriate chapters in Mattison (1983), Dixon (1985), Haley and Berndt (1987), Hayes (1989), Working (1989), and Arnold et al. (1990) for detailed discussions on mammalian reproductive physiology. Only a summary will be included in the following sections.

II. MALE REPRODUCTIVE TOXICITY

A. Spermatogenesis

The testis is composed of a series of highly convoluted seminiferous tubules enclosed in a tunica and supported by connective tissue containing lymphatics, vasculature, phagocytes, and interstitial (Leydig) cells (Steinberger and Steinberger, 1975). Lining the tubules are two distinct populations of cells, the germ cells and the Sertoli cells. As they develop and mature, the germ cells proliferate and migrate from the basement membrane of the tubule toward the lumen. A cross-sectional view of the seminiferous tubule has the appearance of a donut, with a basement membrane around the outer edge separated from the lumen (hole in the center) by a parenchyma consisting of a myriad of morphologically distinct cells. Near the basement membrane are stem cells, immature spermatogonia, and Sertoli cells. Further in from the basement membrane are Sertoli and Leydig cells plus developing spermatogonia, spermatocytes, spermatids, and spermatozoa. Spermatogenesis begins during fetal life, with gonocytes or stem cells being transformed to spermatogonia after birth, although these latter cells lie dormant until puberty when proliferative activity resumes. As rodent species are generally used to assess the effects of toxicants on reproduction, attention will focus on rodents (Steinberger and Steinberger, 1975). Figure 5.2 demonstrates the sequence of spermatogenesis in the laboratory rat, with the time frame for evolution from spermatogonia to spermatozoa. In spermatocytogenesis, the diploid spermatogonia (Type A) divide by mitosis, with each cell undergoing five mitotic divisions to replicate itself, eventually forming a type B spermatogonium which is converted into a primary spermatocyte. This cell type subsequently divides by meiosis to form haploid secondary spermatocytes, with a further meiotic division to form haploid spermatids. The next step, spermiogenesis, involves the differentiation of the spermatids into spermatozoa, metamorphosing from a rounded cell into the characteristically shaped mature spermatozoa having an elongated, condensed nucleus in the head and a flagellum (tail). Once released from the encompassing Sertoli cells into the tubular efferent ducts, the spermatozoa migrate to the epididymis for further maturation where they become fertile and highly motile. They are then released and stored in the seminal vesicles. Spermatozoa are produced continuously; a wave of spermatogonial differentiation occurs approximately every 13 d in the rat to initiate a new "batch" of spermatozoa. Species variability in spermatogenesis is the rule, as is shown in Table 5.3 which lists a number of parameters for seven species. Even within strains of a species, the spermatogenic cycle varies somewhat, i.e., the duration being 48 d in the Long-Evans rat, 51.6 d and 53.2 d in the Sprague-Dawley and Wistar rat, respectively, with an additional 12 d of maturation in the epididymis to acquire fluid and motility and the ability to bind to and penetrate the membranes around the ovum.

Control of spermatogenesis is governed by a "coarse" mechanism maintained via the influence of circulating pituitary gonadotrophins — luteinizing hormone (LH) and follicle-stimulating hormone (FSH). The Leydig cells respond to LH by increasing androgen (principally testosterone) production while the Sertoli cell, the target of FSH, initiates the induction of a number of processes. "Fine" control of spermatogenesis is governed by the Sertoli cell via the secretion of messenger substances to attenuate testosterone production by the Leydig cells and via other FSH-dependent and independent factors that modulate Leydig cell function depending upon the stages of spermatogenesis (Lacy and Pettitt, 1970).

B. Sites of Action/Evaluative Tests

Consider the dynamic situation described above in the presence of an accidental, pulse-type exposure to a toxicant. In the rat, each seminiferous tubule contains approximately 12 complete spermatogenic waves at any time point (Steinberger and Steinberger, 1975). There are cells at all stages of development and maturation in the testis at any one time; some diploid cells are replicating (mitosis), and some are undergoing meiosis to become haploid, while others are maturing and undergoing dramatic morphological changes accompanied by extensive protein synthesis to yield viable spermatozoa. Given the fact that cellular nucleic acids are at their most vulnerable state during cell division, it is highly unlikely that all cells in the testis will be affected equally. Some protection is afforded by the blood-testis barrier, a complex multicellular system of myoid cells encompassing the seminiferous tubules and including the layers of spermatogenic cells within the tubules. The penetration of a chemical will be dependent largely upon the lipophilicity and molecular weight of the agent plus the concentration circulating in the bloodstream following the exposure. However, the testis is not the only target site.

A number of endpoints may be used to assess male reproductive toxicity including such basic parameters as organ (testis, epididymis) weights, evaluation of semen (sperm count, production rate, percent motility, swimming speed, morphology), as well as the histological examination of testicular, epididymal, seminal vesicle, and prostate gland morphology (Zenick et al., 1994). Additional endpoints of toxicity involve sexual behavior and include fertility (mating ratio, pregnancy ratio) and pregnancy outcomes (litter size, live/dead pup ratio, sex ratio, anomalies, postnatal

TABLE 5.3

Species Variability in Parameters Involving Spermatogenesis

Parameter	Mouse	Rat	Hamster	Rabbit	Dog	Monkey	Human
Spermatogenesis duration (days)	26–35	48–53	35	28–40			74
Duration of cycle of seminiferous epithelium (days)	8.6	12.9		10.7	13.6	9.5	16
Life span of:							
B-type spermatogonia (days)	1.5	2.0		1.3	4.0	2.9	6.3
L + Z spermatocytes (days)	4.7	7.8		7.3	5.2	6.0	9.2
P + D spermatocytes (days)	8.3	12.2		10.7	13.5	9.5	15.6
Golgi spermatids (days)	1.7	2.9		2.1	6.9	1.8	7.9
Cap spermatids (days)	3.5	5.0		5.2	3.0	3.7	1.6
Testis weight (grams)	0.2	3.7	1.8	6.4	12.0	4.9	34.0
Daily sperm production							
Per gram testis ($\times 10^6$)	54	14–22	22	25	20	23	4.4
Per individual ($\times 10^6$)	5–6	80–90	70	160	300	1100	125
Sperm reserve in cauda at sexual rest ($\times 10^6$)	49	440	575	1600		5700	420
Sperm storage in epididymal tissue ($\times 10^6$)							
Caput	20		200				
Corpus	7	300	175				420
Cauda	40–50	400	200				
Transit time through epididymis at sexual rest (days)							
Caput and corpus	3.1	3.0		3.0	?	4.9	1.8
Cauda	5.6	5.1		9.7	?	5.6	3.7
Ejaculate volume (ml)	0.04	0.2	0.1	1.0	?	?	3.0
Ejaculated sperm (10^6/ml)	5.0	?	?	150	?	?	80.0
Sperm transit time from vagina to tube	15–60 min	30–60 min		3–4 hr	20 min		15–30 min

Data obtained from various sources including: Altman, P. L. and Dittmer, D. S., *Biology Data Book*, 2nd ed., vol. I, Federation of American Societies for Experimental Biology, 1972,[6] various tables: Eddy, E. M. and O'Brien, D. A., *Toxicology of the Male and Female Reproductive Systems*, Working, P. K., Ed., Hemisphere Publishing Corp., New York, 1989,[14] Chap. 3, pp. 31–100; Blazak, W. F., *Toxicology of the Male and Female Reproductive Systems*, Working, P. K., Ed., Hemisphere Publishing Corp., New York, 1989,[15] Chap. 6, pp. 157–172; Zenick, H. and Clegg, E. D., *Principles and Methods of Toxicology*, 2nd ed., Hayes, A. W., Ed., Raven Press, New York, 1989,[16] Chap. 10, pp. 275–309; Spector, W. S., Ed., *Handbook of Biological Data*, W. B. Saunders Company, Philadelphia, PA; 1956,[5] various tables.

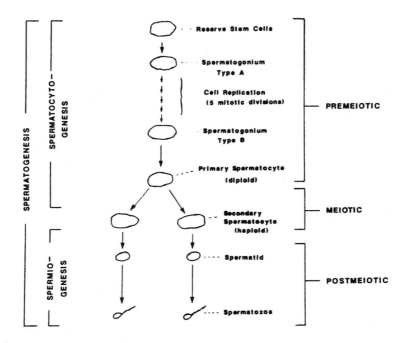

FIGURE 5.2
Mammalian spermatogenesis, showing the premeiotic and meiotic stages of spermatocytogenesis (from reserve stem cells through the primary diploid spermatocyte to the haploid secondary spermatocyte) and the postmeiotic spermiogenesis with the development and maturation of the spermatozoa. Each cycle is completed in a period of 35 to 64 d, depending upon the species, with a new cycle being initiated at the Type A spermatogonium level every 12 to 13 d.

survival, and development. A complete discussion of this topic may be found in Zenick et al. (1994).

The male reproductive cycle is complicated by extensive interorgan involvement including the hormones of the hypothalamus and anterior pituitary, the efferent ducts, epididymis, ductus deferens, accessory sex organs, and the semen (cells and fluid component), as well as the testis. Amann (1982) has presented the most comprehensive summary of sites of action, potentially altered mechanisms, and evaluative tests for reproductive function in the male animal (Table 5.4). A number of *in vitro* and *in vivo* tests can be carried out to determine the status of spermatogenesis.

1. Sperm Production

The first and perhaps the simplest test is an analysis of sperm production, collecting spermatozoa in the most accessible sample at hand: the ejaculate. Viable sperm may also be collected from the cervical mucus of the female following mating. The number of sperm per milliliter of ejaculate will provide a crude measure of deleterious effects on development and maturation, with a significant reduction in numbers suggesting some adverse effect without defining, where in the spermatogenic cycle the toxic action took place. Morphological changes in the head and/or tail, affecting motility and perhaps ovum penetration, may be readily observed under the microscope. However, adverse effects may not be "visible" in terms of morphology or in male fertility but in fetal loss and congenital malformations. A number of *in vitro* assays of functional status including pH, liquifaction, viscosity, respiration, metabolism, acrosomal enzyme level(s) and activity, resistance to stress, etc., can be

TABLE 5.4

Sites and Mechanisms of Action of Reproductive Toxicants in the Adult Male: Approaches for Detecting Altered Reproductive Function

Site of action	Potentially altered mechanisms	Evaluative tests
Hypothalamus	Neurotransmission	None at present
	Synthesis and secretion of GnRH	Hormone assay
	Receptors for LH, FSH, and steroids	Receptor analysis
Anterior pituitary gland	Synthesis and secretion of LH, FSH, and PRL	Hormone assay and GnRH challenge
	Receptors for GnRH, LH, FSH, and steroids	Receptor analysis
Testis	Receptors for LH and PRL on Leydig cells	Receptor analysis
	Testosterone synthesis and secretion	*In vitro* production and hormone assay
	Vascular bed, blood flow	Morphology
	Blood-testis barrier	Morphology
	Receptors for FSH on Sertoli cells	Receptor analysis
	Receptors for steroids	Receptor analysis
	Secretion of inhibin (ABP)	*In vitro* tests
	Sertoli cell function	*In vitro* tests
	Death of reserve spermatogonia	Germ cell counts
	Spermatogonial mitosis	Germ cell counts and % tubules without germ cells
	Spermatocyte meiosis	Spermatid counts and % tubules with luminal sperm
	Spermatid differentiation	Sperm morphology
	Daily sperm production	Spermatid counts
		Seminal evaluation
Efferent ducts	Vascular bed	Morphology
	Resorption	?
Epididymis	Resorption	Sperm maturation
	Concentration of blood constituents	Sperm maturation and biochemical analyses
	Secretion and interconversions	Biochemical analyses
	Enzyme activity	Biochemical analyses
	Transfer of agent to the luminal fluid	Assay for agent
	Smooth muscle contractility	Response to drugs *in vivo* and *in vitro*
	Sperm transport	Sperm in ejaculate
Ductus deferens	Smooth muscle contractility	Response to drugs *in vivo* and *in vitro*
	Sperm transport	Sperm in ejaculate
Accessory sex gland	Secretion of agent	Assay for agent
	Secretion of spermicidal products	Evaluate sperm motility
Semen	Presence of agent	Assay for agent
	Spermicidal components	Evaluate sperm motility

Note: GnRH, gonadotrophin-releasing hormone; LH, luteinizing hormone; FSH, follicle-stimulating hormone; PRL, prolactin.

From Amann, R. P., *Fundam. Appl. Toxicol.*, 2:13–16 (1982). With permission.

carried out on the ejaculate (Table 5.4) (Eliasson, 1978). Hormonal assessment by radioimmune assays and receptor analysis are also useful in targeting sites of toxicant action (Table 5.4).

2. Serial Mating

Repeated mating of agent-treated male animals, usually mice or rats, with untreated, virgin females can be used in assessing male reproductive function *in vivo*. The males(s) which are to receive a range (low, intermediate, high) of dosages may be treated with a single dose or a "pulse" dose over 5 to 7 consecutive days, each male being housed with multiple females (n = 3 or 4) for one or more estrous cycles (approximately 4 d in the rodent) of each female. The females are examined daily for vaginal sperm plugs (indicative of no adverse effects on libido or ejaculation) and the study is continued over the spermatogenic cycle, replacing pregnant females with new, virgin, untreated females. A total of 50 females might be used for each male over the duration of the study. The *fertility index*, defined as the percentage of matings resulting in pregnancy, can be determined over the time period of matings and compared with the time frame of spermatogenesis. As is shown in Figure 5.3, a potential toxicant may affect premeiotic or meiotic-postmeiotic stage cellular events. Congenital malformations and fetal loss would be discovered at necropsy. An immediate reduction in the fertility index after treatment would suggest an adverse effect on epididymal spermatozoa, a somewhat later decrease might indicate damage during the meiotic phase while even a later reduction in the fertility index could indicate severe effects on the spermatogonia and/or the reserve stem-cell population. As can be seen, the time period for each segment of the spermatogenic cycle differs significantly between rats and mice. Corroboration of some of the results can be obtained by a morphological examination of the spermatozoa in ejaculate or vaginal plugs.

3. Extended Mating Study

A variant of the test described above would involve the subchronic administration of the test agent over a period of 6 spermatogenic cycles prior to serial matings with untreated female animals. Each spermatogenic cycle (spermatogonium to primary spermatocyte) starts a new "wave" of synthesis of secondary spermatocytes-spermatids-spermatozoa (Figure 5.2). To ensure that an effect on spermatogenesis has been elicited, treatment of rats, rabbits, or dogs for 58, 48, and 61 d, respectively, would be required since spermatogenesis requires 4.3 to 4.7 cycles of the seminiferous epithelium (Amann, 1982). The 6.0-cycle treatment interval is based on the facts that: (1) several days of treatment will be necessary to achieve a steady-state situation of agent in target sites (a body or organ burden), (2) the test agent may act on specific cell types only at certain stages in the cycle, (3) damage to the germinal epithelium may be evident by the absence of certain germ-cell types, and (4) qualitative changes in germ cells may not be observable until abnormal spermatozoa reach the cauda epididymis and are seen in the ejaculate (Amann, 1982).

This and the previously mentioned test are able to identify *strong, (highly toxic) agents* but these tests will not single out *weak agents*. In most animal species, the number of sperm released in the ejaculate is so high that the fertility index would only be altered significantly either by a severe reduction in the numbers or by extensive morphological/functional damage to the spermatozoa. In contrast, the human has one of the poorest sperm production rates of any mammalian species and spermatogenic damage that would go unnoticed in test animal species could cause reduced reproductive efficiency in the human.

4. Dominant Lethal Assay

A second variant of the serial mating study is the dominant lethal assay in which male animals treated at subtoxic levels (single, pulse dose, or short-term, 7-d treatment) are serially mated with untreated virgin females throughout a complete spermatogenic cycle (Ehling et al., 1978) (Table 5.5). The dosage(s) selected is estimated to cause severe chromosomal damage or lethal germ-cell mutations, resulting in fetal lethality. Positive results should be obtained for both strong and weak toxicants since

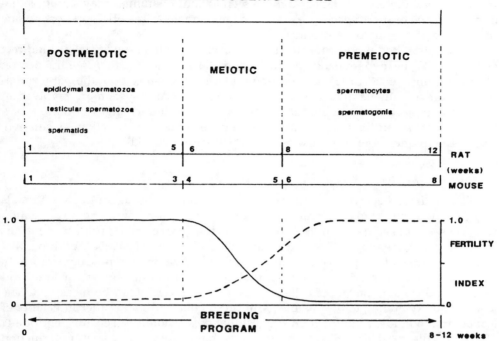

FIGURE 5.3

Treatment of male animals with a reproductive toxicant may result in effects on cells at different stages of development. This schematic diagram illustrates the sequence of events in a dominant lethal assay in which male animals receive a brief (1- to 5-day) exposure to an agent capable of eliciting mutations at some stage of spermatogenesis. The extent of chromosomal damage is subsequently assessed by breeding the treated males serially with virgin females over an extended period of time (8 and 12 weeks for the mouse and rat, respectively). A fertility index (or mutation, malformation, etc.) is developed to reflect the time point of damage to postmeiotic gametes (dotted line) or to premeiotic/meiotic gametes (solid line). Three exposure levels plus controls should be used, each male being mated serially with anywhere up to 50 females over the timespan of the study, usually 3 or 4 females being housed with the male at all times and being removed and replaced as they become pregnant.

TABLE 5.5

Dominant Lethal Assay: Subdivisions of Rodent Spermatogenic Cycle

Portion of cycle	Mouse	Rat
Postmeiotic	1–3[a]	1–5
Meiotic	4–5	6–8
Premeiotic	6–8	8–12

[a] Period of weeks from initiation of spermatogenesis.

it will largely depend on the dosage administered. In this assay, the dams are euthanized at mid-gestation with the numbers of corpora lutea, live, dead, and reabsorbed conceptuses being counted. The antifertility effects of the agent would be obtained from the incidence of pregnancies while the lethal effects would be assessed directly from the increased numbers of early fetal deaths and indirectly from the decreased number of total implantations. Dose-effect relationships will be developed from these parameters. Once again, a sharp alteration in the incidence of the above parameters in relation to those seen in control animals may signify lethal damage to one or more specific cell types in the premeiotic, meiotic, and postmeiotic time frame of spermatozoa production.

Toxicant-related activity may include direct effects with tissue damage or indirect effects on (1) the hypothalamic-pituitary-gonadal axis, (2) hormonal influence on libido and impotence, or (3) the neuromuscular system, since both the parasympathetic and sympathetic divisions of the autonomic nervous system are involved in erection and ejaculation. Reproductive behavior, including changes in mating patterns, a decrease in libido, inability to achieve and maintain erection, ejaculation, coitus, the frequency of intromission, etc., must be monitored.

5. In Vitro Analysis

Studies have been conducted, removing the testes from agent-treated animals or collecting tissue biopsies or micropuncture samples, or by organ homogenization with subsequent separation of the major spermatogenic cell types from suspensions by velocity sedimentation (Lee and Dixon, 1972; Blazak et al., 1985a). With parallel control and treated animals of the same age, such indicators of reproductive toxicity as testicular sperm production rate, epididymal sperm numbers, transit time, and motility (percentage of motile cells and swimming speeds) can be measured. The low variability among adult rats in sperm production rates and other indicators of testicular and epididymal function suggest that these should be sensitive endpoints of toxicity (Blazak et al., 1985a). However, other parameters — i.e., sperm production rate(s), testicular weight, and epididymal sperm numbers — are not well correlated. Careful attention needs to be paid to animal age. An important conclusion drawn from such studies is that spermatozoa production has little to do with reproductive success, with one study showing that nitrobenzene administered at 140 mg/kg/d for five consecutive days caused an 80% reduction in the number of morphologically normal, motile spermatozoa, with a slightly reduced number of implants/pregnant females as the only symptom of reproductive disturbance (Blazak et al., 1985b).

Adult testicular function is largely influenced by the two gonadotrophic hormones, follicle-stimulating hormone (FSH) and luteinizing hormone (LH), both released from the anterior pituitary in response to the actions of the hypothalmic gonadotropin-releasing hormone (GnRH). Each of these glycoproteins has specific targets as is shown in Table 5.6 (Miller et al., 1987; Overstreet and Blazak, 1983). Sensitive radioimmune assays can be used to measure circulating levels of these hormones. Additional hormonal influence comes from testosterone and estradiol originating from the Leydig cells and inhibin from the Sertoli cells, each with its own specific target site, usually in a negative feedback capacity (Table 5.6).

III. FEMALE REPRODUCTIVE TOXICITY

A. Oogenesis

The ovary consists of a collection of growing follicles (the ova plus encasing granulosa and theca cells) lying in a dormant state in supporting tissue. The follicles arise from a population of primordial germ cells formed during embryonic/fetal development along with clusters of interstitial gland cells. These germ cells undergo

TABLE 5.6

Endocrine Control of Testicular Function in Adults

Hormone	Source	Major Target	Direct or Indirect Effect on Target(s)
Luteinizing hormone (LH)	Anterior pituitary	Leydig cells	Stimulate steroidogenesis (testosterone production)
Follicle-stimulating hormone (FSH)	Anterior pituitary	Sertoli cells	Stimulate protein synthesis (e.g., androgen-binding protein)
		Sertoli and/or germ cells	Maturation of spermatids into spermatozoa (spermiogenesis)
Testosterone	Leydig cells	Male accessory glands	Maintain structure and function
		Hypothalamus and pituitary	Negative feedback control on release of FSH and LH
Estradiol	Leydig cells	Anterior pituitary	Negative feedback control on release of FSH and LH
Inhibin	Sertoli cells	Anterior pituitary	Negative feedback control on release of FSH

From Overstreet, J. W. and Blazak, W. F., *Am. J. Ind. Med.*, 4, 5–15, 1983.[17]

numerous mitotic divisions, resulting in several millions of oogonia, the bulk of which become atresic (Figure 5.4). A few oogonia undergo meiotic reduction to the haploid state and become surrounded by a single layer of granulosa cells, this structure being the primordial follicle which remains in an arrested, meiotic, prophase state until after puberty. The other stages of meiosis will not be completed until after puberty and just before ovulation. At puberty, primordial follicles are recruited into a pool of growing primary follicles, though still at an arrested state of prophase meiosis. Other primordial follicles may remain in a dormant state for as long as 35 to 50 years in the human.

During the reproductive life of the multiparous mammal, a group of primary follicles begin to develop at the onset of each menstrual cycle, resulting in an increase in the size of the oocyte and a thickening of the layer of granulosa cells. Further maturation of the primary follicles requires the influence of pituitary follicle-stimulating hormone (FSH) and, later, luteinizing hormone (LH) to form the preovulatory (graafian) follicle which begins to secrete androgens (androstenedione, testosterone) and estrogen (estradiol-17B). At this stage, the remainder of the first meiotic division is completed, the oocyte proceeding through a portion of the second meiotic division before being blocked at the metaphase stage. The maturing follicles recede from the surface of the ovary, accompanied by a large proliferation of the granulosa cells embedding the oocyte at one side of the follicle with the formation of a fluid-filled space, the antrum. A meiotic division occurs in which the secondary oocyte is formed along with the ootid (first polar body). The secondary oocyte contains half the chromosomal complement plus most of the cytoplasm. The ootid is extruded from the follicle. Just prior to ovulation, the follicle swells out on the surface of the ovary as a blister-like protuberance. Ovulation occurs under the influence of steroids and pituitary LH and is accompanied by rupture of the follicle with the discharge of the ovum with the antral fluid and transportation into the fallopian tube. The ruptured follicle collapses, the remaining granulosa and thecal cells being transformed into a gland-like structure, the corpus luteum, that begins to secrete progesterone.

At the time of fertilization, the ovum completes the second meiotic division with the extrusion of a second polar body and the formation of a female pronucleus. With the spermatozoan entering the ovum, the male and female pronuclei combine to produce a diploid cell. With fertilization, the postovulatory corpus luteum responds

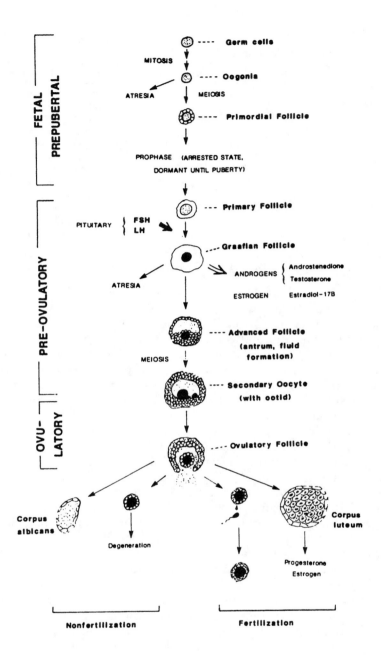

FIGURE 5.4
Mammalian oogenesis, showing the fetal-prepubertal development of the primordial follicles that lie in an arrested state of development until puberty at which time primary follicles begin to develop in response to pre-ovulatory levels of pituitary follicle stimulating hormone (FSH) and luteinizing hormone (LH), with the formation of the graafian follicle and, subsequently, the advanced follicle which undergoes meiosis to produce a haploid oocyte. At the ovulatory stage, one mature ovum is released from each follicle. If the ovum is fertilized, the follicle becomes a steroid-secreting body, the corpus luteum, essential for the maintenance of the pregnancy. If fertilization does not occur, the follicle degenerates into a mass of cells, the corpus albicans.

PREIMPLANTATION EVENTS

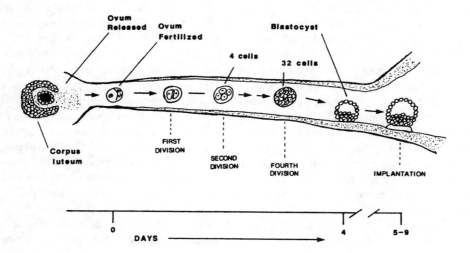

FIGURE 5.5
A schematic diagram illustrates the sequence of events following the successful fertilization of the ovum, denoting the cell divisions over the subsequent 4 d, the formation of the structurally unique blastocyst and the initiation of embryo implantation in the steroid-activated cells of the uterine wall within day 5 to day 9 of fertilization, depending upon the species of mammal.

under the influence of the high levels of circulating LH, the cells synthesizing and secreting progesterone and some estrogen, these being required for decidualization and maintenance of the uterine musculature throught the pregnancy. If fertilization does not occur, the ovulated ovum deteriorates and the empty follicle undergoes luteolysis, degenerating into a fibrous mass of cells called the corpus albicans. The ovulatory cycle will then repeat itself, the time period of the cycle being different for each mammalian species. Once again, species variability in oogenesis is the rule, Table 5.7 listing a number of parameters for eight mammalian laboratory species, including the human for comparison purposes.

With the successful fertilization of the ovum in the upper end of the fallopian tube, the embryo moves downward into the uterus where the myometrial smooth muscle and epithelial layers are being prepared to receive it as a consequence of the influence of progesterone secreted by the corpus luteum (Figure 5.5). By the time the embryo has reached the uterus, it has developed to the blastocyst stage, a sphere of single cells around a fluid-filled cavity in which the impregnated ovum is expanding. The embryo is now ready to implant itself in the receptive uterine wall and to initiate the development of the placental structure in close association with the uterine blood supply of the female for nutritive support (Cross et al., 1994). Considering the various species used in assessing reproductive toxicity, the time sequence is slightly different for each (Table 5.7). In contrast to the human, the gestation period in small mammals is condensed into an extremely short time span, a feature that must be kept in mind because of the very narrow toxic "windows" presented by these species in which the susceptibility of the developing embryo/fetus to chemicals will be enhanced.

B. Sites of Action/Evaluative Tests

Adequate reproductive function is dependent upon an intact hypothalamic-pituitary-gonadal axis. As was observed for the male mammal, a complex interrelationship exists in the female between intrinsic and extrinsic factors for organs/tissues, signifying possible multiple sites of action for toxicants. Complete descriptions of target sites for chemical injury can be found in Mattison et al. (1990) and in appropriate sections of the texts mentioned at the beginning of the chapter. As is shown in Table 5.8, the female reproductive tract is dependent upon neuroendocrine centers (hypothalamus, anterior pituitary) for the secretion of appropriate growth hormones essential for specific action on the postpubertal ovary, the cellular components of the follicle, and, during the pregnancy, the accessory organs (oviduct, uterine muscle) (Amann, 1982). A variety of *in vitro* analyses can be conducted to assess the integrity and function of various aspects of the reproductive organs, particularly the neurohormones, the steroids, and their tissue receptors where highly sensitive radioimmune assays are now available. The biochemical monitoring of uterine and vaginal fluids is being used increasingly to assess the quality of the "environment" of the ovum. In addition, *in vivo* analyses must be performed to assess the overall effects of potential reproductive toxicants on the entire breadth of physiological responses to be examined.

1. Single-Generation Study

As an indicator of whether or not an agent elicits any reproductive toxicity, the agent will be administered at an appropriate dosage range (low, intermediate, high) by a suitable route to groups (n = 5 to 10/treatment group) of young adult, virgin female rodents (mice, rats) for approximately 15 d prior to starting the breeding program with proven, sexually mature, breeding males. As was indicated previously, the dosage range should include a sublethal dose, an intermediate, lower dose, and a no-effect dose. Three or four females are placed with each male, the pregnant (mated) female being removed from the cage upon discovery of a vaginal plug (mice), the presence of sperm in the vagina (rat), or witnessing the occurrence of copulation (rabbit), this date being considered to be day 0 of the pregnancy. Treatment with the same dosage in the same manner will continue throughout the pregnancy. The animals are usually euthanized a day or so before anticipated parturition (days 18, 21, and 29 for mice, rats and rabbits respectively) (Figure 5.6).

The assessment of overall reproductive toxicity is divided into two segments — fertility and teratogenicity — and entails a close inspection of the uterus, the conceptuses, and the ovaries, with the development of quantitative numbers for endpoints of toxicity (Table 5.9). The position and sex of each fetus in each horn of the uterus is noted, beginning at the cervical end and progressing toward the ovarian end. The number of live fetuses, the number of late fetal deaths, and the number of placental (implantation) scars indicative of early fetal deaths/resorption of the conceptus are determined and compared with the number of functional corpora lutea (one ovum, one corpus luteum) in the ovaries. A number of indices will be established (Table 5.10). A *mating index* will be determined by the number of estrous cycles required of each female to produce pregnancy and the number of copulations, giving some indication of reproductive behavior. The *fertility index*, represented by the ratio of the number of females conceiving divided by the number of females exposed to proven, fertile males, is a valuable indicator of overall reproductive capacity. The *gestation index* is determined, that being the number of pregnancies resulting in the

TABLE 5.7
Species Variability in Parameters Involving Oogenesis

Parameter	Mouse	Rat	Guinea Pig	Hamster	Rabbit	Cat	Dog	Monkey	Human
Sexual maturity (days)	28	46–53	84	42–54	120–240	210–245	270–425	1642	
Duration of estrus (days)	9–20 hr	9–20 hr	6–11		30	4	9	4–6	2–8
Ovulation time (days)	2–3 hr	9–20 hr	10 hr		10 hr	24–56 hr	1–3	9–20	15
Ovulation type[a]	S	S	S	S	I	I	S	S	S
No. ova released	8	10	?	7	10	4–6	8–10	1	1
Follicle size (mm)	0.5	0.9	0.8		1.8		10		
Ovum diameter (mm)	0.07–0.087	0.07–0.076	0.075–0.107		0.110–0.146	0.12–0.13	0.135–0.145	0.109–0.173	0.089–0.091
Zona pellucida (mm membrane thickness)			0.012		0.011–0.023	0.012–0.115	0.135	0.012–0.034	0.019–0.035
Transport time (to reach site of implantation) (days)	4.5	3.0	3.5	3.0	2.5–4	4–8	6–8	3.0	3.0
Implantation (days)	4.5–5.0	5.5–6.0	6.0	4.5–5.0	7–8	13–14	13–14	9–11	8–13
Rate of transport of sperm to oviduct (min)	15	15–30	15		5–10				5–60
Rate of transport of embryo to uterus (hr)	72	95–100	80–85		60				80
Fertile life of spermatozoa in female tract (hr)	6	14	21–22	5–12	30–32				24–48
Rate of transport of ova in female tract (hr)	8–12	12–14	20		6–8				24
Segmentation (to form blastocele) (days)	2.5–4.0	4.5	5–6	3.25	3–4				5–8
Primitive streak (days)	7.0	8.5	10.0	6.0	6.5	13.0	13.0	18.0	
Duration of organogenesis (days)	7.5–16	9–17	11–25	7–14	7–20	14–26	14–30	20–45	
Gestational length (days)	20–21	21–22	65–68	16–17	31–32	58–71	57–66	164–168	

Data obtained from various sources including: Ecobichon, D. J., *The Basis of Toxicity Testing*, CRC Press, Inc., Boca Raton, FL, 1992,[2] Chap. 5; Spector, S., *Handbook of Biological Data*, W. B. Saunders Company, Philadelphia, PA, 1956,[5] various tables; Altman, P. L. and Dittmer, D. S., *Biology Data Book*, 2nd Ed., vol. I, Federation of American Societies for Experimental Biology, 1972,[6] various tables; Eddy, E. M. and O'Brien, D. A., Toxicology of the Male and Female Reproductive Systems, Working, P. K., Ed., Hemisphere Publishing Corp., New York, 1989,[14] Chap. 3 pp. 31–100; Manson, J. M. and Kang, Y. J., *Principles and Methods of Toxicology*, 2nd ed., Hayes, A. W., Ed., Raven Press, New York, 1989,[18] Chap. 11, pp. 311–359.

a Ovulation type: I, induced; S, spontaneous.

TABLE 5.8

Sites and Mechanisms of Action of Reproductive Toxicants in the Adult Female: Approaches for Detecting Altered Reproductive Function

Site of action	Potentially altered mechanisms	Evaluative tests
Hypothalamus	Neurotransmission	None at present
	Synthesis and secretion of GnRH	Hormone assay
	Receptors for LH, FSH, and steroids	Receptor analysis
Anterior	Synthesis and secretion of LH, FSH, and PRL	Hormone assay and GnRH challenge
pituitary gland	Receptors for GnRH, LH, FSH, and steroids	Receptor analysis
Ovary	Oocyte toxicity and increased atresia	Counts, morphology
	Abnormal meiosis	?
	Number of LH or FSH receptors in follicular or granulosa cells	Receptor analysis
	E_2 and P_4 synthesis and secretion	Hormone assay or *in vitro* tests
	Sensitivity to luteolysis	*In vitro* tests?
Ovum	Surface proteins interacting with sperm	Biochemical assays
	Altered zona pellucida	Sperm penetration tests
	Metabolic processes	?
	Syngamy	Morphology
	Implantation	Ratio of implantations to corpora lutea
Uterine tube	Fimbriae movement	?
	Ciliagenesis and cilia function	Morphology
	Number of E_2, P_4 receptors	Receptor analysis
	Sperm and ovum transport	Recovery and count
	Fluid environment	Biochemical assays
Uterus	Number of E_2 and P_4 receptors	Receptor analysis
	PGE and PGF_2 secretion	PG assay
	Protein and glycoprotein secretion	Biochemical assays
	Sperm survival, transport	Recovery and count
	Luminal fluid	Biochemical analysis
	Exposure of sperm and the embryo to agent in secretions	Assay for agent
	Parturition	Incidence of dystocia
Cervix	Barrier to sperm	*In vitro* tests
Vagina	Exposure to sperm to agent in secretions	Assay for agent
Mammary gland	Shedding of agent in milk	Assay for agent
	Altered milk composition	Biochemical analyses
	Decreased milk yield	Measure (weight of young, growth)

Note: GnRH, gonadotrophin-releasing hormone; LH, luteinizing hormone; FSH, follicle-stimulating hormone; PRL, prolactin; E_2, estradiol; P_4, progesterone; PG, prostaglandin.

From Amann, R. P., *Fundam. Appl. Toxicol., 2:13–16 (1982). With permission.*

birth of live litters. Dose-effect relationships are developed for each parameter. In reproductive studies, good record-keeping is essential, and Tables 5.10 and 5.11 illustrate the scope and the details of the information required as endpoints of toxicity testing (OECD, 1996). All conceptuses undergo gross examination for visible birth defects (terata) and are necropsied for microscopic examination for the presence of organ and skeletal defects.

One variant of the single-generation test takes into account that there may be physiological, neurobehavioral, or biochemical deficits caused by the toxicant that would not be evident from a morphological examination. In this modified protocol (Figure 5.6), each dam, pretreated for 15 d before breeding, is allowed to give birth to the litter, the litter size is adjusted (8 pups/dam), and they are reared to weaning age; all the while, the dam is receiving the test agent. At weaning, the dams and offspring are euthanized for autopsy. In this manner, the perinatal and postnatal vigor and viability of the pups, i.e., weight gain and development, and maternal

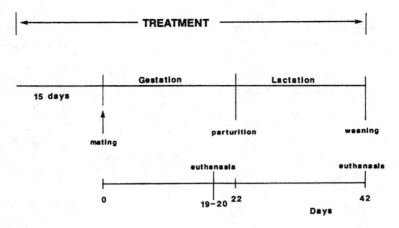

FIGURE 5.6

A schematic diagram depicting a single generation reproductive study in which virgin female rodents (mice, rats) are exposed to the test agent for 15 d prior to mating, are exposed to the same dosage of agent throughout pregnancy and are either (1) euthanized on the day before parturition (day 19 or 20) for examination of the offspring, or (2) allowed to give birth normally and with continuing treatment allowed to raise the young until weaning at which time the offspring may be euthanized or subjected to biochemical, physiological, or behavioral assessment.

TABLE 5.9

Endpoints of Reproductive Toxicity in Female Rodents

Preconception evaluation
Animal weight
Mating behavior
Conception rate (preimplantation, fertilization)
Postconception evaluation
Implantation number
Corpora luteal number
Size of litter
Deaths (embryonic, fetal)
Live fetuses
Incidence of malformations (external, internal)
Maternal weight gain
Date of delivery to be compared with date of conception
Postnatal evaluations
Pup weight, crown-rump length
Number of pups born, numbers alive and dead
Frequency of malformations (external, internal)
Vitality and viability of newborn pups
Problems at parturition
Maternal-newborn relationship
Ability of mother to rear young — lactation
Postnatal growth and development
Survival incidence from delivery to day 21
Developmental landmarks — time of eye opening, hair growth, pinna opening, vaginal opening
Functional testing — day 21 or later

behavior (rearing ability, lactational capacity) can be assessed in relation to the dosage level of test agent.

A second but more complex variant of the single-generation test is one in which suitable numbers of both the males and females have been treated with an appropriate

TABLE 5.10

Fertility and Reproductive Indices Used in Single and Multigeneration Studies

Index	Derivation
Mating	$= \dfrac{\text{No. confirmed copulations}}{\text{No. of estrous cycles required}} \times 100$
Male fertility	$= \dfrac{\text{No. males impregnating females}}{\text{No. males exposed to fertile, nonpregnant females}} \times 100$
Female fertility	$= \dfrac{\text{No. of females confirmed pregnant}}{\text{No. of females housed with fertile male}} \times 100$
Female fecundity	$= \dfrac{\text{No. of females confirmed pregnant}}{\text{No. of confirmed copulations}} \times 100$
Implantation	$= \dfrac{\text{No. of implantations}}{\text{No. of pregnant females}} \times 100$
Preimplantation loss	$= \dfrac{\text{Corpora lutea} - \text{No. of implants}}{\text{No. of Corpora lutea}} \times 100$
Parturition incidence	$= \dfrac{\text{No. of females giving birth}}{\text{No. of females confirmed pregnant}} \times 100$
Live litter size	$= \dfrac{\text{No. of litters with live pups}}{\text{No. of females confirmed pregnant}} \times 100$
Live birth	$= \dfrac{\text{No. viable pups born/litter}}{\text{No. pups born/litter}} \times 100$
Viability	$= \dfrac{\text{No. of viable pups born}}{\text{No. of dead pups born}} \times 100$
Survival	$= \dfrac{\text{No. of pups viable on day 1}}{\text{No. of viable pups born}} \times 100$
Pup death (day 1–4)	$= \dfrac{\text{No. of pups dying, postnatal days 1–4}}{\text{No. of viable pups born}} \times 100$
Pup death (days 5–21)	$= \dfrac{\text{No. of pups dying, postnatal days 5–21}}{\text{No. of viable pups born}} \times 100$
Sex ratio (at birth)	$= \dfrac{\text{No. of male offspring}}{\text{No. of female offspring}} \times 100$
Sex ratio (day 4) (day 21)	$= \dfrac{\text{No. of male offspring}}{\text{No. of female offspring}} \times 100$

TABLE 5.11

Tabular Summary Report of Effects on Reproduction/Development

OBSERVATIONS	DOSAGE			
	0 (control)	mg	kg	bw	d
Pairs started (N)				
Female showing evidence of copulation (N)				
Females achieving pregnancy (N)				
Conceiving days 1–5 (N)				
Conceiving days 6–...ᵃ (N)				
Pregnancy = 21 days (N)				
Pregnancy = 22 days (N)				
Pregnancy = 23 days (N)				
Dams with live young born (N)				
Dams with live young at day 4 pp (N)				
Corpora lutea/dam (mean)				
Implants/dam (mean)				
Live pups/dam at birth (mean)				
Live pups/dam at day 4 (mean)				
Sex ratio (m/f) at birth (mean)				
Sex ratio (m/f) at day 4 (mean)				
Litter weight at birth (mean)				
Litter weight at day 4 (mean)				
Pup weight at birth (mean)				
Pup weight at day 4 (mean)				
ABNORMAL PUPS				
Dams with 0				
Dams with 1				
Dams with 2				
LOSS OF OFFSPRING				
Pre-implantation (corpora lutea minus implantations)				
Females with 0				
Females with 1				
Females with 2				
Females with 3				
Pre-natal (implantations minus live births)				
Females with 0				
Females with 1				
Females with 2				
Females with 3				
Post-natal (live births minus alive at post natal day 4)				
Females with 0				
Females with 1				
Females with 2				
Females with 3				

Note: (N) = number.

dosage range of test agent; the males to 60 d, the females for 15 d prior to initiating the breeding program. Each treated male is mated with two females at each dosage level; the female, while still being treated, is allowed to go to term, to deliver the litter, and to rear the offspring to weaning, at which time the dams and offspring are euthanized for autopsy. The parameters listed in Table 5.9 can be ascertained, but the results are complicated by the fact that no decision can be made whether toxicity was elicited in the male gametes or in those of the female. Only the general effects of the agent can be deduced. However, one could gain some insight into the paternal contribution to the reproductive toxicity by continuing to mate the treated males with untreated females and measuring the same parameters.

2. Multiple-Generation Studies

It has been demonstrated that reproductive toxicity, in the form of behavioral, physiological, and/or biochemical anomalies, may not occur in the treated animals, but may be "visited upon" the daughters, this phomenon being in keeping with an earlier statement that the developing ovaries of the fetal daughter contain all of the ova used during that individual's reproductive life. In addition, there may be morphological or structural anomalies produced in reproductive organs, etc., that would not become apparent until the daughter (or son) began a reproductive life. The best example in the human is, perhaps, diethylstilbestrol (DES) which has been proven not only to be carcinogenic (vaginal, clear-cell, adenocarcinoma) in postpubertal young women, but to have been responsible for genitourinary tract anomalies in both males and females born to women treated with DES during pregnancy (Bibbo et al., 1977; Herbst et al., 1971; Kaufman et al., 1980; Poskanzer and Herbst, 1977).

With the above single-generation protocol, there was no means of testing the behavioral, physiological, or biochemical consequences of exposure to reproductive toxicants since, either at birth or at weaning, all were euthanized for in-depth study. In modifying the protocol to allow the survival of the newborn until they reach maturity and begin reproducing, these endpoints of toxicity could be explored over any number of generations. The standard protocol usually involves two or three generations as is shown in Figure 5.7. Multigeneration studies are used with agents that are considered to accumulate in the body, particularly food additives, trace metals, pesticides, environmental contaminants, etc. acquired involuntarily over a lifetime of exposure.

Groups of breeding-age females (the F_0 generation, n = 10/treatment group) may be treated with a range of dosages of the test agent for a period of 15 to 60 d before mating with proven, fertile males. Treatment of the dam is continued throughout the pregnancy and the postpartum lactational period so that the young — the F_{1A} generation — have been exposed both transplacentally and via the milk to the test agent. The F_{1A} progeny are euthanized at weaning for necropsy and a detailed examination for both gross and microscopic anomalies. Approximately 2 weeks after weaning, the F_0 dam, still receiving the test agent, is rebred to produce a second litter, the F_{1B} generation. At weaning, a number of the females of the F_{1B} litter are selected for further reproductive studies, are treated with the same dosage of the test agent, and at an appropriate age, are bred to begin the next cycle and the production of an F_{2A} generation. The F_{2A} offspring are euthanized at weaning age, and the F_{1B} dam is rebred to provide a second litter — the F_{2B} generation — that provides the source of continuously exposed females to begin the next generation, the F_{3A} and F_{3B} progeny.

In addition to the pre- and post-conception parameters listed in Table 5.9, the investigator has the opportunity to assess the post-parturition care of the progeny by the dam (newborn-maternal relationships, ability to rear the young, lactational adequacy, etc.) as well as the viability and vitality of the young, postnatal growth and development, and anatomical and functional integrity. Within 6 weeks of birth, both males and those females not selected for reproductive studies can be utilized in experimental paradigms to assess sensory, motor, and cognitive neurological function,

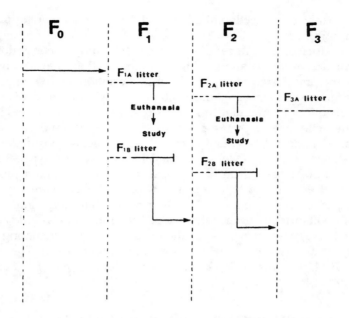

FIGURE 5.7

A typical three-generation reproductive study in which the agent-exposed F_0 female rodents are bred to control, untreated males with the production of F_{1A} litters that are euthanized at birth for morphological examination. Having rested the F_0 females for 2 weeks while continuing treatment, they are rebred with untreated males to produce F_{1B} litters which the treated females are allowed to rear. Females from the F_{1B} litters, having been exposed to the test agent both transplacentally and via the milk, form the source of females for the next, the F_2 generation and begin receiving the test agent at weaning, throughout maturation and their reproductive stage. The F_{2A} litters are euthanized at birth, the F_{1B} female rested and rebred to produce F_{2B} litters, providing a source of continuously agent-exposed females for the subsequent F_3 generation.

hepatic and renal function, etc., making full use of the progeny from F_1, F_2, and F_3 generations to detect any adverse health effects arising in a dose-dependent manner from exposure to the test agent.

How many generations should be studied? A strong case can be made for a complete investigation of two generations based on both (1) the biological aspect that the gametes of the progeny (male and female) of the F_1 generation have been exposed continuously to the test agent since the earliest stages of *in utero* development through to the reproductive period, and (2) the tragic example of DES-induced morphological genitourinary anomalies in both males and females born to DES-treated mothers. Any effect on the early germ cells should be detected as should effects on these cells at later stages. The two-generation study, if an appropriate dosage range has been chosen, should allow an investigator to predict reproductive hazards associated with the chemical with some confidence. A case could be made for a three-generation study if, by some unusual circumstances, only the early stage germ cells were selectively damaged without an effect on later cell stages.

3. Fertility Assessment by Continuous Breeding

Designed to provide an overview of reproductive success and the possible impairment of any one of a number of reproductive endpoints without delineating the exact mechanism, this variant of a multigeneration study involves a repeated forced breeding regimen throughout the reproductive lifetime of the female animal.

The protocol permits the detection of delayed effects which are not apparent during the first few matings.

Usually conducted with mice, pregnant females may be continuously treated with the agent before (14 d) and during gestation or they may receive a "pulse" exposure at some preselected time period during gestation. Following the rearing of the litters, the female offspring are housed continuously with untreated fertile males, removed when noticeably pregnant, allowed to deliver their young, and immediately returned to the males again. Over a period of 50 weeks, a number of litters will be born, the total number of live young born per female being recorded as a measure of total reproductive capacity (McLachlan and Dixon, 1973; Dixon, 1982). With procarbazine, an antineoplastic drug, a single exposure administered prenatally was sufficient to affect the fertility of the female offspring. Effects were not immediately noticed, but by 20 weeks of repeated breeding, there were reductions in the cumulative number of offspring per breeding group. Similar protocols could be developed to test the effects of agents on male reproduction by continuously mating the exposed animals with untreated virgin females (Lamb and Chapin, 1985). The males would be treated for 70 d, the time period of one spermatogenic cycle, prior to mating.

IV. PREIMPLANTATION STUDIES

Up to this point, we have examined techniques by which the effects of toxicants on male and female gametes and on the developing conceptus have been studied. However, recent epidemiological studies have indicated that 60 to 75% of all fertilized oocytes die, with some 50% of that loss occurring before implantation (Kline and Stein, 1985; Warburton, 1987). Linked to this observation is the fact that chromosomal aberrations are found in 45 to 65% of all first-trimester spontaneous abortions (Boue et al., 1975; Kline and Stein, 1985). Considerable attention has been focused on the possible action of drugs and "environmental" chemicals on the embryo in the period prior to implantation in the uterine wall (Figure 5.5). Previously, investigators had to follow a pregnancy through to term and study the reproductive outcome. Unfortunately, the dying, preimplantation, fertilized oocyte leaves no trace of it ever having been there except for a functional corpus luteum, the indicator that an ovum was released. However, there are new manipulative techniques for harvesting preimplantation fertilized oocytes, exposing them briefly to potential toxicants, and either culturing them *in vitro* or reintroducing the treated embryos into foster mothers and allowing them to develop to term. A recent review gives a fascinating insight into these techniques (Spielmann and Vogel, 1989). Such techniques are feasible with the embryos of mice, rats, and rabbits. The preimplantation development in the mouse is more comparable to the human situation than is the rabbit (McLaren, 1985). However, considerable research has been conducted with rabbit blastocysts since they are much larger; they are composed of more than 10,000 cells, whereas the mouse, rat, and human blastocyst contain only about 100 cells (Bavister, 1987). The preimplantation period is unique in that cleavage-stage embryos can be cultured *in vitro* for several days, even to the point of hatching from the zona pellucida and "implanting" on the wall of the culture flask. A summary of the findings of such investigators is presented in Table 5.12, suggesting that this is a viable technique of examining a very important period in development.

The development of the fertilized ovum up to the time of implantation reveals a period of tremendous cellular activity and differentiation (Figure 5.5). Following fertilization, the rodent oocyte undergoes four rapid mitotic divisions in less than 3

TABLE 5.12

Principles of Drug Action During Early Pregnancy

1. Embryotoxic effects of the treatment of pregnant animals before preimplantation can be detected before implantation.
2. During the preimplantation period, treatment of the mother may inhibit embryonic development in a dose-dependent manner, not in an "all-or-nothing" fashion.
3. Different groups of cells in blastocysts (mouse) exhibit different sensitivities to the agent in a dose-dependent manner.
4. The effects of embryotoxic drugs in the embryo can be detected shortly after treatment.
5. Ultraviolet irradiation of preimplantation embryos (mouse) provides evidence of at least two active DNA-repair mechanisms (excision and postreplication repair).
6. The onset of the activity of both Phase I and Phase II drug-metabolizing enzymes coincides with the formation of the blastocyst cavity.
7. Contribution of drug metabolism in preimplantation embryos is negligible compared to the amounts of agent (and metabolites) available from the maternal system through tubal and uterine secretions.
8. There are no special barriers to protect preimplantation embryos (rabbit), with drug acquisition being dependent upon molecular weight and lipid solubility.
9. A low percentage of term malformations can be induced by exposure of the dam to genotoxic chemicals shortly after fertilization and during the preimplantation period.
10. Malformations can be induced by retroviruses in culture with preimplantation embryos and by insertional mutagenesis in transgenic mice, transferring the embryos to foster mothers.

Data from Spielmann and Vogel (1989).

d, giving rise to a 32-cell embryo that by day 4 becomes a blastocyst consisting of an inner cell mass, a cavity, and an encompassing trophoblast cell layer. At day 4, the blastocyst "hatches" from the covering zona pellucida and by day 5 to day 9, depending on the species, has implanted on the endometrial layer of the uterine surface and has initiated the development of microvilli to make contact with the maternal blood supply in the uterine wall, eventually to form the placenta. The trophoblast layer, the yolk sac in rodent species, remains important for nutrition right up to the time of the completion of the placental structures and acquisition of nutrients from that source. The presence of rapidly dividing cells is synonymous with heightened susceptibility to agents capable of eliciting damage to nuclear material.

The mechanisms of action of toxicants can be studied following the treatment of the mother early in pregnancy by morphological, cytological, and cytogenetical parameters. Morphological endpoints can be examined by flushing the cleavage-stage embryo from the oviducts and uterus, explanting them *in vitro*, and examining the following endpoints: (1) development to the blastocyst stage, (2) hatching from the zona pellucida, (3) attachment to the surface of the culture dish, and (4) the outgrowth of three different cell types (trophoblasts, the inner cell mass composed of entoderm, and ectoderm) (Spielmann and Vogel, 1989). Cytological endpoints include the cell number/embryo as an indicator of inhibited embryonic growth, particularly the cells of the inner cell mass which appear to be more sensitive to toxicants than the trophoblast cells. Cytogenetical endpoints include: (1) the detection of micronuclei (suggestive of chromosomal aberrations) in preimplantation embryos during the interphase of the cell cycle, (2) the determination of sister chromatid exchanges, incorporating bromodeoxyuridine into the replicating DNA, and (3) chromosomal aberration tests during the first cell cycle following exposure to the test agent (most cells carrying the structural aberration will be eliminated in the second cycle). It is important to appreciate that the *in vitro* development of early embryos appears to closely mimic the *in vivo* situation (Bavister, 1987).

A number of protocols have been described for the study of toxicant action *in vivo* early in pregnancy in suitable rodent species, the most complete being that of

Cummings (1990) (Figure 5.8). In the first protocol, the positive mating is considered as day 0 of the pregnancy and treatment with the agent is initiated within 24 h (day 1) through day 8 (Figure 5.8A). At necropsy on day 9, a spectrum of endpoints can be evaluated to assess the impact of the test agent on the cleavage-stage embryo, on implantation (day 4), and also on the postimplantation period of decidual development. A refined variant of this protocol is shown in Figure 5.8B where the treatment period can be split into two phases: early administration (day 1 through day 3) to assess preimplantation susceptibility, and the second phase, beginning on day 4 through day 8, to examine postimplantation effects. All animals will be euthanized on day 9. These two protocols, taken in context with the day 1 through day 8 protocol, would differentiate whether or not the agent interfered with the process of implantation.

A third protocol (Figure 5.8C) involves a study of decidual cell response (DCR), manually stimulating the uterine cervix on proestrus/estrus (day 0) to initiate a pseudopregnancy following which the test agent is administered on day 1 through day 8. On day 4, decidual induction is performed by surgically traumatizing the entire length of the uterine lining of one horn, leaving the other horn to serve as a control. On day 9, DCR will be evident by a marked increase (tenfold) in uterine weight compared to the control horn. Microscopic examination of the traumatized uterine horn will reveal a rapid development and differentiation of the endometrium similar to that observed early in pregnancy.

The rate at which the embryo is transported in the oviduct is extremely important because synchronization between the development of the embryo and that of the endometrial lining of the uterus is crucial for a successful implantation. Potential reproductive toxicants may accelerate or retard embryo transport resulting in premature or delayed arrival at the prepared endometrium. As is shown in the fourth protocol (Figure 5.8D), treatment of the newly pregnant animal begins at 9:00 a.m. on day 1 through day 3, with representative groups of animals being euthanized at 3:00 p.m. of day 1 and at 9:00 a.m. and 3:00 p.m. of day 2 and day 3. At necropsy, the uterine horns are divided into appropriate segments, the embryos being flushed from each segment with buffered saline, counted, stained, and examined microscopically for the stage of development (number of cells per embryo). Quantitation of the number of embryos, distance traveled, and development may be related in a dose-dependent manner to the single dose of test agent administered on day 1.

Validation of such techniques as those described in Figure 5.8 is essential before the protocols can be applied beyond the experimental stages of determining sites and mechanisms of reproductive failure. Validation of Cummings' protocols has been carried out by testing bromoergocryptine, an agent known to inhibit pituitary prolactin secretion (Cummings et al., 1991). Bromoergocryptine affected embryo implantation at least through day 4 of gestation, but had no impact on embryo transport rate, suggesting adverse maternal effects which were reflected in reduced serum progesterone levels and impaired uterine function.

While these are interesting techniques for studying the mechanisms of reproductive toxicity in early pregnancy, they cannot be used for risk evaluation since possible effects cannot be examined at term. However, techniques have been developed and tested whereby the externalized "exposed," cleavage-stage embryo can be reintroduced and allowed to implant in the sensitized uterus of a foster mother. One example of the dichotomy of agent-induced reproductive events can be demonstrated with methylnitrosourea (MNU) which, if given to pregnant mice on days 2, 3, or 4, caused extensive malformations (exencephaly, cleft palate, abnormal tails, vertebrae, ribs, long bones, and renal anomalies) plus a decreased survival rate at 21 days of age (Takeuchi, 1984; Vogel et al., 1989). When blastocysts were exposed

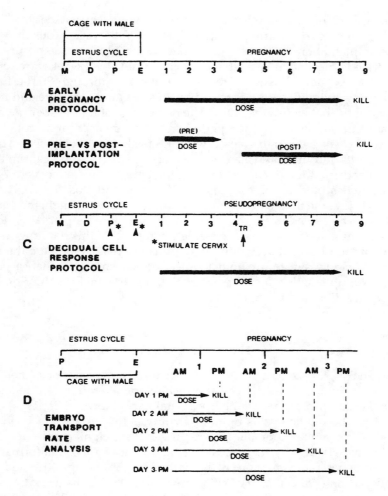

FIGURE 5.8

A schematic diagram illustrating experimental protocols to study toxicological mechanisms of implantation failure *in vivo* in rodents, modified from Cummings (1990), with permission. Treatment throughout day 1 to day 8 of pregnancy (*Protocol A*) or treatment through day 1 to day 3 or through day 3 to day 8 (*Protocol B*) will allow assessment of pre- and postimplantation effects of the test agent. *Protocol C* is designed to assess the possible biological effects of the test agent on the decidual cells of the uterus in an induced pseudopregnancy, treatment with the agent being initiated from day 1 through day 8. *Protocol D*, spanning only the first 3 d of the pregnancy, is designed to monitor the effects of treatment on the rate of transport of the preimplantation embryos in the uterine horns by euthanizing treated pregnant animals every 12 h from day 1 through day 3 with microscopic examination of the opened uterus for the distance travelled by the embryos. See text for additional details. (Modified from Cummings, A., *Fundam. Appl. Toxicol.*, 15: 571–579, 1990. With permission.)

directly to MNU, no malformations were found in term fetuses, but mortality was significantly increased (Iannaccone, 1984). Other studies have demonstrated that the embryo is more susceptible to genotoxic agents before implantation than afterwards (Spielmann and Vogel, 1989).

The value of integrating *in vivo* and *in vitro* reproductive studies and the need for multiparameter analysis can be appreciated in the rather interesting set of experiments exploring the mechanism(s) by which methyl chloride induced dominant lethality (Working et al., 1985a, 1985b). Bred to male Fischer 344 rats exposed to

3000 ppm methyl chloride 6 h/d for 5 days, females showed elevated rates of postimplantation embryonic loss during the first 2 weeks following exposure and high levels of preimplantation embryonic loss from weeks 2 to 8 postexposure. *In vitro* analysis revealed a decline in vas deferens sperm counts by 2 weeks after exposure, with sperm counts being drastically reduced in weeks 3 through 8. The frequency of intact sperm was significantly depressed by 2 weeks after exposure and remained low throughout the balance of the study. The percentage of motile sperm was markedly decreased throughout the study period and abnormal sperm morphology was enhanced from week 1 through week 5 with the peak effect being seen at week 3. From these results, fertility could also be considered to play a significant role. Experiments were conducted in which preimplantation embryos were recovered and cultured from females bred to exposed males (Working and Bus, 1986). The results showed that, during the time when preimplantation losses were high, the percentage of unfertilized ova equaled or exceeded the percentage of preimplantation loss measured in the dominant lethal assay. A consideration of all of this data suggested that the preimplantation losses detected in the dominant lethal assay were the result of failure of fertilization due to a cytotoxic effect on sperm rather than a genotoxic effect. The postimplantation losses were attributed to a methyl chloride-induced inflammatory reaction in the epididymis.

V. TERATOGENICITY

A teratogen is an agent that induces structural malformations, metabolic or physiological dysfunction, psychological or behavioral alterations, or deficits in the offspring, either at birth or in a defined postnatal period (Schardein, 1985). Perhaps as important in the public eye as reduced fertility is the problem of birth defects, malformations, congenital anomalies, or teratogenesis, heightened by the fact that so little is known about why they occur. In the human, 20% of malformations are due to known genetic transmission, with another 3 to 5% being attributed to chromosomal aberration (Wilson, 1977). While environmental factors are known to contribute to malformations, i.e., radiation (<1.0%), infections (2 to 3%), maternal metabolic imbalance (1 to 2%), and drugs and environmental chemicals (4 to 6%), the remainder, some 65 to 70% of all malformations, arise from unknown causes. More recent data confirm the earlier observations, teratogens (drugs, chemicals, etc.) accounting for 3.4% of malformations, with some 43% occurring from unknown causes (Nelson and Holmes, 1989) (Table 5.13). While there was early recognition of the induction of congenital malformations in the human by certain chemicals (nitrogen mustard, androgenic hormones, aminopterin, viruses, and environmental contaminants such as methyl mercury), these agents were known to be potent toxicants. The tragedy surrounding the thalidomide-induced phocomelia in the late 1950s generated a fear that commonly used drugs that were considered safe were capable of eliciting disastrous effects on the unborn. This raised the spectre of the unknown about foods, food additives, pesticide residues, environmental contaminants, etc., with public opinion taking the extreme point of view that everything was hazardous. The criteria for the recognition of a new teratogen in humans are listed in Table 5.14. In the 1960s, regulatory agencies began to request the inclusion of teratogenicity studies in the toxicity data package submitted for evaluation. In 1973, a joint Canadian–U.S. working group formulated guidelines for the testing of chemicals for mutagenicity, teratogenicity, and carcinogenicity (Health and Welfare, Canada, 1973). Teratological assessment is required by all regulatory agencies around the world today.

TABLE 5.13

Causes of Malformations Among Affected Infants

Causes	No. of Infants	Percent
Genetic causes		
Chromosomal	157	10.1
Single mutant genes	48	3.1
Familial	225	14.5
Multifactorial inheritance	356	23.0
Teratogens	49	3.2
Uterine factors	39	2.5
Twinning	6	0.4
Unknown causes	669	43.2

From Nelson and Holmes, *New Engl. J. Med.*, 320, 19–23 (1989). A study of 1549 anomalies out of 69,277 infants.

TABLE 5.14

Criteria for Recognizing a New Teratogen in the Human

1. An abrupt increase in the frequency of a particular defect or association of defects (syndrome)
2. Coincidence of this increase with a known environmental change, such as widespread use of a new drug
3. Known exposure to the environmental change at a particular stage of gestation yielding a characteristically defective syndrome
4. Absence of other factors common to all pregnancies yielding infants with the characteristic defect

Data from Wilson (1977).

A teratogenic response depends upon the administration of a *specific treatment* of a *particular* dose of agent to a genetically *susceptible species* when the embryos are in a *susceptible stage of development*. There is little need to dwell on the aspects of specific treatment and particular dose since by now the reader should be cognizant that biological effects should be dose-related. Physical agents, perhaps with the exception of radiation, rarely enter the fetal compartment, affecting the developing embryo only when levels are toxic to the maternal organism. On the other hand, chemical agents, most being moderately lipid soluble, readily penetrate the placenta, affecting the developing organism and causing deviant development (death, malformations, functional deficits, retardation of growth). A critical factor in teratogenesis is the rapidly changing rate(s) of cell division, with increased rates of replication enhancing the possibilities of mutations. For example, in developing rats, there are 10 mitotic divisions of cells between days 8 and 10 of gestation, resulting in $N \times 2^{10}$ new cells (N being the number of cells at the start of organogenesis). The teratogenic threshold, the dose at which an agent induces malformations, can be above, equal to, or most often, below the embryolethal threshold.

Susceptible species and stage(s) of development require elaboration. As might be expected, neither are species nor strains within species equally susceptible or sensitive to a particular agent, some responding more extensively than others, presumably as a consequence of genetic factors associated with rate(s) and route(s) of biotransformation of the chemical to reactive intermediates. In some instances, selective biotransformation plays a key role, with only those species in which the "correct" metabolite is formed being affected. This was the case with thalidomide, with the human, the monkey, and the rabbit producing a teratogenic intermediate — possibly a polar metabolite or an arene oxide — while other species did not (Williams et al., 1965; Gordon et al., 1981; Blake et al., 1982). An agent that is teratogenic in some species may exert little or no effect in others or, if similar teratogenic effects are seen, the frequency may be quite different. Additionally, abnormalities produced in one species may differ completely from those induced in another. Given this complex situation, what species are used as surrogates for the human?

As with other reproductive studies, the mouse, the rat, and the rabbit have provided the bulk of information on the teratogenic potential of chemicals because of (1) their genetic homogeneity, (2) the low incidence in most strains of spontaneous congenital anomalies, (3) the cost and ease of handling, breeding, and rearing these animals, and (4) the large litters born to the females. While animal experiments give only an approximation of possible effects in the human, Tuchmann-Duplessis has stated that not a single chemical exists that is teratogenic in the human that has not produced malformations in rodents (Tuchmann-Duplessis, 1972). A World Health Organization (WHO) expert panel suggested that, in addition to studies carried out in rodents and lagomorphs, teratogenicity studies should be done in the dog, the cat, the pig, or the monkey, prior to the extrapolation of results to the human (WHO Scientific Group, 1967). Most protocols call for teratogenicity studies in two species, one being a nonrodent, usually the rabbit but they could include the dog or cat.

As should be obvious from the previous sections of this chapter, it is impossible to design a single set of experimental approaches to explore all of the multilevel interrelationships between the mother and the developing embryo. The task is too complex and the solution to this difficulty has been to "break up" reproduction into manageable segments. We have examined how male and female gamete production can be studied independent of one another, yet combined with breeding studies to assess the overall effect of toxicant exposure on reproduction. The fate of pre- and postimplantation embryos can be studied independently by *in vitro* and *in vivo* techniques including breeding studies. In all of these scenarios, one of the endpoints of reproductive outcomes is the incidence, type, and severity of birth defects recorded at the necropsy of the offspring. However, teratogenicity can be studied independently of all of the other influences of hormonal, nutritional, and cytotoxic effects that might be contributing to the malformation incidence. One needs to begin with a healthy, normal conceptus *in situ* in a normal, healthy, untreated pregnant female bred with a normal, untreated male. In teratogenicity studies, one is dealing with two biological systems: the maternal organism and the embryo.

In the human, the period in which agents can affect the morphological development of the embryo is short, largely being completed by the eighth week of pregnancy at just about the time the woman becomes aware that she is pregnant. As is shown in Figure 5.9, the sequence of embryonic events during this 56-d period is such that each organ/system undergoes a critical stage of differentiation at a precise moment and that at these times, the susceptibility of the embryo is greatest, and specific damage to organs/tissues can occur (Tuchmann-Duplessis, 1975). Thus, the teratogenic period is equivalent to the period of primary organogenesis and gives rise to the concept of a "toxic" or "target" window for each organ system during which time period groups of cells are organizing, are rapidly dividing, and are susceptible to chemical injury. As can be seen, many of these target windows are quite narrow, requiring delivery of an appropriate target tissue concentration of agent at a specific time in order to be certain of eliciting a biological effect. The fetal period, beginning at the end of the 8th week of gestation, is one in which little further differentiation of organs occurs other than closure of the palate, the reduction of the umbilical hernia (at the 9th week), and the differentiation of the external genitalia (12th week) (Tuchmann-Duplessis, 1980).

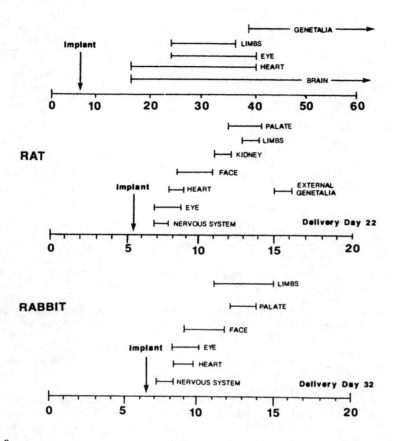

FIGURE 5.9

A comparison of critical periods of embryogenesis in the human, the rat, and the rabbit, indicating the concept of narrow "target windows," the time intervals during which organogenesis of specific tissues/organs occurs, these being crucial periods of cellular hypersusceptibility to chemical-induced cytotoxicity and the subsequent appearance of anomalies or birth defects. Note that the period of susceptibility in the human occurs in the first 60 d of the pregnancy, at a time when the woman would be unaware of the pregnancy. In the animal surrogate models, the extremely short duration of the "target windows" point out the necessity of exposing the animals to the appropriate concentration of test agent at the correct time in order to be assured that the agent will or will not exert an effect on a particular organ system. In the standard teratological study protocol, healthy pregnant females are exposed to an appropriate dosage range (three levels plus controls) from day 6 through day 15 (for mice and rats) or from day 6 through day 18 (for rabbits). Modified from Tuchmann-Duplessis (1975).

Turning to these surrogate animal models used in teratogenicity studies where the pregnancy is contracted into a period of 21 d (rat, mouse) or 32 d (rabbit), the "target windows" for some organ systems are sometimes no longer than a 24-h period (MacKenzie and Hoar, 1995) (Figure 5.9). The period of organogenesis, between the time of implantation (day 4.5 to 6.0 for mouse and rat; day 7 for rabbit) and approximately day 15 (mouse, rat) or day 18 (rabbit), is the time frame in which the test agent must be administered. The time intervals for exposure during primary organogenesis in other species are shown in Table 5.15.

The standard protocols involve breeding the untreated animals and ascertaining day 0 (by vaginal plug in mouse or rat, evidence of breeding in rabbit) and initiating

TABLE 5.15

Species Differences in Gestational Endpoints

Species	Implantation (day)	Primary organogenesis (days)	Average gestation (days)
Human	7–8	10–56	270
Rat	5.5–6	6–15	21–22
Mouse	4.5–5	6–15	19–20
Hamster	4.5–5	4–14	16
Rabbit	7	6–18	32
Guinea pig	6	6–20	67
Rhesus monkey	9	9–40	165
Dog	13–14	—	63
Pig	10–12	7–35	114

TABLE 5.16

Mammalian Neurobehavioral Test Battery

Parameter	Conduction of Study
Surface righting (postnatal days 4 and 7)	Righting reflex, placing the pups on their backs on a smooth surface and recording the time interval required to turn over with all four feet on the surface
Negative geotaxis (postnatal days 4 and 7)	Pups placed in a head-down position on a 30 inclined plane, measuring the time interval required for them to reorientate themselves to a head-up position
Cliff avoidance (postnatal day 7)	Pups placed on a platform 10 cm above a table top and positioned so that the forelimbs and snout are at a point where an imaginary line of the table edge is between the eye orbits. The time required to retreat backwards is recorded
Swimming behavior (postnatal days 4 and 14)	Pups are placed in a water tank (23°C), swimming behavior being rated for direction (straight, circling, floating), head angle out of water (ears out, ears half out, nose and top of head out, unable to hold head up), limb movements (all limbs, back limbs)
Olfactory orientation (postnatal day 14)	Pups placed in the connecting arm of a two-compartment box, one compartment containing fresh (unused) wood chips and the other used chips (home) with which the animal is familiar. The time required for the animal to find the "home" box is measured.

From Tanaka et al., *Food Chem. Toxicol.*, 30, 1015–1019 (1992). With permission.

treatment of the pregnant females at control, low, intermediate, and high dosage levels (n = 10 female rabbits or 20 female rats/treatment group) from day 6 through day 15 if the species is the mouse or rat and from day 6 through day 18 if the rabbit is used. The pregnant dams are euthanized 1 d prior to parturition and are necropsied, and the fetuses are examined for visible anomalies before dissection and microscopic examination of fixed and stained sections for internal defects. Great care is taken at necropsy to identify each fetus and its position in the uterine horn, beginning at the cervical end and proceeding to the ovarian end of the fallopian tubule. This is done on the off-chance that a gradient concentration of the test agent might be found in the uterine vessels, being highest at the cervical end, with those fetuses being more severely affected than the fetuses at the distal end. Some fetuses will be cleared with alcoholic potassium hydroxide and subsequently stained with alizarin red to examine skeletal defects. Dose-effect relationships will be established for defects and level(s) of treatment.

Alcohol, solvent and drug abuse, metal (mercury, lead, manganese) exposure, etc., have been associated with transplacental transport of the agents, with subtle neuroteratogenicity being observed only later. With the euthanasia of all offspring before parturition, there is no opportunity to study the appearance of functional deficits, particularly those associated with the nervous system still developing well into the postnatal period. Frequently, teratogenic protocols are modified to permit some treated pregnant animals to birth and rear their young, selective testing of neurobehavioral function(s) being conducted during and after weaning. Table 5.16 describes one functional and behavioral test battery (Tanaka et al., 1992). Other innovative tests of sensory, motor, and cognitive functions may be included.

VI. EMBRYO CULTURE

The culturing of preimplantation rodent embryos has already been described, these embryos proceeding quite normally *in vitro* up to the point of initiating implantation on the surface of the incubation flask. Embryonic development during the postimplantation phase of primary organogenesis involves a number of precisely timed cellular events including cell proliferation, migration, association, differentiation, and cell death. The exact mechanism by which an agent elicits a teratogenic effect cannot be closely monitored *in vivo* during organogenesis without destruction of the embryo. However, new techniques have been developed whereby a postimplantation embryo can be surgically removed from the uterus and can be cultured successfully *in vitro* for several days in suitable media. Such preparations can be used to screen chemicals *in vitro* for teratogenic potential.

The properties of an ideal *in vitro* teratogenicity screening technique would include (Wilson, 1978):

1. The use of biological subjects available in large numbers
2. Subjects undergoing progressive development
3. Relevance to known mechanisms of teratogenicity
4. Being easily performed, yielding interpretable results
5. An intact organism capable of absorbing, circulating, and excreting chemicals
6. Responsiveness to a wide variety of agents
7. Using doses of test agent approximately equivalent to those found at sites of action *in vivo*
8. Yielding a minimum number of false negative results
9. Control over dosage and the time of exposure
10. Elimination of maternal factors that might interfere with the test system's response to the agent

In general, the protocols call for the surgical removal of the postimplantation embryos of mice or rats at approximately day 8 of gestation, the dissection of extraneous tissue from the embryo — although leaving the yolk sac placenta intact — and transfer to a suitable medium such as serum at 37°C in an oxygenated environment (Sadler et al., 1982). Given the disadvantages that life support can be maintained for only a certain length of time *in vitro* until the cell systems become too complex, i.e., from approximately day 8 through day 13, this is the time period of primary organogenesis, and the major organ systems appear to develop quite normally in this artificial environment. This *in vitro* system provides an ideal technique by which to study mechanisms of action through continual microscopic monitoring of the developing embryo.

The responsiveness of the day 8 to day 12 rodent embryo to agents that are teratogenic or cytotoxic per se is quite remarkable (Homburger and Goldberg, 1985). Where test agents may require metabolic activation to reactive intermediates, this can be achieved by either (1) incubating the embryo in serum with test agent plus the usual hepatic S9 fraction with cofactors, or (2) administering the test agent to an animal, allowing it to biotransform the agent, and subsequently harvesting enough blood from the treated animal to permit culturing the embryo in the serum in order to ascertain if there is any circulating teratogenic intermediate(s) present. This latter technique has proven useful in assessing the fact that blood serum from female monkeys and women having histories of repeated fetal wastage failed to promote normal growth and development of rat embryos in culture (Klein et al., 1982; Carey et al., 1983; Muechler et al., 1984). The results of such studies suggested the presence of "endogenous" teratogenic factors in the sera of these individuals. Considerable mechanistic research has involved the use of various anticancer drugs, these agents being known to react with nucleic acid per se or following suitable metabolic activation (Homburger and Goldberg, 1985). While *in vitro* development of cultured rodent embryos does not extend beyond day 13, an endpoint at which the placenta takes on a more dominant nutrient acquisition role and the yolk sac is relegated to a minor role, most of the major organ systems will have responded to a teratogenic agent if it is positive. One should not be unduly concerned that development after day 14 cannot be examined.

VII. HARMONIZATION

With the number of potential protocols possible under Segment I, II, and III reproductive studies (Figure 5.1), it is not surprising that various national and international regulatory agencies have developed different, quite specific, testing criteria and minute details of study design (Speid et al., 1990; MacKenzie and Hoar, 1995). Considerable effort is being expended to harmonize guidelines for toxicity testing among agencies, permitting industry to avoid costly replication of studies having only minor deviations in design which would result in rejection of the studies when submitted to certain national agencies in support of product registration. Ideally, there should be one set of international guidelines, eliminating redundancy although maintaining flexibility. Nowhere has harmonization been more active than in reproductive toxicity testing (Manson, 1994). While the guidelines have not been finalized, there is general international agreement on "most probable option" designs for fertility and developmental toxicity studies.

As summarized by Manson (1994), the purpose of the fertility study is to evaluate treatment effects on gametogenesis, mating behavior, fertility, and viability of the conceptus. The study designs, shown in Figure 5.10, are for separate-sex studies. Females are treated for 2 weeks prior to mating, throughout mating, to the time of implantation (gestational day 6) at which time the treatment is discontinued, the females being euthanized at mid-pregnancy or at term to assess agent-induced effects on pre-implantation and post-implantation survival (Figure 10A). Male rodents are treated for 4 weeks before mating (Figure 10B), this exposure period being considered sufficient to detect functional effects on male fertility and mating behavior. At necropsy after 4 weeks, male reproductive organ weight, histology, and sperm (both

FERTILITY STUDIES

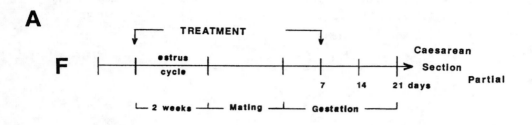

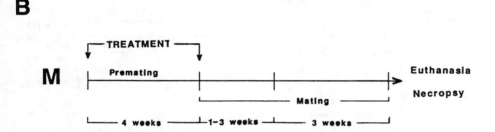

FIGURE 5.10
A schematic diagram of fertility studies in: A, female rodents treated for 2 weeks prior to and throughout mating up to implantation (gestational d 6), with euthanasia taking place at mid-pregnancy or at term to assess agent-induced effects on pre- and/or postimplantational loss; B, male rodents, treated for 4 weeks before mating, with necropsy after 6 weeks to assess agent-induced effects. Data from Manson (1944).

testicular and epididymal) counts are determined in order to assess agent-related effects. The pregnant females mated with the treated males may be euthanized at parturition for study.

The international guidelines for both range-finding and for developmental toxicity studies require treatment of pregnant females from the beginning of implantation (gestational day 6), through weaning (lactational day 21) (Figure 5.11). A range-finding study for a new agent may be essential with euthanasia of all animals at postpartum day 21 (Figure 5.11A). For developmental toxicity, the dams are allowed to birth and rear their offspring, with testing for postnatal functional development, including neurobehavioral as well as reproductive toxicity and the production of an F_2 generation. A variant of this study design permits caesarean-section of a portion of the treated, pregnant animals before parturition. The international guidelines require 20 pregnant animals per treatment group, with 40 for studies in which there are both caesarean-section and maternal delivery components.

VIII. SCREENING TESTS

Whole animal teratogenicity tests are expensive and time-consuming. Ideally, what would be useful is some type of short-term *in vitro* test system that could be used to screen chemicals rapidly for teratogenic activity, allowing investigators to proceed with more detailed, in-depth investigations on the positive ones. Such a test system should (Fabro, 1985):

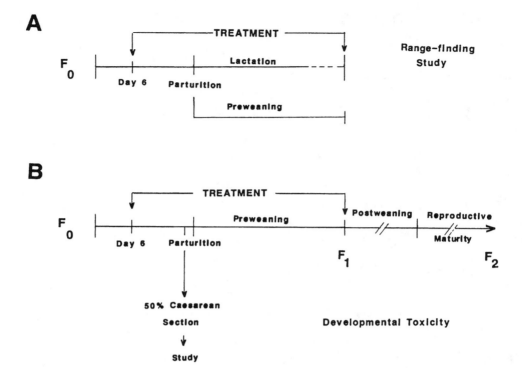

FIGURE 5.11
A schematic diagram of the international guidelines for developmental studies in female rodents with:
A, a range-finding study where dams and offspring are euthanized at postpartum day 21, having been
treated from gestational day 6 through weaning; and B, a developmental study where treatment is
continuous from gestational day 6 through to weaning, with some animals being euthanized at partition
while others are allowed to deliver, their litters (F_1) being studied until they attain reproductive maturity.
Data from Manson (1994).

1. Produce quantifiable results
2. Give an estimate of the hazard of a chemical to humans
3. Test most of the developmental events which, if disrupted, could produce a poor
   pregnancy outcome
4. Be easy to perform and to evaluate
5. Be accurate and inexpensive
6. Be capable of testing large numbers of chemicals rapidly

Additional desirable features of an ideal screening test include the following: (1) use
of an intact organism capable of absorbing, circulating, and excreting chemicals, (2)
give few "false negative" results, and (3) react to varied types of agents.

The pre- and postimplanatation embryo techniques described above have been
used as screening techniques for potential teratogens. Extensive use has been made
of embryonic tissue (limb bud mesenchymal cells, neuroepithelium, renal cells, chick
neural crest cells, etc.) for both organ culture and primary cell culture techniques,
these tissues being quite content *in vitro*, with development/growth as well as
biochemical and morphological differentiation proceeding satisfactorily (Welsch, 1987).
Cell differentiation, migration, and intercellular communications can be examined.

Not surprisingly, a number of nonmammalian cell systems have been tested as potential methods of detecting cytotoxic/teratogenic agents in embryonic development (Segment II). One such assay has involved the *Hydra attenuata*, a small freshwater coelenterate that can be dissociated by homogenization, the cells being incubated in a medium with clusters of cells developing into a complete adult organism in the absence of cytotoxic agents while producing peculiar disorganized structures in the presence of such agents (Johnson et al., 1982; Johnson and Gabel, 1983). Indeed, the hydra has been used as an "artificial" embryo since during the regeneration into a totally new adult hydra, they pass through an ordered ontogenic sequence of most of the developmental phenomena including cell migration, differentiation, induction, etc., expected of any developing system. A comparison of developmental toxicity indices in mammals and hydra reveal an astonishingly good correlation for a wide range of chemicals (Johnson and Gabel, 1983; Johnson and Christian, 1985). The evaluation of equimolar concentrations of chlorophenols in the cultured hydra assay and in postimplantation whole rat embryo culture revealed a good linear correlation between the two assays for a developmental hazard index, making these assays useful for the rapid detection and ranking of hazardous chemicals in complex mixtures of chemical wastes (Mayura et al., 1991). A second nonmammalian system involves the embryo of the amphibian *Xenopus laevis*: the FETAX (frog embryo teratogenesis assay: *xenopus*) quantitative estimation of teratogenic hazard (Fabro, 1985). Cultured over a 96-h period of exposure to the test agent, xenopus embryos undergo growth and development, structural changes, motility, and pigmentation, all endpoints that can be measured as indices of teratogenic hazard (Brown and Fabro, 1982). This assay system has proven to be useful in the detection of a variety of moderate-to-strong teratogens and its performance can be enhanced with the inclusion of a suitable metabolic activation system to biotransform weak teratogens into more potent intermediates (Dawson et al., 1989; Fort et al., 1988; Fort and Bantle, 1990).

Unfortunately, while some of these systems appear to be valid tools for screening potential teratogens, regulatory agencies have been reluctant to break away from the standardized *in vivo* testing protocols since these newer test systems have not been validated. There is also the problem of extrapolation from these tests to the human, considerably more difficult than using the routine animal tests for teratogenic human risk assessment. In addition, there are real concerns of litigation if a product, tested by a new but not widely accepted method, should be shown to elicit adverse effects on developing embryos, effects that might have (or have not) been identified by a "tried-and-true" standard technique. To date, no one is willing to risk this. Teratogenicity tests should be able to answer these three questions (Fabro, 1985):

1. Can the agent induce developmental defects (teratogenic potential)?
2. What are the effective doses (teratogenic potency)?
3. Are the effective doses below adult toxic doses (teratogenic hazard)?

It is a matter of time, but advances will be made in the area of screening assays and their validation. The reader may recall that, not too many years ago, the Ames test for mutagenicity was an unvalidated oddity. It became a validated standard screening technique, albeit overworked and frequently misinterpreted.

REFERENCES

Amann, R.P. Use of animal models for detecting specific alterations in reproduction. *Fundam. Appl. Toxicol.* 2: 13-16 (1982).

Bavister, B.D. *The Mammalian Preimplantation Embryo.* Plenum Press, New York (1987).

Bibbo, M., Gill, W., Azizi, F., Blough, R., Fang, V., Rosenfield, R., Schumacher, G., Sleeper, K., Sonek, M., and Weid, G. Follow-up study of male and female offspring of DES-exposed mothers. *Obstet. Gynecol.* 49: 1-8 (1977).

Blake, D.A., Gordon, G.B., and Spielberg, S.P. The role of metabolic activation in thalidomide teratogenesis. *Teratology* 25: 28-29A (1982).

Blazak, W.F., Rushbrook, C.J., Ernst, T.L., Stewart, B.E., Spak, D., Dibiasio-Erwin, D., and Black, V. Relationship between breeding performance and testicular/epididymal functioning in male Sprague-Dawley rats exposed to nitrobenzene (NB). *Toxicologist* 5: 121 (Abstract No. 484) (1985a).

Blazak, W.F., Ernst, T.L., and Stewart, B.E. Potential indicators of reproductive toxicity: testicular sperm production, and epididymal sperm number, transit time and motility in Fischer 344 rats. *Fundam. Appl. Toxicol.* 5: 1097-1103 (1985b).

Boue, J.G., Boue, A., and Lazar, P. Retrospective and prospective epidemiological studies of 1,500 karyotyped spontaneous human abortions. *Teratol.* 12: 11-26 (1975).

Brown, N.A. and Fabro, S. The *in vitro* approach to terato-genicity testing. In *Developmental Toxicology.* Snell, K. (Editor). Croom Helm, London (1982), pp. 33-57.

Carey, S.W., Klein, N.W., Frederickson, W.T., Sackett, G.P., Greenstein, R.M., Sehgal, P., and Elliott, M. Analysis of sera from monkeys with histories of fetal wastage and the identification of teratogenicity in sera from human chronic spontaneous aborters using rat embryo cultures. *Trophoblast Res.* 1: 347-360 (1983).

Cross, J.C., Werb, Z., and Fisher, S.J. Implantation and the placenta: key pieces of the development puzzle, *Science* 266, 1508-1518 (1994).

Cummings, A. Toxicological mechanisms of implantation failure. *Fundam. Appl. Toxicol.* 15: 571-579 (1990).

Cummings, A.M., Perreault, S.D., and Harris, S.T. Use of bromoergo-cryptine in the validation of protocols for the assessment of mechanisms of early pregnancy loss in the rat, *Fundam. Appl. Toxicol.* 17: 563-574 (1991).

Dawson, D.A., Fort, D.J., Newell, D.L., and Bantle, J.A. Developmental toxicity testing with FETAX: evaluation of five compounds. *Drug Chem. Toxicol.* 12: 67-75 (1989).

Dixon, R.L. Potential of environmental factors to affect development of reproductive systems. *Fundam. Appl. Toxicol.* 2: 5-12 (1982).

Dixon, R.L. (Editor). *Reproductive Toxicology.* Raven Press, New York (1985).

Ehling, U.H., Machemer, L., Buselmaier, W., Dycka, J., Frohberg, H., Kratochvilova, J., Lang, R., Lorke, D., Muller, D., Peh, J., Rohrborn, G., Roll, R., Schulz-Schencking, M., and Wiemann, H. Standard protocol for the dominant lethal test on male mice. *Arch. Toxicol.* 39: 173-185 (1978).

Eliasson, R. Semen analysis. *Environ. Health Perspect.* 24: 81-85 (1978).

Fabro, S. On predicting environmentally-induced human reproductive hazards: An overview and historical perspective. *Fundam. Appl. Toxicol.* 5: 609-614 (1985).

Fort, D.J. and Bantle, J.A. Analysis of the mechanism of isoniazid-induced developmental toxicity with frog embryo teratogenesis assay: xenopus (FETAX). *Teratogen. Carcinogen. Mutagen.* 10: 463-476 (1990).

Fort, D.J., Dawson, D.A., and Bantle, J.A. Development of a metabolic activation system for the frog embryo teratogenesis assay: Xenopus (FETAX). *Teratogen. Carcinogen. Mutagen.* 8: 251-263 (1988).

Gordon, G.B., Spielberg, S.P., Blake, D.A., and Balasubramanian, B. Thalidomide teratogenesis: Evidence for a toxic arene oxide metabolite. *Proc. Natl. Acad. Sci.* 78: 2545-2548 (1981).

Haley, T.J. and Berndt, W.O. (Editors). *Handbook of Toxicology.* Hemisphere Publishing Corporation, Washington (1987).

Hayes, A.W. (Editor). *Principles and Methods of Toxicology.* Second Edition. Raven Press, New York (1989).

Health and Welfare Canada. The Testing of Chemicals for Carcinogenicity, Mutagenicity and Teratogenicity (1973).

Herbst, A.L., Ulfelder, H., and Poskanzer, D.C. Adenocarcinoma of the vagina. Association of maternal stilbestrol therapy with tumor appearance in young women. *New Eng. J. Med.* 284: 878-881 (1971).

Homburger, F. and Goldberg, A.M. (Editors). *Concepts In Toxicology. In Vitro Embryotoxicity and Teratogenicity Tests.* Karger, New York (1985).

Iannaccone, P.M. Long term effects of exposure to methyl-nitrosourea on blastocysts following transfer to surrogate female mice. *Cancer Res.* 44: 2785-2789 (1984).

Johnson, E.M. Perspectives on reproductive and developmental toxicology. *Toxicol. Indus. Health* 2: 453-482 (1986).

Johnson, E.M. and Christian, M.S. The hydra assay for detecting and ranking developmental hazards. In *Concepts in Toxicology. In Vitro Embryotoxicity and Teratogenicity Tests.* F. Homburger and A.M. Goldberg (Editors). Karger, New York (1985), pp. 107-113.

Johnson, E.M. and Gabel, B.E.G. An artificial "embryo" for detection of abnormal developmental biology. *Fundam. Appl. Toxicol.* 3: 243-249 (1983).

Johnson, E.M., Gorman, R.M., Gabel, B.E.G., and George, M.E. The *Hydra attenuata* system for detection of teratogenesic hazards. *Teratogen. Carcinogen. Mutagen.* 2: 263-276 (1982).

Kaufman, R.H., Adam, E., Binder, G.L., and Gerthoffer, E. Upper genital tract changes and pregnancy outcome in offspring exposed *in utero* to diethylstilbestrol. *Am. J. Obstet. Gynecol.* 137: 299-308 (1980).

Klein, N.W., Plenefish, J.D., Carey, S.W., Frederickson, W.T., Sackett, G.P., Burbacher, T.M., and Parker, R.M. Serum from monkeys with histories of fetal wastage causes abnormalities in cultured rat embryos. *Science* 215: 66-69 (1982).

Kline, J. and Stein, Z. Very early pregnancy. In *Reproductive Toxicology.* Dixon, R.L. (Editor). Raven Press, New York (1985), pp. 251-265.

Lacy, D. and Pettit, A.J. Sites of hormone production in the mammalian testis, and their significance in the control of male fertility. *Brit. Med. Bull.* 26: 87-91 (1970).

Lamb, J.C., IV and Chapin, R.E. Experimental models of male reproductive toxicity. In *Endocrine Toxicology.* Thomas, J.A., Korach, K.S. and McLachlan, J.A. (Editors). Raven Press, New York (1985), pp. 85-115.

Lee, I.P. and Dixon, R.L. Antineoplastic drug effects on spermatogenesis by velocity sedimentation cell separation. *Toxicol. Appl. Pharmacol.* 23: 20-41 (1972).

MacKenzie, K.M. and Hoar, R.M. Developmental Toxicology. In *CRC Handbook of Toxicology,* Derelenko, M.J. and Hollinger, M.A. (Editors), CRC Press, Boca Raton, Ch. 12, pp. 403-450 (1995).

Manson, J.M. Testing of pharmaceutical agents for reproductive toxicity. In *Developmental Toxicology,* Second Edition, Kimmel, C.A. and Buelke-Sam, J. (Editors), Raven Press, New York, Ch. 15, pp. 379-402 (1994).

Mattison, D.R. (Editor). *Reproductive Toxicology.* Alan R. Liss, Inc., New York (1983).

Mattison, D.R., Plowchalk, D.R., Meadows, M.J., Al-Juburi, A.Z., Gandy, J., and Malek, A. Reproductive toxicity: Male and female reproductive systems as targets for chemical injury. *Med. Clin. of N.A.* 74: 391-411 (1990).

Mayura, K., Smith, E.E., Clement, B.A., and Phillips, T.D. Evaluation of the developmental toxicity of chlorinated phenols utilizing *Hydra attenuata* and postimplantation rat embryos in culture. *Toxicol. Appl. Pharmacol.* 108: 253-266 (1991).

McLachlan, J.A. and Dixon, R.L. Reduced fertility in female mice exposed prenatally to procarbazine. *Fed. Proc.* 32: 745 (Abstract No. 2988) (1973).

McLaren, A. Early mammalian development. *Prog. Clin. Biol. Res.* 163A: 29-35 (1985).

Miller, R.K., Kellogg, C.K., and Saltzman, R.A. Reproductive and perinatal toxicology. In *Handbook of Toxicology,* Haley, T.J. and Berndt, W.O. (Editors), Hemisphere Publishing Corp., Washington, Ch. 7, pp. 195-309 (1987).

Mosher, W.D. and Pratt, W.F. Fecundity and infertility in the United States, 1965-1982. NCHS Advance Data 104. Publication PHS 85-1250. Washington, D.C. U.S. Public Health Service (1985), p. 1-8.

Muechler, E., Mariona, F.G., Miller, R.K., Gilles, P.A., Rhinehardt, E.A., Klein, N.W., and Greenstein, R.M. The culture of rat embryos and sera from women with histories of spontaneous abortion. *Fertil. Steril.* 41: 225 (Abstract No. 51) (1984).

Nelson, K. and Holmes, L.B. Malformations due to presumed spontaneous mutations in newborn infants. *N. Engl. J. Med.* 320: 19-23 (1989).

Organization for Economic Cooperation and Development (OECD). Proposal for New Guidelline 416-Two-Generation Reproduction Toxicity Study. OECD Draft Document, April 1996.

Overstreet, J.W. and Blazak, W.F. The biology of human male reproduction: an overview. *Am. J. Ind. Med.* 4: 5-15 (1983).

Poskanzer, D. and Herbst, A. Epidemiology of vaginal adenosis and adenocarcinoma associated with exposure to stilbestrol *in utero. Cancer* 39: 1892-1895 (1977).

Sadler, T.W., Horton, W.E., and Warner, C.W. Whole embryo culture: a screening technique for teratogens? *Teratogen. Carcinogen. Mutagen.* 2: 243-253 (1982).

Schardein, J.L. *Chemically Induced Birth Defects.* Marcel Dekker, New York (1985).

Smith, J.M. and Costlow, R.D. Recognition, evaluation and control of chemical embryotoxins in the workplace. *Fundam. Appl. Toxicol.* 5: 626-633 (1985).

Speid, L.H., Lumley, C.E., and Walker, S.R. Harmonization of guidelines for toxicity testing of pharmaceuticals by 1992. *Reg. Toxicol. Pharmacol.* 12: 179-211 (1990).

Spielmann, H. and Vogel, R. Unique role of studies on preimplantation embryos to understand mechanisms of embryo-toxicity in early pregnancy. *Crit. Rev. Toxicol.* 20: 51-64 (1989).

Steinberger, E. and Steinberger, A. Spermatogenic function of the testes. In *Handbook of Physiology. Section 7. Endocrinology Vol. V. Male Reproductive System*. Hamilton, D.W. and Greep, R.O. (Editors). American Physiological Society, Washington, D.C. (1975), pp. 1-19.

Takeuchi, I.K. Teratogenic effects of methylnitrosourea on pregnant mice before implantation. *Experientia* 40: 879-881 (1984).

Taaka, T., Takahashi, O., and Oishi, S. Reproductive and neuro-behavioral effects in three-generation toxicity study of piperonyl butoxide administered to mice. *Food Cosmet. Toxicol.* 30: 1015-1019 (1992).

Tuchmann-Duplessis, H. Teratogenic drug screening. Present procedures and requirements. *Teratology* 5: 271-286 (1972).

Tuchmann-Duplessis, H. *Drug Effects on the Fetus*. ADIS Press, Sydney (1975).

Tuchmann-Duplessis, H. The experimental approach to terato-genicity. *Ecotox. Environ. Safety* 4: 422-433 (1980).

Vogel, R., Granata, I., and Spielmann, H. Cytogenetic studies on preimplantation mouse embryos exposed to methylnitrosourea *in vitro*. *Reprod. Toxicol.* 3: 23-30 (1989).

Warburton, D. Reproductive loss: how much is preventable? *New Eng. J. Med.* 316: 158-160 (1987).

Welsch, F. (Editor). *Approaches to Elucidate Mechanisms in Teratogenesis*. Hemisphere Publishing Corp., Washington (1987).

WHO Scientific Group. Principles for the testing of drugs for teratogenicity. WHO Tech. Rep. No. 364 (1967), pp. 1-18.

Williams, R.T., Schumacher, H., Fabro, S., and Smith, R.L. The chemistry and metabolism of thalidomide. In *Embryopathic Activity of Drugs*. Robson, J.M., Sullivan, F.M., and Smith, R.L. (Editors). Little, Brown and Co., Boston (1965), pp. 167-193.

Wilson, J.G. Teratogenic effects of environmental chemicals. *Fed. Proc.* 36: 1698-1703 (1977).

Wilson, J.G. Survey of *in vitro* systems. Their potential use in teratogenicity screening. In *Handbook of Teratology*. Vol. 4. Wilson, J.G. and Fraser, F.C. (Editors). Plenum Press, New York (1978).

Working, P.K. (Editor). *Toxicology of the Male and Female Reproductive System*. Hemisphere Publishing Corp., New York (1989).

Working, P.K. and Bus, J.S. Failure of fertilization as a cause of preimplantation loss induced by methyl chloride in Fischer 344 rats. *Toxicol. Appl. Pharmacol.* 86: 124-130 (1986).

Working, P.K. Bus, J.S., and Hamm, T.E., Jr. Reproductive effects of inhaled methyl chloride in the male Fischer 344 rat. I. Mating performance and dominant lethal assay. *Toxicol. Appl. Pharmacol.* 77: 133-143 (1985a).

Working, P.K., Bus, J.S., and Hamm, T.E., Jr. Reproductive effects of inhaled methyl chloride in the male Fischer 344 rat. II. Spermatogonial toxicity and sperm quality. *Toxicol. Appl. Pharmacol.* 77: 144-157 (1985b).

Zenick, H., Clegg, E.D., Perreault, S.D., Klinefelter, G.R., and Gray, L.E. Assessment of male reproductive toxicity. A risk assessment approach. In *Principles and Methods of Toxicology*. Third Edition, Hayes, A.W. (Editor), Raven Press, New York, Ch. 27, pp. 937-988 (1994).

Chapter 6

MUTAGENESIS — CARCINOGENESIS

I. INTRODUCTION

Major consequences of cellular cytotoxicity are mutations in the deoxyribonucleic (DNA) or ribonucleic (RNA) acids, giving rise to adverse reproductive outcomes, as discussed in the previous chapter, or in carcinogenicity. Theories have been advanced that the process of mitogenesis, defined as the induction of increased cell proliferation, may be responsible for such events, based on the fact that a dividing cell is much more at risk of mutating than is a quiescent one, there being an increased chance of reproducing un- or misrepaired nucleic acids (Ames and Gold, 1990; Cohen and Ellwein, 1990). However attractive, mitogenesis is not the only cause of cancer, occurring frequently under the control of endogenous agents in the absence of cancer (Weinstein, 1991).

Genotoxic agents may be defined as "any agent which, by virtue of its physical and chemical properties, can induce or produce heritable changes in those parts of the genetic apparatus that exercise homeostatic control over somatic cells, thereby determining their malignant transformation" (Druckery, 1973). In the broadest meaning, "malignant" could refer to genetic alterations or mutations resulting both in defects in reproductive outcomes and in carcinogenicity. Interaction of agents, both physical and chemical, with nucleic acids results in the disruption of the transfer of genetic information and the production of either a lethal effect with subsequent death of the cell(s) or weak-to-severe damage to one or more cellular functions at the level of ribonucleic acid (RNA), membranes, proteins, and enzymes. These experiments are extremely complex to conduct in intact animals, generally requiring long-term, multigeneration studies. Except for the dominant lethal test discussed in the previous chapter, few results could be ascribed with any certainty to particular damage to the nucleic acids in terms of a dose-effect relationship other than for extremely potent agents. Therefore, considerable interest has focused on a variety of short-term, *in vitro* test systems using microorganisms, plants, insects, and cultured mammalian cells that have been developed to screen potentially mutagenic, teratogenic, and/or carcinogenic agents. Such screening assays allow the rapid assessment of large numbers of chemicals in a relatively short period of time, as well as providing some indication of possible mechanism(s) of action. Positive results in such systems might eliminate the need for the more costly, time consuming *in vivo* studies.

TABLE 6.1

Chemical-Induced Alterations in Cellular Nucleic Acids Resulting in a Defective Genetic Code

Biological effect	Site of action
Point mutations	• Base-pair transformations
	1. *Transition — one purine base substituting for another purine base*
	2. *Transversion — a purine base substituting for a pyrimidine base (or vice versa)*
	• Chemical effects
	1. *Base conversion*, i.e., cytosine to uracil or adenine to hypoxanthine
	2. *Alkylation* by carbonium ions, electrophilic-nucleophilic interaction producing methylated bases
	• Abnormal analogs — anticancer agents
Frameshift mutations	• The deletion (or addition of one or a few nucleotide pairs sufficient for the genetic code out of sequence
Clastogenesis (chromosomal aberrations)	• Deletions, insertions, translocations, rearrangements, etc. that are detectable by light microscopy as breaks, gaps, exchanges, isolated piece
Chromosomal mutations	• Incorrect reincorporation of broken portions

II. MUTAGENESIS

Mutations can be considered hereditary changes produced in the genetic information encoded in the deoxyribonucleic acid (DNA) in cells. A mutation may also be defined as a stable heritable change in a DNA nucleotide sequence which may be detected as a phenotypic change (Venitt, 1981). A variety of reactions can take place to yield a defective genetic code, as is outlined in Table 6.1, the net result being a misreading or misinterpretation of the DNA triplet code or even disruption of entire sections of the chromosomes. It should be appreciated that few positive agents induce only one type of mutational change. A spectrum of damage may be seen, dependent upon (1) the level of exposure, (2) the primary DNA alteration, and (3) subsequent secondary effects caused by the response of the organism to the initial alteration in the DNA (Venitt, 1981). A mutagenic agent may be expected to cause profoundly different mutational effects in organisms of different genetic background.

As will be seen below, the short-term tests use *prokaryotic* and *eukaryotic* cells in culture. The former, including bacteria and blue-green algae (cyanobacteria), do not have a true nucleus, the nuclear material being dispersed throughout the cell cytoplasm, and such cells reproducing by cell division. Eukaryotic cells, characteristic of cells of higher organisms, possess a true nucleus bounded by a nuclear membrane and reproduce by mitosis. Many of the bacterial test systems use *auxotrophic* organisms which cannot grow unless some nutrient, usually an amino acid or a sugar, is included in the minimal medium since they cannot synthesize this nutrient. In effect, the auxotrophic organism is already a mutant bacterium with a highly specific defect in a locus, a freak if you will. Its counterpart — the normal or "wild-type," nonmutated, *prototrophic* organism — need not be supplied with the essential nutrient substance, being capable of synthesizing its own supply from components in the minimal medium. The basis of the bacterial tests involve either (1) a reverse-mutation from the nutrient-dependent strain to a "wild-type" capable of sustaining itself on minimal medium, or (2) a forward-mutation whereby additional, agent-induced changes in the genetics of the cell result in a new easily identified and scored phenotype. Forward mutations present a larger genetic target for the chemical to act upon, with mutations occurring at several loci within one gene or being spread over several genes and the relatively easy identification of a new phenotype. Reverse mutation assays, using organisms with mutations at an easily detected locus, provide quite a

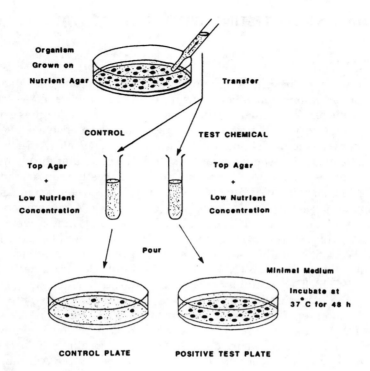

FIGURE 6.1

The basic microbial mutagenicity assay (the plate test) capable of detecting a direct-acting mutagen. Suitable quantities (10^8 organisms/ml) of a mutant tester strain organism (*Salmonella typhimurium, Escherichia coli*), grown on nutrient agar, are incubated in test tubes with low nutrient agar plus top agar in the presence and absence of different concentrations of test chemicals. The tubes are decanted onto plates of minimal medium and incubated at 37°C for 48 h. Generally, a dose-related growth of colonies on the minimal medium is indicative of a mutagenic action by the test agent, converting the mutant organisms from an *auxotrophic* form where a specific nutrient (amino acid, sugar) is required to a *prototrophic* form that can synthesize the required nutrient from the simple chemicals in the minimal medium.

small, specific, and selective target site for the chemical to act on, whereby the second, agent-induced mutation must abolish or modify the effect(s) of the preexisting mutation (Venitt, 1981).

The basis of the bacterial mutagenicity assay is shown in Figure 6.1. For a direct-acting mutagen, the reverse-mutation "plate test" — also called the "plate-incorporation" or "agar overlay" test — requires that test tubes of the suitable bacterial strain (n = 10^8 organisms/ml) be mixed with known concentrations of the test agent and be incubated in melted top agar containing a small quantity of the nutrient essential for the growth of the auxotrophic organism. This permits the auxotrophic bacterium to divide for several generations in the presence of the test chemical. The incubated mixture is then decanted onto the surface of an agar plate containing glucose and simple salts, the essential nutrient being omitted from this agar (minimal agar). With the depletion of the small amount of essential nutrient, all of the auxotrophic organisms stop growing except those affected by the test agent which have reverted (back-mutated) to prototrophy, these organisms forming colonies, each one being the progeny of a single revertant, "wild-type" bacterium. Up to concentrations where the mutagen causes extensive or even lethal damage to the genome of the auxotrophic bacteria, the number of revertants usually increases proportionally to the amount of test agent in the incubation medium.

III. MUTAGENICITY TESTING WITH PROKARYOTIC CELL SYSTEMS

A. The Ames Test

Based on the hypothesis that carcinogens are initially mutagens — some causing base-repair substitutions and others causing frameshift mutations — and that carcinogenesis is the result of somatic mutations, Ames and his colleagues experimented with microbial assay systems that would be rapid and inexpensive to use as efficient screening techniques to detect potentially hazardous chemicals (Ames et al., 1973a). Positive results in such screening assays would be a signal that the chemical should undergo further testing in more time-consuming and costly mammalian systems.

The most extensively used bacterial assay system has been the one using mutant tester strains of *Salmonella typhimurium* developed by Dr. Ames and co-workers in the early 1970s (Ames et al., 1972a, 1972b). The original strains were genetically defective for histidine (his-), the organisms being unable to synthesize this chemical. One strain (TA1535) could be used to detect mutagens that caused base-pair substitutions, while two other strains (TA1537, TA1538) would detect frameshift mutations (Ames et al., 1975b). The sensitivity of the organisms to genetic damage was greatly increased by the incorporation of two additional mutations: one, *uvrB*, caused the loss of the excision repair system (the organism could no longer repair some of the damage to DNA); the second, *rfa*, resulted in the loss of the lipopolysaccharide membrane barrier coating the surface of the bacterium (making the bacterium more permeable to chemicals in solution) (Ames et al., 1973a, 1973b; Ames et al., 1975b). Two additional strains (TA100 and TA98) were developed by transferring an antibiotic resistance R factor plasmid (pKM101) to TA1535 and TA1538 strains, respectively (McCann et al., 1975b). These modified strains were now capable of detecting classes of carcinogens not previously detectable with strains in use, plus they had increased sensitivity to the point of detecting weakly mutagenic agents (Table 6.2). For routine mutagenicity testing, it is recommended that the three standard strains (TA1535, TA1537, TA1538) plus the two R-factor strains (TA98 and TA100) be used (Ames et al., 1975b; Maron and Ames, 1983). Rapid screening can be carried out using the TA100 and/or the TA1535 strains, the latter having a much lower spontaneous mutation rate for mutagens that do not preferentially revert TA100 (Ames et al., 1975b; McCann et al., 1975b). By altering the genome of the tester strains by deletions or additions of genetic information, the sensitivity of the strains was increased and the detection rate of carcinogens as mutagens rose from approximately 70% to over 90% (McCann et al., 1975a, 1975b). The assay system does not respond to known noncarcinogens. The utility of this microbial test system in detecting carcinogens/mutagens from various sources and in every sort of biological fluid (blood, urine, saliva) as well as air, soil, water, and food has been discussed extensively (Ames, 1979, 1983; McCann et al., 1975b; McCann and Ames, 1976).

1. The Spot Test

As a tool for the rapid screening of large numbers of chemicals for mutagenic potential, the spot test is the simplest technique. It consists of the incubation of a suitable tester strain of *Salmonella typhimurium* (TA98, TA100 or TA1535) in a plate-incorporation test (minimal medium to which is applied an agar overlay containing the organisms and a minimal amount of histidine to initiate growth but not to sustain it), placing the test agent (a few crystals or microlitres or a filter paper disk soaked with a solution of known concentration of the chemical) directly on the agar, followed

TABLE 6.2

Genotype of *Salmonella typhimurium* TA Strains Used in Mutagen Testing Systems

Strain	His	LPS	Repair	R-factor	Plasmid pKM101	Nature of Mutation
			Mutation Nomenclature[a]			
TA97	hisD6610	rfa	uvrB	+R	+	+4 near CCC
TA98	hisD3052	rfa	uvrB	+R	+	−1 near CG
TA100	hisG46	rfa	uvrB	+R	+	AT → GC
TA102	pAQ1 hisG428/Δhis	rfa	+	+R	+	GC → AT ochre
TA1535	hisG46	rfa	uvrB	−R	−	AT → GC
TA1537	hisC3076	rfa	uvrB	−R	−	+1 near C...C
TA1538	hisC3052	rfa	uvrB	−R	−	−1 near CG...CG

[a] Strains are all histidine deficient (his-), being unable to synthesize this chemical due to mutations at given loci as indicated; LPS, the rfa mutation resulting in the loss of a lipopolysaccharide from the membrane coating the bacterium which allows easier penetration of chemicals through the membrane envelope; Repair, uvrB, a mutation resulting in the loss of a DNA-repair system; R-factor, strains having (+) or deficient (−) in an antibiotic resistance-factor plasmid pKM101.
From Ames et al. (1975b).

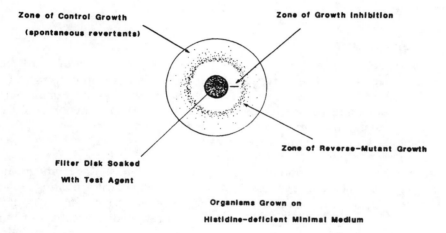

FIGURE 6.2
The rapid "spot" test conducted with suitable tester strain organisms grown in low nutrient medium with top agar, decanted onto minimal medium, and once the "lawn" of bacteria is established, exposed for 48 h to the test agent in solution on a filter disk. The diffusion of the chemical through the agar medium guarantees that the organisms are exposed to a range of concentrations of test agent. A zone of growth inhibition, possibly due to cytotoxicity (lethal mutations), will be observed beyond which a ring of prototrophic colonies will be established, indicating a mutagenic action on the auxotrophic organisms. A few spontaneous revertant colonies will be visible at the periphery of the plate. With single plates and different strains of auxotrophic organisms exposed to the same concentration of test agent on the filter disk, the most sensitive tester strain can be selected for more detailed studies.

by a subsequent period of incubation during which the agent will diffuse through the agar. Water-soluble agents have difficulty in penetrating the agar. Some preliminary indication of the toxicity of the chemical for the bacterial strain can be obtained by the size of the zone of growth inhibition of the background "lawn" of bacteria and/or the growth of revertant bacteria around the application site (Figure 6.2) (Ames et al., 1975b; McCann and Ames, 1976). In this manner, a range of concentrations of chemical is tested on one petri dish since the chemical diffuses outward through the agar becoming more diluted with distance. If a different tester strain is applied to each plate in this screening assay, the most sensitive strain can be selected to obtain a proper dose-response relationship in an expanded study.

2. The Original Ames Test

The initial test system used suitable amounts (10^8 organisms/ml final concentration) of a selected tester strain incubated in test tubes with molten top agar, a small amount of histidine, and a range of concentrations of the test chemical. The incubation mixture was applied uniformly over a petri dish containing minimal medium agar (no histidine), followed by incubation at 37°C for 48 h (Figure 6.1). Replicate plates (N = 3 or 4) were "carried" for each concentration of test agent plus a suitable number of control plates. After 48 h, the revertant colonies on the control and "chemical-exposed" plates were counted and the thin background lawn of small colonies surviving on the small amount of histidine was examined (Ames et al., 1975b; Maron and Ames, 1983). The corrected number of revertant colonies (total number minus the spontaneous revertant colonies) was plotted on graph paper against each concentration of test agent (microgram/ml) in the incubation medium to yield a dose-response relationship which, usually, was linear over a portion of the dosage range.

3. The Standard Ames Test

As was stated by Ames et al. (1973a), the principal limitation of any bacterial system for detecting mutagenicity was that bacteria do not duplicate mammalian metabolism in activating chemicals. It is well known that not all carcinogens are active per se but undergo Phase I biotransformation, usually involving the cytochrome P-450 related monooxygenases, into highly reactive intermediates, the ultimate carcinogens. In the original Ames assay, only direct-acting carcinogens would be detected; procarcinogens, requiring metabolic activation beforehand, would not be detected since bacteria cannot perform this task very efficiently. Homogenates of mammalian liver, an excellent source of the necessary chemical-activating enzymes, have been used by other investigators to convert procarcinogenic agents into ultimate carcinogens (Garner et al., 1972; Malling, 1971). With the addition of rat or human hepatic homogenates to the incubation mixture (organisms, top agar, histidine, test chemical, buffer), many suspect carcinogens became positive mutagens by virtue of "activation" to reactive intermediates capable of interacting with the bacterial genome.

Since the enzymatic activity is highly variable between individual livers within and between species, any investigator would appreciate a standardized enzyme preparation for the activation of procarcinogens/promutagens to mutagenic intermediates. The ideal preparation would be one possessing the maximum amount of enzymatic activity that could be stored for prolonged periods of time in aliquots small enough that a single tube from a large pool of prepared material could be removed from storage and used for an entire day, with the unused portion being discarded. To acquire this source of monooxygenase activity, young adult male rats (strain of choice) of 200 to 300 g body weight are treated with a single injection (ip) of a commercial mixture of polychlorinated biphenyls (Aroclor 1254, diluted in peanut or corn oil to a concentration of 200 mg/ml) at a dosage of 500 mg/kg. The animals receive water and food *ad libitum* for 5 consecutive days until 12 h before euthanasia, at which time food is removed. The animals are killed by a blow to the head followed by decapitation. Homogenates of the liver (30% w/v) are prepared,

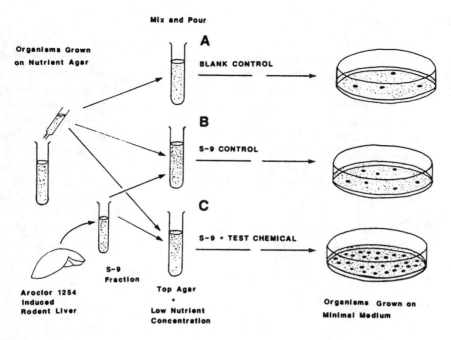

FIGURE 6.3

The "Ames Test" showing the incubation of mutant tester strain organisms (10^8 organisms/ml) in test tubes containing (A) low nutrient medium plus agar, (B) this medium plus the S-9 fraction from Aroclor 1254-induced rat liver, and (C) this medium plus the S-9 fraction plus the test chemical (range of concentrations). The mixtures are poured over minimal medium agar and incubated at 37°C for 48 h. The presence of the S-9 fraction insures that promutagens are biotransformed into reactive intermediates or proximate mutagens. Over a range of concentrations of test agent, the number of colonies should increase in a dose-dependent manner, signifying a mutation to prototrophy.

a supernatant fraction called the S-9 is obtained by centrifugation of the homogenate at $9000 \times g$ for 10 min, is pooled and then subdivided into 1.0- to 2.0-ml aliquots in well sealed glass tubes, and is kept frozen at –80°C (Ames et al., 1975b; Maron and Ames, 1983). While many chemicals administered to rats will induce the activity of cytochrome P-450-related monooxygenases, they tend to induce only specific functions that may or may not use the procarcinogen(s) as a substrate. In contrast, Aroclor 1254 induces the complete range of monooxygenase functions (Ecobichon and Comeau, 1974; Ames et al., 1975b).

As is shown in Figure 6.3, an aliquot of 0.2 to 0.3 ml of the S-9 fraction is added to the incubation mixture (organisms [10^8 organisms/ml], test agent, molten top agar) in a buffer containing 8.0 mM MgCl$_2$, 33 mM KCl, 5.0 mM glucose-6-phosphate, 4.0 mM TPN and 100 mM sodium phosphate pH 7.4. This is mixed quickly (within a minute) and poured on the minimal medium agar plate. Following incubation for 48 h at 37°C, the revertant colonies on the plate are counted, with the numbers being corrected for spontaneous revertants detected on control plates and revertants found in S-9 fraction control plates carried through the experiments (Ames et al., 1975b; Maron and Ames, 1983). This system has become a validated standard assay around the world and is capable of detecting mutagenic carcinogens in tobacco smoke condensates, hair dyes, "natural" health foods, environmental samples, etc. (Ames, 1979, 1983; Ames et al., 1975a, 1975b; Kier et al., 1974).

B. Host-Mediated Assay

Considering the fact that the isolated hepatic S-9 fraction may not contain all of the enzymatic activity required to activate procarcinogens, investigators have altered the *in vitro* test by incubating the indicator organisms in an animal previously treated with the chemical. Generally, the animal (the host) receives an oral or ip dosage of the test chemical followed by an injection of the tester strain in suspension into the peritoneal cavity. Following a suitable period of "incubation" of the organisms — hopefully in the presence of reactive intermediates formed by the animal's enzymes — samples of the peritoneal fluid and organisms are retrieved and applied to a minimal medium agar plate. Significant growth of colonies would indicate reverse-mutation of the organisms to a prototrophic form. Additional controls must be included since there may be components in the rodent's diet that will cause mutations. While this technique would appear to be a useful adjunct to the other tests, trials have indicated that certain classes of carcinogens are not detected by this assay system and that it should not be used in the preliminary screening of potential carcinogens (Simmon et al., 1979).

C. Coliform Assays

The organism *Escherichia coli* has been introduced into the variety of short-term *in vitro* test systems. Auxotrophic tester strains such as the tryptophan-dependent WP2 mutant, the p3478 (pol A-) strain deficient in DNA polymerase, the 343/113 strain for point mutations at several loci, the WP2 excision repair mutant with or without the R-factor plasmid pKM101, etc., have all been adapted into plate-incorporation assay systems quite similar to those described for *Salmonella typhimurium*. Reverse- and forward mutations are examined with the production of prototrophic, "wild-type" organisms and new easily identified phenotypes, or the differential killing of repair-deficient strains. As with the standard Ames assay, the experiment is done with and without the S-9 mammalian liver fraction, thereby allowing the investigator to distinguish between direct-acting compounds and those requiring metabolic activation (Brusick et al., 1980; Purchase and Ashby, 1982).

An interesting variant of the coliform reverse-mutation assay is the SOS chromotest where the tester strain, *E. coli* PQ37, after incubation with a test substance in the presence and absence of the S-9 liver fraction, may show enhanced beta-galactosidase (an induction assay) and alkaline phosphatase (a control for protein synthesis) activity (LeCurieux et al., 1994). This assay system lends itself to automation, using microplates and an automatic microplate reader to quantitate the color generated by the enzymatic reactions.

IV. MUTAGENICITY TESTING WITH EUKARYOTIC CELL SYSTEMS *IN VITRO*

Genetic defects in man can be created by the induction of point mutations in the genome, chromosomal structural aberrations, and aneuploidy (any deviation from an exact multiple of the haploid number of chromosomes). Therefore, test systems to detect the mutagenic potential of chemicals should cover all of these aspects. The previously described microbial assay systems are based on reactions related to the direct alteration of DNA or the interference with DNA metabolism. The segregation of chromosomes is dependent upon an intact spindle fiber production for mitosis, the molecular target and essential component being tubulin (Picket-Heaps et al., 1982; Zimmerman, 1983). Thus, tests based on point mutations, deficiencies in DNA-repair systems, etc., would not reveal chemical-induced chromosomal malsegregation associated with tubulin during meiosis and mitosis. Tests for chromosomal damage require a more "advanced" organism than bacteria. Fungi fulfil this requirement in that they provide the advantages of the prokaryotic organism (rapid growth, large test population) with a genome that is organized into chromosomes requiring a mitotic apparatus similar to that found in higher mammalian cells (Styles, 1981). With such cell systems, it is possible to monitor mutagenic effects at both the gene and chromosomal level, examining point mutations as well as mitotic gene conversion and nondisjunctions (recombination, chromosomal loss). Organisms in common use for such test systems include the yeasts, *Saccharomyces cerevisiae, Schizosaccharomyces pombe,* the bread-mold *Neurospora crassa,* and the fungus, *Aspergillus nidulans* (Zimmerman, 1983).

Extensive studies have been done on yeast genetics and there are detailed genetic maps on the organism and a host of biochemical markers (Parry and Parry, 1984). *S. cerevisiae* is stable in either a haploid or diploid state. It can be cultured on defined media, with control over growth conditions permitting the study of chemical-induced effects during meiotic and mitotic cell division. All fungi, including yeasts, maintain the nuclear membrane throughout cell division. Studies have demonstrated that yeasts can be used to study chemical-induced mitotic aneuploidy, point mutation, mitotic recombination, and mitotic chromosome loss (Parry et al., 1981; Zimmerman, 1983).

A.   *Saccharomyces* Forward-Mutation Assay

A variety of forward-mutation systems have been used with yeast cultures, the most extensively studied one being based on the induction of defective alleles of the gene for adenine synthesis. The test uses strains of *S. cerevisiae* carrying a defective mutation of the adenine-1 and adenine-2 genes and growth in culture results in the production of red-colored colonies as a consequence of the accumulation of an intracellular pigmented intermediary (aminoimidazole carboxylic acid ribonucleotide) in the adenine biosynthetic pathway (Parry and Parry, 1984). Chemical-induced forward mutations (base substitutions, frameshifts, deletion of DNA) may alter genes that precede the red pigment step in synthesis, the organism becoming doubly defective, the colonies that grow in culture being white (uncolored) when grown on a low adenine medium.

B.   *Neurospora Crassa* Reverse- and Forward-Mutation Assays

Early studies with this fungus were in an assay system using an adenine-requiring strain (the double mutant 70007, 38701) to measure reverse-mutation from adenine dependence to independence (Kølmark and Westergaard, 1949). With a low rate of spontaneous reversion, strain 38701 was useful in the identification of very weak mutagens, and extensive studies were carried out in the 1940s and 1950s with this strain. See DeSerres and Malling (1983) for a historical review of this test system. The subsequent development of a double mutant strain, adenine dependent and also requiring the sugar inositol (strains 38701, 37401), allowed the study of reverse mutations at two loci (Kølmark, 1953). The assays are conducted in much the same manner as those discussed for bacteria, with the defective organisms being incubated with the test chemical and small amounts of the required nutrients and then cultured on minimal medium deficient in the required nutrients. The reverse mutation to prototrophic organisms independent of the required nutrient would be indicated by the growth of colonies.

Forward-mutation assays were developed using two strains of *Neurospora* (ad-3A, ad-3B mutants) that not only had an adenine dependence but, during growth, acquired a reddish-purple pigment in the vacuoles of the mycelium (DeSerres and Kølmark, 1958; DeSerres and Malling, 1971). A positive test following chemical exposure resulted in "wild-type" conidia producing white colonies. In a second major advance with this organism, a two-component heterokaryon was developed that was heterozygous in the ad-3 region (+/ad-3A, +/ad-3B strains), this proving useful not only to detect ad-3 mutants arising from point mutations at the ad-3 loci but also to detect multilocus deletions (DeSerres and Malling, 1983). Since the ad-3A and ad-3B loci are closely linked, such multilocus deletions might involve either or both loci simultaneously.

While both yeast and fungal test systems have been used for a long time, they have not proven to be as popular as the bacterial systems among investigators. Supporters of the fungal assay systems are of the opinion that they should be an integral part of any comprehensive testing scheme, not just an optional alternative (Zimmerman, 1983). Others feel that the fungal sytems offer no clear-cut advantage over bacterial systems, some chemicals being positive in fungi and negative in bacteria and vice versa (DeSerres and Malling, 1983). Metabolism would appear to play an important role, with some mutagens not being activated by fungi (false negative results), while in other cases, fungi lack enzymes found in mammalian cells and generate false positive results since the organisms cannot destroy the test chemical. Fungal cells can be combined with a variety of activation systems to get around the problem of promutagen biotransformation (Zimmerman et al., 1982).

C. MAMMALIAN CELL TEST SYSTEMS

The previously described test systems have all involved *in vitro* assays, the microorganisms having little capability to biotransform/activate agents, requiring the inclusion of activating systems, and, in general, being quite dissimilar to mammalian cells. Looking at test systems using eukaryotic cells higher than bacteria, yeasts, and fungi, one encounters a wide variety of assays utilizing various mammalian cells *in vitro*, both established cell lines and primary cultures of tissue cells derived from treated animals. Some of these cell systems, particularly those from rodents, are capable of limited biotransformation activity while others, those derived from human cells or long-established cell lines, must be enhanced by the addition of activating systems such as the S-9 fraction of rodent liver or co-culturing with primary cultures of rodent hepatocytes. These test systems permit a closer examination of the mechanisms of action responsible for gene mutation and chromosomal aberrations. Rather than focus on the cell systems used, since many are interchangeable, the approach will be to explain the functional aspect(s) of the assays.

1. DNA Damage/Repair

Chemical-induced damage to the nucleic acids of mammalian cells generally results in a valiant effort by the cells' enzymatic systems to repair the defect(s), resulting in the unscheduled synthesis of DNA (Williams, 1977; Kornburst and

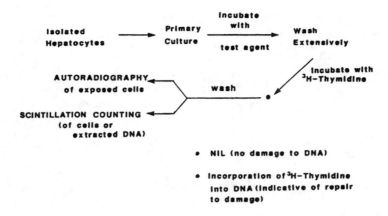

FIGURE 6.4
A bioassay for unscheduled DNA synthesis. Isolated primary culture hepatocytes are grown on glass slides in medium containing a range of concentrations of the test agent. Following a suitable time period of incubation, the slides are washed extensively to remove the unabsorbed chemical, and the slides are incubated with tritiated thymidine. If the test agent has caused damage to the cellular DNA, repair mechanisms will be activated, the enzymes incorporating the radiolabel into the nucleic acid. Suitable techniques of quantitating the radiolabel (autoradiography, scintillation counting of cells or extracted DNA) will give an indication of the extent of the repair process and will reflect the amount of damage to the DNA.

Barfknecht, 1985). The assessment of cellular effects can be made at the level of the DNA. As is shown in Figure 6.4, isolated, metabolically active hepatocytes, obtained from collagenase-perfused rodent liver and cultured on glass coverslips, are incubated briefly in "clean" medium or in medium containing a range of concentrations of test chemical. Following this step, the cells are repeatedly washed to remove traces of the test agent before placing them in medium containing tritiated thymidine. Unscheduled DNA synthesis, indicative of functional DNA repair mechanisms, will result in the incorporation of radiolabeled thymidine into the nucleic acid. Following fixation and drying of the cells, they may be exposed to photographic emulsion and, after several weeks of exposure, the radioactive "grains" in the nucleus can be counted and the numbers adjusted for the "grains" detected in the nuclei of control cells. A more rapid technique involves washing the radiolabeled, thymidine-exposed cells and either (1) counting the tritium in a known volume of cells by scintillation techniques or (2) extracting the DNA and estimating the amount of thymidine incorporated per unit weight of DNA in control and chemical-exposed cells.

Human cells (lymphocytes, fibroblasts, etc.) may also be used in this assay, but since they do not have highly active biotransformation enzymes, the assay is usually carried out in the presence and absence of an activating system such as the S-9 fraction of rodent liver.

A variation of this test system involves treating the animal with the potential toxicant and, following a suitable time period, euthanizing the animal and preparing primary hepatocyte cultures for a pulse exposure to incubation medium containing tritiated thymidine and completion of the assay as described above.

2. Forward Mutations in Chinese Hamster Cells

Clones and subclones of Chinese hamster ovary (CHO) and pulmonary (V79) cells, having stable karyotypes with 20 and 21 chromosomes, respectively, will grow actively in culture, doubling their number every 12 to 16 h and exhibiting plating

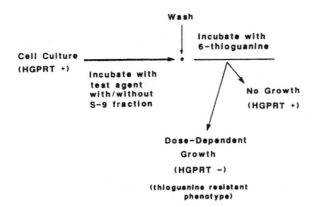

FIGURE 6.5

Chinese hamster ovary (CHO) cell mutagenesis. Cells positive for the enzyme hypoxanthine-guanine phosphoribosyl- transferase (HGPRT+) are cultured in medium containing various concentrations of the test agent in the presence and absence of the S-9 fraction from rodent liver. Following a washing step to remove unabsorbed test agent, the cells are incubated with 6-thioguanine, an inhibitor of HGPRT. The absence of subsequent growth signifies that the test agent did not cause a mutation at the HGPRT locus, the cells still being HGPRT+. Further growth of the cells is indicative of a mutation resulting in a 6-thioguanine resistant phenotype, the cells being deficient in the enzyme (HGPRT-) and capable of replication without the enzyme.

efficiencies of 75 to 95% (Krahn, 1983). These cell lines have been available since the late 1950s. One genetic marker, common to both cell lines, is the enzyme hypoxanthine-guanine phosphoribosyl- transferase (HGPRT), controlled by an X-linked gene. Agents such as 6-thioguanine and 8-azaguanine are cytotoxic to cells possessing HGPRT. Resistance to these agents denotes a mutation at the HGPRT locus and either an absence of activity (HGPRT-) or such low activity that hypoxanthine is not incorporated into the cellular macromolecules. The mutation is quite stable. As these cell lines do not possess active Phase I microsomal monooxygenases, the S-9 fraction is generally included in the assay. However, consideration must be given to the fact that these cell lines do possess Phase II detoxifying enzymes, principally glutathione-sulfotransferase (GST) and glutathione (GSH), providing some potential to detoxify reactive intermediates.

In the assay, CHO or V79 cells positive for HGPRT (HGPRT+) are incubated with the test agent in the presence and absence of an aliquot of the S-9 fraction of rodent liver (Figure 6.5). After a suitable time period, the cells are washed to remove the test agent and are recultured in medium containing 6-thioguanine or 8-azaguanine. Mutations at the HGPRT locus, causing a HGPRT-deficient cell (HGPRT-), are reflected in the ability of the deficient cells to grow in the presence of the guanine analog, the increase in the number of colonies being related to the amount of chemical.

3. Mouse Lymphoma Cell Assay

An established line of mouse lymphoma cells heterozygous for the enzyme thymidine kinase (L5178Y/TK±) has proven useful in the *in vitro* study of mutagenic carcinogens (Amacher and Turner, 1983). Chemical-induced mutations at the locus result in the loss of thymidine kinase activity with the formation of a homozygous strain (TK-/-). Both the TK± and TK-/- strains can grow on normal medium, but the incorporation of 5-bromo-2-deoxyuridine (BrdU) into the medium results in cytotoxicity to the TK± cells, growth and replication occurring only in the enzyme-deficient cells.

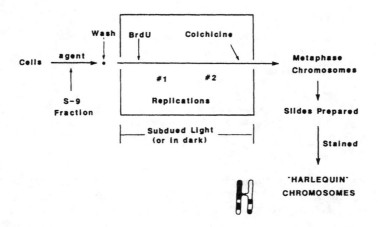

FIGURE 6.6

The sister chromatid exchange (SCE) assay. Suitable cultured cell lines (Chinese hamster ovary (CHO) or pulmonary (V79) cells) are incubated with test agent in the presence and absence of aliquots of S-9 fraction for 2 h. Following a washing to remove unabsorbed test agent, the cells are transferred to medium containing 6-bromo-deoxyuridine (BrdU) and are allowed to pass through two DNA replications (24 to 30 h) before colchicine is added to arrest the cells at the metaphase stage of chromosomal replication. Slides are prepared and stained with a fluorescent dye, exposed to ultraviolet light, and then stained with Giemsa. Damage caused by the exposure to the test agent (breaks, fragments, etc.) will be reflected in the exchange of chromosomal "pieces" between chromosomes, the effect seen under a microscope being that of a variegated pattern of light and dark staining sections, giving the chromosome a "harlequin" appearance.

As was described for the above mammalian cell test systems, the heteroygous (TK±) cells are incubated with the test agent in the presence and absence of an activating enzyme system for a suitable time period, followed by thorough washing to remove unabsorbed test chemical and a subsequent incubation in medium containing BrdU. The mutagenic potential of the test agent (or reactive intermediates) will be indicated by a dose-dependent increase in the number of colonies of mutant (TK-/-) cells in the medium.

4. Sister Chromatid Exchanges — Chromosomal Aberrations

This *in vitro* test system has been used extensively as a short-term assay to detect *clastogenic* (chromosome-breaking) chemicals. The results have demonstrated a good correlation between mutagenic carcinogens that elicit sister chromatid exchanges (SCEs) and which induce gene mutations in other short-term assays (Wolff, 1983). The utility of the assay is such that it can be adapted for a variety of cell lines including CHO and V79 lines, mouse lymphoma cells, human lymphocytes, and even primary cultures of cells (lymphocytes) recovered from humans or animals exposed to hazardous chemicals (Fucic et al., 1990; Oestreicher et al., 1990; Pelclova et al., 1990). The assay is capable of detecting both direct-acting chemicals and those requiring metabolic activation.

As is shown in Figure 6.6, suitable test cell populations are cultured in medium containing a range of concentrations of the test chemical, essential co-factors, and aliquots of S-9 fraction of rodent liver for approximately 2 h. Subsequently, the cells are washed free of test agent and are transferred into a medium containing 5-bromodeoxyuridine (BrdU) and allowed to pass through two DNA replications, a time period of 24 to 30 h depending on the cell system. Colchicine is added to the incubation for 3 h before the end of incubation. All of these steps must be carried

TABLE 6.3

Selection Criteria for IPCS Collaborative Study on
Higher Plant Genetic Systems

1. Ease of use
2. Well-developed methodology
3. Used by a number of investigators
4. A large data base on chemical mutagens
5. Adaptability of protocols to different climatic conditions
6. Ease of distribution of source material

Data from Grant (1994).

out in the absence of direct artificial or natural light, with such exposure causing degradation of the BrdU-substituted DNA. The cells, containing metaphase chromosomes, are fixed and stained with a fluorescent dye (Hoechst 33258), washed with distilled water, exposed to UV light, and subsequently stained with Giemsa (5%) for 3 min. The exchanges of chromosomal "pieces" in the second division are visible microscopically as "harlequin chromosomes," the BrdU being found in one polynucleotide strand in control (unaffected) chromosomes but scattered in both polynucleotide strands where SCE has occurred. The extent of the exchange(s) is scored numerically for 50 cells at each level of exposure (Dean and Danford, 1984).

V. MUTAGENICITY TESTING WITH EUKARYOTIC CELLS *IN VIVO*

A. Mutagenicity Testing in Higher Plants

Plant bioassays have been in existence for many years for the detection, screening, and monitoring of environmental, chemical-induced, cytogenetic aberrations and gene mutations (Grant, 1994; Grant and Salamone, 1994). Many such tests have been recommended to regulatory authorities as alternative, first-tier, assay systems for the detection of possible genetic damage resulting from environmental pollution. The advantages of these assays, listed in Table 6.3, make them ideal for screening potential mutagens, clastogens, and carcinogens (Grant, 1994).

As has been indicated, some of the *in vitro* assays described above can be adapted to conduct the initial phases of the experiment *in vivo*, treating animals with the test chemical, allowing them to "incubate" the agent and convert it to reactive intermediates that will elicit chromosomal damage, this stage being followed by the euthanasia of the animals and the harvesting of the desired cells for subsequent *in vitro* assessment of the effects. However, there are other mutagenicity tests that examine chromosomal aberrations *in vivo*.

In the Gene-tox program of the U.S. EPA, nine plant genotoxicity assays for seven plant species were evaluated, having met the requirements that the species were used in a number of different laboratories and that there was a large data base permitting comparisons between laboratories and assay systems. The results for the test battery (Table 6.4) revealed a high sensitivity with few false negatives and were considered to be appropriate tests in the prediction of carcinogenicity (Ennever et al., 1988). More recently, the International Program on Chemical Safety (IPCS) initiated a collaborative study on higher plant genetic systems for screening and monitoring environmental pollutants, choosing the *Arabidopsis thaliana* white embryo and the Tradescantia stamen hair tests for gene mutation assays, while the *Vicia faba* root tip and the Tradescantia micronucleus tests were chosen for chromosomal aberration

TABLE 6.4

Test Battery for U.S. EPA's Gene-Tox Program

Assay System	Parameter Measured
Allium cepa	Chromosome aberration assays
Arabidopsis thaliana	Mutation assays
Barley (*Hordeum vulgare*)	Chromosome aberration assays
	Chlorophyll-deficient mutation
Soybean (*Glycine max*)	Chlorophyll spot mutations
Tradescantia	Assays for gaseous mutagens
	Cytogenetic tests
Vicia faba	Cytogenetic tests
Zea mays	Specific locus mutation assays

From Grant, (1994).

assays (Grant and Salamone, 1994). Experiments conducted with the known mutagens (methyl nitrosourea, maleic hydrazide, sodium azide, and azidoglycerol) demonstrated the utility of these assays to detect mutagens and clastogens. A recent paper has described a sensitive sister chromatic exchange test, using the chromosomes of root-tip meristem cells of germinating spruce fir (*Picea abies*) seedlings (Schubert and Rieger, 1994). Much more will be seen of such versatile assays being used as first-tier screening procedures for environmental contaminants, hopefully with government recognition.

B. Mutagenicity Testing in *Drosophila Melanogaster*

The major advantages of the fruitfly as a test organism in genetic studies have been enumerated: a sexually reproductive eukaryotic species, germ cell stages paralleling those of mammals, genetically well known, three major large chromosomes, many mutations with visible effects as useful markers, special chromosomes with combinations of markers and rearrangements, short generation time, and large numbers of progeny (Valenica, 1983). An additional feature is the fact that this organism is capable of metabolizing a wide range of chemicals, making it suitable for the study of the conversion of promutagens to mutagens.

One test system makes use of the fact that males of one strain carry a gene for yellow body color on the X chromosome. Males of two days of postpartum age are exposed to the test chemical, dissolved at different concentrations in sucrose-water, with appropriate controls being carried throughout the study. Surviving males are mated with females. If there are no yellow-bodied males in the progeny, one can assume that a lethal mutation has occurred. Below the lethal concentration(s) of test agent, numbers of distinctive yellow-bodied males should be seen, inversely proportional to the dose to which the parent male was exposed.

For screening large numbers of chemicals, the sex-linked recessive lethal test (SLRL) in the fruit fly is the best choice, this assay screening some 800 loci and detecting lethal effects associated with either intragenic mutations (point mutations, small deletions) or chromosomal rearrangements in an animal where the spontaneous mutation rate per locus is comparable to rates found for human loci (Lee et al., 1983; Valencia, 1970). Assays using appropriate strains of fruitfly will detect not only strong mutagens but also weak agents. A variety of endpoints can be assessed, with effects on the X and Y chromosomes being visible as phenotypic changes in body color, shape and color of the eye, changes in bristles on the thorax, etc. A number of biological parameters have been investigated in germ cells or somatic tissue of

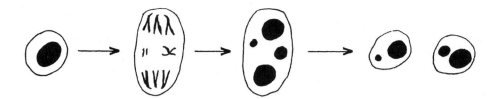

Agent-Treated

Stem Cell or

Lymphocyte

Binucleated Cells

With Micronuclei

FIGURE 6.7

The formation of binucleated daughter cells following the mitotic division of a cell (stem cell, lymphocytes, etc.), with the appearance of one or more small nuclei (micronuclei) as well as the normal, large nucleus when appropriately stained with May-Grunwald-Giemsa. Micronuclei may be formed as a consequence of: (1) mutations to kinetochore proteins, centromeres, and/or spindle apparatus, leading to unequal chromosome distribution or whole chromosome loss at anaphase, or (2) unrepaired DNA breaks resulting in acentric chromosomal fragments (Fenech, 1993).

Drosophila for links between initial alkylating patterns and the kinds of genetic effects observed. In germ cells, these include:

1. Mutation induction relative to cytotoxicity.
2. The proportion of chromosomal aberrations to that of recesssive lethal mutations.
3. The ability of alkylating agents to cause delayed mutations (expressed by the ratio of F_2 lethals to F_3 lethals.
4. The role of repair processes.
5. The influence of expression time on the formation of chromosomal aberrations.
6. The induction of mutations relative to quantitative DNA binding.

In somatic cells, the proportion of somatic recombinations vs. somatic mutations has been measured (Vogel, 1983).

While not yet adopted as an OECD Test Guideline, considerable interest has been expressed in the somatic mutation and recombination tests (SMART) developed to induce genetic alterations in somatic cells of *Drosophila melanogaster* (Vogel, 1992). The reticence of OECD to develop this test was related to the lack of expertise and experience in member countries (OECD, 1995). The white/white+ (w/w+) eye mosaic system has been shown to detect a broad spectrum of genetic alterations, with interchromosomal mitotic recombination being a major event (Vogel and Nivard, 1993). It is a fast and low cost *in vivo* assay and has been evaluated with good results for approximately 200 chemicals including pesticides and promutagens (Vogel and Nivard, 1993; Aguirrezabalaga et al., 1994). Details for the conduction of this assay are described in the previous references.

C. The Micronucleus Test

Micronuclei arise from chromosomal fragments that are not incorporated into daughter cell nuclei at mitosis because they lack a centromere and are not "pulled" to the appropriate pole of the spindle (Heddle, 1973; Schmidt, 1975). After the telophase stage in mitosis, the undamaged chromosomes as well as the acentric fragments give rise to daughter nuclei (Figure 6.7). The detached, broken segments, even entire lagging chromosomes, are also included in the daughter cells, usually being transformed into one or several micronuclei that are generally much smaller (1/5 to 1/20) than the principal nucleus. With appropriate staining, these small bodies are visible by light microscopy.

Micronuclei can occur in any cell type of proliferating tissue (Adler, 1984). A variety of nucleated cells, harvested from agent-treated animals, can be used in this assay. The mouse is a favored animal species, with fetal hepatic cells, maternal bone marrow erythroblasts (young erythrocytes), lymphocytes, pulmonary alveolar macrophages, etc., being useful populations of cells (Adler, 1984; Cole et al., 1983; Fenech, 1993; Sahu and Das, 1995). Fetal tissues are very vulnerable to chromosomal damage by electrophilic chemicals, the damaged DNA in mitotically active fetal cells being more likely to undergo replication than in adult tissues (Cole et al., 1983). Suitable cells can also be obtained by bronchiolar lavage, from the buccal cavity and from the urine. If cytotoxicity has occurred as a consequence of exposure to a mutagenic chemical, such cells may contain micronuclei, indicative of chromosomal damage. Recent papers have described the use of fish which, of course, have a nucleated erythocyte, as suitable species to monitor micronucleus formation as an endpoint of environmental pollution (Metcalf, 1988; Al-Sabti and Hardig, 1990).

Details are given by Adler (1984) for the metaphase analysis and the micronucleus analysis of bone marrow cells (Figure 6.8). Single or repeated treatment of mice with a range of concentrations of test chemical coupled with multiple posttreatment sampling intervals should be adequate to determine the mutagenic potency of the agent. The animals are killed and the femurs are dissected out and cut open at the distal (knee) end, inserting a needle on a syringe (1.0 ml) containing 0.4 ml of Hank's balanced salt solution (HBSS), keeping the bone below the surface of HBSS in a centrifuge tube and forcing the marrow out through the opening around the needle by flushing with the contents of the syringe. After repeated aspiration and flushing, the bone should be visibly empty of marrow. The free cells are centrifuged (5 min at 1000 rpm) and the supernatant HBSS is discarded, being resuspended in a hypotonic solution for 15 min (mice), 20 min (Chinese hamster), or 30 min (rat). At the end of this period, the cells are centrifuged again, the supernatant is discarded, and the cells are agitated with the dropwise addition of freshly prepared cold fixative (methanol:glacial acetic acid, 3:1). The fixative is changed twice after a 10-min period and, on addition of a third volume, the cells are refrigerated for 60 min. The fixative should be changed again just before the preparation of the slides. A drop of the cell suspension is applied to the surface of a clean, grease-free glass slide, allowing the fixative to evaporate quickly to stick the cells firmly to the glass surface. The slide can be stained with 5% Giemsa, with 2% acetic orcein, or with the combined Giemsa and May-Gruenwald stain.

The cells of interest are those young erythrocytes that have just expelled their main nucleus. With the combined Giemsa and May-Gruenwald stain, the polychromatic erythrocytes (PCEs) stain a bluish to purple color due to the high content of RNA in the cytoplasm while the mature normochromatic cells (NCEs) stain reddish to yellow. The ratio of NCE to PCE is determined by counting a total of 2000 erythrocytes per slide within "fields" examined. An increase in PCEs signals a stimulation of proliferative activity due to an early phase of cell depletion. Depression of bone marrow proliferation results in a markedly reduced number of PCEs and adversely affects the micronucleus yields. The main purpose of the test is to determine the number of micronucleated PCEs. The extensive review by Adler (1984) should be consulted before attempting this assay because artifacts abound.

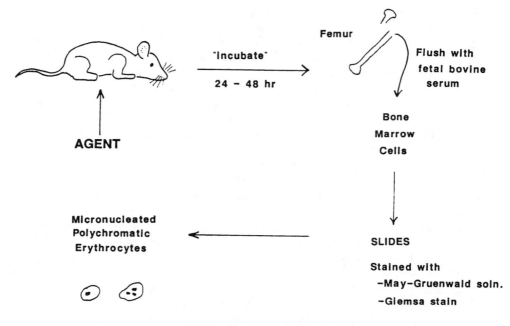

MICRONUCLEUS ASSAY

FIGURE 6.8
The bone-marrow micronucleus test in which suitable experimental animals are treated with single or repeated doses of the test agent, euthanized within 24 to 48 h of exposure, the femur being removed by dissection and opened to permit a thorough flushing out of the bone marrow cells with Hank's balanced salt solution. The harvested cells are centrifuged and subsequently spread on a slide, staining with May-Grunwald-Giemsa to highlight the nuclear material for examination by light microscopy (Adler, 1984).

For those species possessing nucleated erythrocytes (fish, birds, etc.), the micronucleus assay is much more simple, a sample of heparinized blood being smeared and air-dried on a glass slide. Following fixation in absolute ethanol, the smears are stained for 15 min with 10 to 20% Giemsa prepared in Sorenson buffer solution and, once dried, can be coverslipped (Al-Sabti and Hartig, 1990). The Giemsa stains the nuclear material much more darkly than the cytoplasm and the micronuclei can be readily seen by light microscopy. Usually, a thousand erythrocytes per specimen/slide are analyzed to determine the frequency of cells with one or more micronuclei.

D. The Dominant Lethal Assay

While this *in vivo* test in male rodents is properly a test of the potential of an agent to cause lethal mutations in the genome thereby interfering with reproductive success, the assay was considered under reproductive tests in Chapter 5.

VI. THE IMPOSSIBILITY — A TEST FOR ALL MUTAGENS!

A clear-cut indication of mutagenic potential may be exceedingly difficult to attain, particularly for weak mutagens. The vagaries of any individual *in vitro* or *in vivo* mutagenicity test including variability in sensitivity, the complexity of the organism

TABLE 6.5

A Battery of Tests for the Evaluation of Mutagenic Potential of Chemicals

Type	Test system/assay	Function
Bacterial	Ames *Salmonella* — liver S9	Reverse-mutation
	Escherichia coli	Reverse-mutation
Mammalian (*in vitro*)	Mouse lymphoma L5178Y(TK +/−)	Forward-mutation
	Chinese hamster ovary (CHO) HGPRT	Forward-mutation
	Pulmonary V79 cells HGPRT	Forward-mutation
	Mammalian cell lines	Chromosomal aberrations
	Mammalian cell lines	Sister-Chromatid exchange (SCE)
Mammalian (*in vivo*)	*Drosophila melanogaster*	Sex-linked recessive lethal assay
	Rodent bone-marrow stem cells	Chromosomal aberrations
	Rodent bone-marrow stem cells	Micronucleus formation
	Rodent (mouse, rat) dominant lethal assay	Lethal mutation

Data from National Research Council, *Toxicity Testing, Strategies to Determine Needs and Priorities*, National Academy Press, Washington, D.C. (1984).

and its genetics, and the different ways in which an agent may affect the DNA, all conspire to yield vague answers as well as false positive and false negative results. To circumvent inconclusive results, most regulatory agencies have suggested that agents should be assessed by a battery of tests discussed in this section. The COMA Mutagenicity Committee (U.K.) recommended that the combination include tests for: (1) the detection of gene mutation in bacteria, (2) chromosomal damage to mammalian cells *in vitro* (metaphase analysis), (3) the induction *in vitro* of gene mutation in mammalian cells or a test *in vivo* in *Drosophila melanogaster*, and (4) a chromosomal metaphase analysis test *in vivo* or the micronucleus test (Jones, 1981). The U.S. EPA proposed a battery of eight different kinds of tests from groups designed to: (1) test gene mutation, (2) detect chromosomal aberrations, and (3) detect primary DNA damage (U.S. EPA, 1978). The Organization for Economic Cooperation and Development (OECD) adopted requirements for ten tests (Table 6.5) that it considered to be representative of well-established and reproducible test systems (OECD, 1984). Decisions to proceed with the further evaluation of a chemical rest on the outcomes of these tests, taken in context with the mechanism(s) of action of the agent.

The examination of mutagenic potential in such a battery of tests frequently reveals a spectrum whereby positive results are indicated by most of the microbial assay systems; equivocal results are observed in fungi and negative results are found in mammalian cell systems (Purchase and Ashby, 1982; Zeiger, 1987). A variety of factors contributing to these heterogeneous results include:

1. The greater sensitivity of cytoplasm-dispersed nucleic acids in prokaryotic cells to any agent that can penetrate the cell membrane

2. The absence of cellular detoxifying mechanisms in prokaryotic cells

3. Limitations in the efficiency of DNA repair mechanisms in prokaryotic cells or the inability of such mechanisms to repair extensive damage

4. The presence of detoxifying enzymes in eukaryotic cell systems

5. Variable levels of sensitivity to certain classes of mutagenic agents, depending upon the mechanism(s) of action

6. The lack of interlaboratory consistency in dose-effect relationships for one test as well as between tests

TABLE 6.6

Criteria for the Performance of Mutagenicity Tests

Criterion	Definition
Sensitivity	$\dfrac{\text{Number of carcinogens found positive}}{\text{Number of carcinogens tested}}$
Specificity	$\dfrac{\text{Number of noncarcinogens found negative}}{\text{Number of noncarcinogens tested}}$
Accuracy (with the tested population)	$\dfrac{\text{Number of correct test results}}{\text{Number of chemicals tested}}$
Predictive value	$\dfrac{\text{Number of carcinogens found positive}}{\text{Number of positive results obtained}}$
Prevalence	$\dfrac{\text{Number of carcinogens}}{\text{Number of chemicals tested}}$

Data from Purchase and Ashby (1982).

In developing a battery of short-term carcinogenicity/mutagenicity test systems, the performance of the tests with a number of chemicals should be assessed in terms of the criteria listed in Table 6.6 (Purchase and Ashby, 1982). Interpretation of a set of results should always bear in mind the known mechanisms by which other chemicals induce mutagenicity in the particular cell system(s) being used (Williams, 1989).

VII. CARCINOGENICITY

Cancers have been an age-old problem and a leading cause of death. They are a major concern to the public who hear that some 70 to 90% of all human cancers are attributable to environmental causes (Higginson, 1968). However, this statement was misinterpreted by the media and subsequently by the public to refer only to environmental pollution, whereas Higginson included lifestyles, hobby activities, diet, etc. — a definition of total environment rather than just those by-products of industries found in the out-of-doors (Higginson, 1981). A review of early occupational health literature reveals that cancers associated with particular chemicals have been known since at least 1775 when Percivall Pott reported on the incidence rate of scrotal cancer among London chimney sweeps, attributing it to chronic exposure from childhood to soots from combustion products of coal (Kipling and Waldron, 1975). Epidemiological studies in the 1800s identified specific chemical-related tumors in certain occupations, i.e., radioactivity (lung cancer in uranium miners), copper and arsenic (scrotal cancer in smelter workers), aromatic amines (bladder cancer in dye workers), asbestos (pulmonary fibrosis and cancer in workers), and, more recently, vinyl chloride (hepatic cancer in plastics industry workers) (Saffioti and Wagoner, 1976). Emphasis has been placed upon epidemiological studies establishing an association between chemicals and diseases, including carcinogenesis, among exposed workers. However, such studies are after the fact. The ethics of waiting until enough positive proof of an association has been obtained before "moving" on a chemical to reduce or eliminate exposures is questionable, hence, the interest in short-term predictive assays to identify chemicals of potential hazard, the *in vitro* mutagenicity tests being one such group of test systems. In 1918, using the epithelium of the rabbit ear as a test site, Japanese scientists demonstrated that chemical substances causing cancer in humans also caused cancer in animals, thereby providing another means of testing chemicals (Yamagiwa and Itchikawa, 1918). Currently, most substances known to be carcinogenic to humans have been found to cause cancer in animals (Wilbourn et al., 1986). However, the converse is not true, only some 10% of mammalian (animal) carcinogens elicit cancer in humans.

Cancer can be considered as normal cell growth, differentiation, and development in the absence of control. Evidence points conclusively to the phenomenon that malignant cells of most neoplasms show chromosomal aberrations, suggesting that a chemical carcinogen must interact with DNA before the mutagenic\-carcinogenic process can begin (Yunic, 1983). Current theories consider carcinogenesis to be a multistage process (Figure 6.9). The first stage involves some specific genetic damage to the cell — induced by a genotoxic chemical, physical, or biological agent — converting the normal cell into an intermediate "initiated" cell containing a permanent (heritable) defect that is replicated faithfully in the progeny. These are now preneoplastic cells. As was suggested in the model of Moolgavkar and Knudson (1981), these altered cells may undergo normal apoptosis (programmed, physiological, cell death) or, being unique, may attract the attention of an alerted immune system and be scavenged by T-cells and macrophages (Bursch et al., 1992; Vaux and Strasser, 1996). The development of distinct clones of these altered cells is controlled by "promoters," agents influencing growth-hormone production, regulating gene expression, and frequently interfering with cell differentiation, giving rise to the proliferation of immature cells (Scott et al., 1984; Shields and Harris, 1990). Some of the DNA alterations may result in the expression of dormant genes (promotion genes), activation of proto-oncogenes, or suppression of growth control (suppressor) genes. For example, over 50% of human tumors show defects in the p53 codon, a gene responsible for the synthesis of p53 protein which normally suppresses runaway cell growth (Ames et al., 1995; Hollstein et al., 1991). Such defects result in either no p53 protein being synthesized or the synthesis of an ineffective nonsense protein, with a subsequent uncontrolled division of the initiated cells. Progression, the final stage of cancer development, is characterized by changes in the phenotypic appearance of the cells and growth rate, brought about by the activation of promotional genes or proto-oncogenes or by the inactivation of suppressor genes (Cohen and Ellwein, 1990,1991; Moolgavkar and Knudson, 1981; Shields and Harris, 1990). Some proportion of the malignant cells may be susceptible to destruction by the activated immune system, but cell production eventually overwhelms the immunodefence, forming the primary malignancy and eventually, secondary or metastatic malignancies. It should be appreciated that many mammalian cells already exist in an "initiated" state, dormant viral oncogenes having been incorporated into the genome of the cells for generations, existing as proto-oncogenes, and only awaiting activation by another chemical, usually a radical, whereby a second genetic error occurs (Bishop, 1982; Cohen and Ellwein, 1991; Stowers et al., 1987).

The operational definition of a carcinogen is "an agent having the ability to induce tumor formation as evidenced by (1) an *increased incidence* over that seen in control individuals, (2) a *decrease in the latency period* of appearance, (3) the *production of tumor types not seen* in control individuals, and (4) an *enhanced multiplicity* of tumors at different sites. Such agents may be considered as **genotoxic** or **ultimate** carcinogens, acting either directly with DNA through strong covalent bonds (adducts) or requiring prior conversion by cellular enzymes from unreactive procarcinogens to reactive intermediate or **proximate** carcinogens capable of covalent binding to DNA.

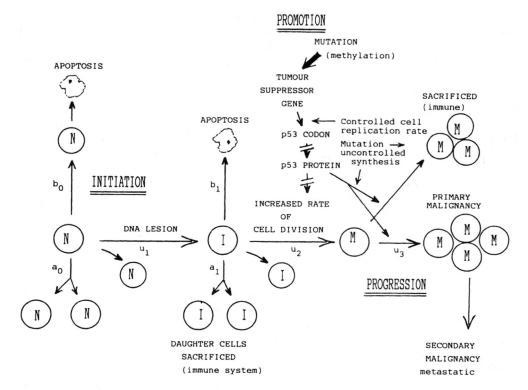

FIGURE 6.9

A modification of the Moolgavkar and Knudson (1981) model of multistage carcinogenesis showing initiation (the initial transformation of a normal cell, (N) to an initiated cell (I) bearing a DNA lesion, with the subsequent promotion to a malignant (M) cell being controlled by a second cellular insult causing (1) activation of a proto-oncogene or (2) a defect in a tumor suppressor (p53) gene which normally controls cell replication rates through the p53 protein this gene synthesizes. Progression to primary or secondary malignancies requires the uncontrolled replication of the malignant cell. The existence and persistence of each cell type is governed by individual birth and death rates (constants a, b, u), with opoptosis and immunological destruction exerting control over the population of cells.

Most chemical carcinogens belong to the latter group, requiring metabolic activation before exhibiting any carcinogenic potential. Dosage is extremely crucial: too little being without effect since normal detoxification mechanisms will efficiently destroy the agent, whereas too much agent will overwhelm the activation/detoxification mechanisms, with toxicity other than carcinogenesis being seen since too little reactive, proximate carcinogen will have been formed. A second group of carcinogens, the **epigenetic or nongenotoxic** carcinogens, do not appear to damage DNA but enhance the growth of tumors by some mechanism of *promotion* (enhanced absorption, increased (or decreased) biotransformation, reduced elimination of the carcinogenic agent) or *cocarcinogenesis* (hormonal action on cell proliferation, inhibition of intercellular communication to reduce restraints imposed by neighboring normal cells, immunosuppression of protective mechanisms). The term *"tumor promoter"* should be limited to the discussion of two-stage model systems in which tumor development is examined after the application of an initiating agent (Perera, 1991). The term *"nongenotoxic carcinogen"* should be used to designate an Ames-negative agent capable of causing the development of malignant tumors in 2-year bioassays when the animals are exposed to the agent alone (Perera, 1991). It is obvious that mechanisms by which agents induce carcinogenesis are intricate and complicated

(Ashby and Purchase, 1992; Farber, 1987; Weisburger and Williams, 1980,1991; Williams, 1990). How, then, does one test chemicals of various structures for their potential to elicit cancers and the mechanisms by which they act?

VIII. TESTING STRATEGIES FOR LIMITED BIOASSAYS

In the previous section, a testing tier or battery was examined in which prokaryotic and eukaryotic cells were used to assess the mutagenic potential of carinogens, with damaged DNA or altered chromosomes (genome) being endpoints indicative of the ability of the chemical to change genetic material. These tests provided results for the initial level of decision making, the detection of direct-acting genotoxic carcinogens, and in some cases, indirect-acting procarcinogens (Weisburger and Williams, 1981; Williams and Weisburger, 1981). A more recent test battery, for genotoxic carcinogens, includes a group of three tests, the Ames test in *Salmonella typhimurium*, the Williams test with evidence of DNA repair in hepatocytes (Williams et al., 1982), and direct documentation of DNA adduct formation in the ^{32}P postlabeling technique (Randerath et al., 1989; Weisburger, 1994). While these test systems provide a rapid assessment of possible mutagenicity, they are fraught with methodological difficulties, including the interpretation of results to higher life forms and the uncertainty that they actually reflect the properties of the suspect agent. Ideally, one would like additional test systems, possibly *in vivo*, where the concerns about agent biotransformation to reactive (or more reactive) intermediates could be addressed. Preferably, such tests would be of an intermediate duration and not as time consuming (>2 years) or as expensive as the classical chronic rodent studies. Strategies have been developed whereby use is made of the properties of rapidly regenerating tissues (*in vivo*) or of particular strains of rodents — possibly already bearing initiated, preneoplastic cells — that have a high susceptibility to tumor formation (Williams, 1989, 1990).

A. Rat-Liver Altered Foci Induction

In this test system, the regenerative capability of rat liver, following partial hepatectomy, is utilized to test the effects of initiator (direct-acting) carcinogens and/or cancer-promoting chemicals on rapidly replicating cells, the endpoint of analysis being the formation of foci of phenotypically-altered cells indicative of a preneoplastic lesion that could progress to cancer. A significant feature of the regenerating hepatocytes is that they possess elevated levels of Phase I biotransforming enzyme activity compared to normal hepatocytes, thereby enhancing the biotransformation of procarcinogens. The preneoplastic foci may progress directly to cancers and/or may first produce hyperplastic nodules that subsequently proceed to tumors (Pereira, 1982b). These foci are recognized histochemically as cellular aggregates displaying altered enzymatic activity or containing abnormal levels of cellular constituents different from neighboring normal cells. One such enzymatic marker is gamma-glutamyl transpeptidase (GGTase) found in distinctly higher levels in foci, hyperplastic nodules, and hepatocellular carcinomas. In other assay systems, marked decreases in glucose-6-phosphatase and adenosine triphosphatase are detected in the foci compared to levels found in surrounding normal hepatocytes. In one assay, the inability of foci to accumulate iron is used as a histochemical endpoint (Weisburger and Williams, 1981). The use of these early hepatocellular lesions instead of

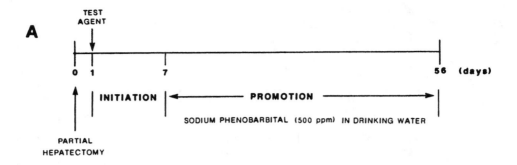

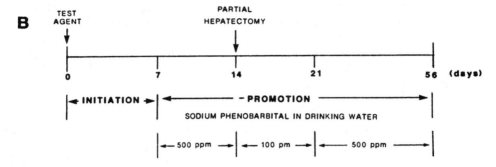

FIGURE 6.10
The rat liver altered foci assay. (A) The broad spectrum assay, partial hepatectomy is conducted in the rat, removing 60 to 70% of the hepatic lobes. At 1 d after the hepatectomy, the test agent is administered. At 6 d after treatment, and until the termination of the experiment at day 56, the effects of the test agent are promoted by incorporating sodium phenobarbital (500 ppm) in the drinking water, a procedure quaranteeing that the hepatic enzymes are maximally induced. In (B) Initiation by the test agent and an initial phase of promotion with sodium phenobarbital precede the partial hepatectomy. After the surgery, the phenobarbital level in the drinking water is decreased for 7 d because of the toxicity of this chemical in animals unable to efficiently biotransform it. At 7 d after surgery, the level of sodium phenobarbital can be safely increased again for the duration of the experimental period. Following euthanasia of the animals on day 56, the livers are sectioned, mounted on slides, and stained appropriately to detect the foci of altered cellular phenotypes (increased or decreased enzyme activity, altered iron incorporation, etc.). The effects of the test agent is quantitated on the basis of the number of foci produced. Modified from Pereira (1982b).

malignant tumor formation permits a marked reduction in the time period required for the assay as well as an increase in the sensitivity of the assay (Pereira, 1982b). There are several variants of the assay protocol depending upon the mechanism of action of the chemical, i.e., initiator, promoter, or cocarcinogen (Figure 6.10).

In one protocol, the broad spectrum assay, partial hepatectomy is carried out surgically by aseptic techniques, approximately 60 to 70% of the lobes of the rat liver being removed some 18 to 24 h prior to the administration of the test chemical (Figure 6.10A). At 6 d posttreatment, the animals receive sodium phenobarbital, a known tumor promoter, in their drinking water (500 ppm, µg/l) *ad libitum*, with this treatment continuing for 7 weeks to elicit maximum enzyme induction in the liver. Foci of altered hepatocytes are visible as early as 3 weeks after treatment and are well developed in large numbers by 7 to 12 weeks. The animals are euthanized at some suitable time point, and the regenerating livers are removed, sliced for histochemical staining, fixed, and examined by light microscopy for the number of histochemically distinct foci.

In the two-stage protocol, initiation and promotion stages are separated (Figure 6.10B). Treatment with the test agent is initiated; treatment with sodium phenobarbital in the drinking water is begun 7 d after the test agent and the partial hepatectomy is carried out after a further 7 d. Note that for 1 week following the partial hepatectomy, the barbiturate concentration is reduced to 100 ppm (because of increased toxicity) and is subsequently raised to 500 ppm for the remainder of the study period.

While this test system will detect direct-acting carcinogens and procarcinogens requiring metabolic activation, the technique can be modified to detect promoters. Phenobarbital is one such agent, although its action appears to be restricted to the liver where it exerts an enzyme-inducing function (Carthew et al., 1995). Other chemicals could be tested as promoters in the same fashion, substituting them for phenobarbital in the drinking water or incorporating them into the food. Fasting of the animals during the initiation stage will also enhance the development of hepatic preneoplastic lesions (foci) (Schmitt et al., 1993).

B. Tumor Induction

Rodents, like other mammals including the human, usually show a low background incidence of spontaneous tumor production due to a variety of unidentified causes usually labeled as "environmental" (Page, 1977). Genetics plays an important role since there are certain strains of rodents showing a marked predisposition toward the production of specific tumor types at particular sites, the incidence(s) being as high as 30 to 50% in "normal" untreated animals. This is suggestive of a significantly altered genome and an already "initiated" animal strain. Dermal, pulmonary, and hepatic neoplasms in mice and breast cancer in female Sprague-Dawley rats are specific examples (Williams and Weisburger, 1981).

While no one in their right mind would consider using one of these tumor-susceptible strains in an extended chronic study, they have their uses in limited bioassays for carcinogens, promoters, and cocarcinogens. All four of the criteria for declaring a chemical to be a carcinogen can be studied with these animal models at less cost and with a saving of time. The latency period for tumor development can be drastically reduced in such chemical-treated animals, tumors appearing within 3 to 6 months of initiating treatment whereas, in the control group, the same tumors would not appear until much later. The results are generally presented as the incidence (percentage) of animals with tumors compared to controls at some point in the study interval. With certain chemicals, a multiplicity of tumor types at different sites may also be observed. These limited bioassays are not used in a battery of tests but one or more might be selected depending upon information (structure, disposition in body, mechanism of action, etc.) available for the chemical. The four most commonly used test systems have shown sensitivity to chemicals of diverse structure (Williams, 1990).

In such studies, the test chemical may be administered in the diet as in subchronic and/or chronic studies (Chapter 4, Figures 4.1 and 4.2). Chemicals that act as initiators or promoters cannot be differentiated in the straightforward bioassay since a promoter might be influencing the susceptible or abnormal genome predisposing the animal to tumor induction, i.e., the proto-oncogene theory. However, a "two-stage protocol" requiring an initiator or a promoter of tumorigenicity can be developed, with the test chemical acting as either one or the other. Experiments of this

TABLE 6.7

Criteria for the Development of a Carcinogen-Testing Matrix

Tier	Purpose	Criteria
1	Screening	Needs are satisfied by the various bacterial mutagenicity using systems. They are responsible to initiating chemicals and not sensitive to chemicals that influence the development of cancer, i.e., the promoters.
2	Confirmation	Matrix of *in vivo* mouse-skin assay, rat-liver altered foci assay, and mouse lung adenoma plus *in vitro* cell transformation and *in vivo* micronucleus, bone-marrow cytogenetics, DNA damage and repair and SCE assays.
		Tests must be clearly related to carcinogenesis, removing from consideration any chemical falsely identified as positive in Tier 1 tests. The tests must also identify all or almost all chemical carcinogens.
3	Risk estimation	Long-term, "lifetime" testing in suitable species (rodent) to give results that can be used to predict the risk associated with a chemical.

Data from Bull and Pereira (1982).

type are frequently seen in skin painting studies (Mohtashamipur et al., 1990; Shukla et al., 1996). A known carcinogen such as dimethyl- or diethyl-nitrosamine or 7,12-dimethylbenz(a)anthracene may be administered at low initiating doses followed by the subsequent administration of the test chemical, the effect(s) (incidence, decrease in latency, new types, multiplicity) being compared between untreated, initiator-treated, and initiator/promoter-treated groups. The mouse dermal tumor assay is frequently used for this differentiation in mechanism of action (Pereira, 1982a). Another variant involves an initiation-selection-promotion protocol where an initiator such as diethylnitrosamine is administered as a single dose followed, in 2 weeks' time, by a selection procedure (feeding a diet containing 2-acetylaminofluorene[2-AAF] for 2 weeks with a necrogenic dose of carbon tetrachloride by gavage midway through the 2-AAF treatment) and followed by a promotion period of some 23 weeks during which the basal diet contained a chemical considered to be a promoter (Abdellatif et al., 1990).

Limited *in vivo* bioassays augment the results from the *in vitro* microbial and mammalian cell test systems and that of the rat liver foci assay in the decision-making process (Williams and Weisburger, 1981; Weisburger and Williams, 1991). Positive results in two or more of the *in vitro* assays plus a positive result in the *in vivo* limited bioassay group would signify that a chemical was highly suspect as a potential carcinogenic risk to humans, particularly if the results were obtained at low-to-moderate dosages (Weisburger and Williams, 1981,1991). Such a chemical would be considered to be a genotoxic carcinogen. Chemicals showing negative results in the microbial/mammalian cell battery and positive results in the limited bioassay systems would be considered as potential promoting agents, with further testing as nongenotoxic agents being required (Perera, 1991).

In developing a testing matrix for carcinogenesis, one has to consider specific attributes and criteria that the bioassays must meet (Table 6.7) (Bull and Pereira, 1982). The evaluation of carcinogenicity of large numbers of chemicals can be accomplished by a three-tier decision tree. Tier 1 — **screening** — can be accomodated by the bacterial mutagenesis testing systems plus those mammalian cytogenic systems that detect clastogens (chemicals breaking DNA). Tier 2 — **confirmation** — of the Tier 1 assays, has been less rigorously developed, but the U.S. EPA have proposed a Carcinogenesis Testing Matrix that consists of (1) mouse skin initiation/promotion, (2) Strain A mouse lung adenoma, (3) rat liver foci, (4) cell transformation, and (5) *in vivo* sister chromatic exchange (Bull and Pereira, 1982). The results from a combination of these bioassays should confirm the Tier 1 results. Tier 3 — **risk estimation** — involves the eventual testing of the chemical in long-term bioassays in order to obtain values useful in predicting risk to the human.

IX. LONG-TERM CARCINOGENICITY STUDIES

Equivocal or inconclusive results obtained from the *in vitro* tests and the limited *in vivo* bioassays can result in a decision to initiate an extended, "lifetime," chronic carcinogenicity study in suitable rodent (mouse, rat, hamster) species (Gregory, 1988). Such studies should not only identify the "complete carcinogen" (initiator and/or promoter) but also those agents acting possibly through the poorly understood epigenetic mechanisms (Williams and Weisburger, 1981; Williams, 1990). In the long-term carcinogenicity study, the four parameters (incidence, reduced latency, new type(s), multiplicity of tumors) in the operational definition of a carcinogen can be explored in conjunction with dosage in the anticipation that dose-effect relationships can be established for one or all of the parameters.

Carcinogenicity studies of up to 2 years' duration are usually conducted in the males and females of two species of rodent (18 months in mice and 24 months in rats) and frequently in different strains within a species based on the known inter-strain variability in response to chemicals. All of the arguments concerning the use of outbred vs. inbred or hybrid strains, the robust nature, sensitivity vs. insensitivity, biotransformation, pharmacokinetics, etc., must be considered (see Chapter 2). The aims of the study are to determine the incidence of tumor production in relation to a range of doses of the test agent administered in the drinking water or diet over the test period without a significant incidence of other types of toxicity being detected. Ideally, no toxicity other than carcinogenicity should be observed since one is attempting to ascertain the potential of the chemical to elicit cancers at a low-level lifetime exposure. An important endpoint in this type of study is to determine the lowest dose at which no carcinogenicity is observed, a no observable effect level (NOEL). Various protocols have been designed for the conductance of long-term carcinogenicity studies. Considerable thought and planning must occur before initiating such studies and a consideration of the comments of Roe (1981) would be beneficial.

The simplest protocol is to expose the animals (n = 50 animals of each sex per treatment group and adequate numbers of control animals) to the range of doses (minimum 3 levels) via an appropriate route over the study period, ascertaining within and between groups the number of macroscopically visible swellings with confirmation of their neoplastic nature by microscopy as the "lumps and bumps" appear. In addition, the usual monitoring of growth and development, food/water consumption, mortality, morbidity, and periodic hematological/biochemical evaluation of blood samples, urinalysis, etc., is carried out. A second type of protocol would be similar to that shown for the chronic study in Figure 4.9 where subgroups representative of the animals in each treatment group would be euthanized at pre-selected time intervals throughout the study period in order to examine, by microscopy, the morphological appearance and development of tumors in target tissues throughout the stages of initiation/promotion, cellular changes, preneoplastic lesions, and the neoplasms.

The exorbitant costs of conducting an independent chronic 1-year study and a 2-year carcinogenic study has resulted in the two being incorporated together, with

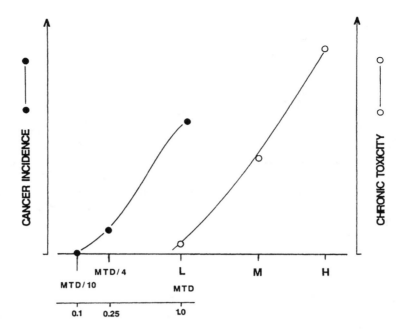

FIGURE 6.11

A theoretical example of a combined chronic toxicity-carcinogenicity study in which a range of doses was selected to address the two endpoints of toxicity. A low dose (L) was selected at the maximum tolerated dose (MTD) level. At the low (L), moderate (M), and high (H) dosages, a dose-dependent incidence in toxicity was observed (o—o). At the pre-selected low (L or MTD), the MTD/4 and MTD/10 dosages, a dose-related incidence of cancer was observed (●—●). If only the MTD, MTD/4 and MTD/10 dosages had been used in an independent carcinogenicity study, the dose-effect curve would have been that observed in the insert figure.

the inclusion of an additional number of dosages lower than those eliciting some noncarcinogenic, toxic endpoint (Rao and Huff, 1990). There are advantages to this approach. The starting point for the selection of these lower dosages begins with the estimated maximum tolerated dose (MTD), usually derived from a 90-d subchronic study. The MTD is defined by the U.S. EPA as "the highest dose that causes no more than a 10% weight decrement, as compared to the appropriate control groups; and does not produce mortality, clinical signs of toxicity, or pathological lesions (other than those that may be related to a neoplastic response) that would be predicted to shorten the animals' natural life span." Usage of the MTD is defended by such philosophical statements as: (1) whether compounds cause cancer or other chronic diseases under extremely high exposure conditions, (2) to minimize the chance that a weak carcinogen might remain undetected, (3) to permit the use of maximum levels of compounds proposed as food additives or pesticides in order to maximize intended benefits to food manufacturing or to agriculture, and (4) to compensate for the relatively small numbers of animals being tested and the limitations in statistical power of the bioassay to detect significant increases in cancer incidence (Carr and Kolbye, 1991).

Figure 6.11 depicts a theoretical scenario of a carcinogenicity study incorporated with a chronic toxicity study. At the estimated MTD (the preselected low dosage) and the moderate and high dosages, there is a significant dose-related incidence of target organ toxicity. For the carcinogenicity assessment over 18 or 24 months, usually two additional dose levels lower than the MTD are arbitrarily selected, the 0.25 MTD and the 0.1 or 0.125 MTD. It is important to remember that one is not dealing with a linear relationship between dosage and effect, although the NOEL for tumor formation would have been obtained.

Considerable controversy exists around the use of the MTD, with some scientists claiming that it is not high enough to elicit the anticipated effects. Others state that, if the test chemical is a weak toxicant as is seen with many food additives and pesticides, the MTD becomes exceedingly high, disrupting normal biotransformation and causing cellular injury, toxic hyperplasia, and toxicity-induced carcinogenesis through abnormal cell proliferation (Carr and Kolbye, 1991). This raises the concerns expressed earlier about "mitogenesis increasing carcinogenesis" (Ames and Gold, 1990). An alternative to the MTD would be to determine a level of exposure, called a pharmacokinetic adjusted dose (PAD), through pharmacokinetic assessment during the conduction of subchronic studies. A level of exposure may be obtained that does not exceed the primary metabolic "breakpoint," thereby avoiding unnecessary use of potentially problematic, secondary metabolic pathways, and/or oxidative stress and peroxisome proliferation in the animals (Kavlock, 1991; Moody et al., 1991). The information required from a suitable subchronic study would include:

1. Whether steady-state tissue concentrations were attained
2. The time required to achieve a steady state with the dosage regimen
3. The total metabolic load
4. Changes in metabolic and pharmacokinetic characteristics with time, dose, and dose schedule

With this information, the MTD can be replaced by a more meaningful minimal toxic dose (minTD), the above-mentioned PAD, or the highest subtoxic dose (HSTD) that can be tolerated by the test animals over a long period without observed toxicity or morphological changes (Carr and Kolbye, 1991).

An excellent example where these principles were applied was during the classic reevaluation of 2,4-dichlorophenoxyacetic acid (2,4-D), particularly the carcinogenicity studies conducted by Hazelton Laboratories America, Inc. for the Industry Task Force on 2,4-D Research Data (Expert Panel Report on Carcinogenicity of 2,4-D, 1987). The highest dose level was 45 mg/kg/day, this being a concentration that was tolerated by the rats for the duration of the study. When no significant carcinogenicity was found, critics complained that higher doses should have been used. However, such levels would have compromised the general wellbeing of the test animals since it was known that (1) at 50 mg/kg/day or higher, there was a break in the linear pharmacokinetics, where excretion was not proportional to intake, and (2) doses of 60 mg/kg/day or higher caused damage to the renal tubular epithelium. Similar problems are encountered with 2,4,5-trichlorophenoxyacetic acid (2,4,5-T), the blood plasma kinetics for this herbicide being presented in Chapter 2, Figure 2.5. A somewhat similar situation was reported for the dose-dependent fate of vinyl chloride and carcinogenesis (Watanabe and Gehring, 1976).

Whatever type of protocol is used, all dead animals, those seriously moribund, those surviving at the end of the study period, and/or those euthanized at preselected time intervals will be subjected to an extensive postmortem examination, with organs being weighed, examined for gross anomalies ("lumps and bumps") and samples of tissues preserved for light and electron microscopic study. The sites and numbers of benign (adenomas) and malignant (carcinomas) tumors are tallied for each animal in the study, are examined in the light of the criteria in the operational definition of a carcinogen, and then a decision is made concerning the carcinogenic potential of the test agent. As was stated previously, the NOEL value or a good estimate of it should be obtained from the study, this being the "number" upon which regulatory agencies will begin to assess the hazard of the test agent to human health. This topic will be addressed in the concluding chapter.

Concerns have been voiced by scientists, regulators, politicians, and the public that potential carcinogens are usually tested one by one rather than in combinations like the real life situation to which all are exposed, i.e., low levels of a mixture of potential carcinogens in air, water, food, etc. Few studies have attempted to address this situation. A recent heroic study of 102 weeks' duration, feeding a combination of 40 carcinogens at low levels (each at 1/50 of the TD_{50}, is a case in point (Takayama et al., 1989). There was a significant number of hepatic neoplastic nodules and follicular cell tumors of the thyroid, evidence of some target-organ selectivity/preference of the mixture. However, agents possibly associated in synergistic or additive carcinogenic effects could not be identified, a situation that is likely to prevail as others attempt this type of study.

REFERENCES

Abdellatif, A.G., Préat, V., Vamecq, J., Nilsson, R., and Roberfroid, M. Peroxisome proliferation and modulation of rat liver carcinogenesis by 2,4-dichlorophenoxyacetic acid, 2,4,5-trichlorophenoxyacetic acid, perfluorooctanoic acid and nafenopin. *Carcinogenesis* 11: 1899-1902 (1990).

Adler, I.-D. Cytogenetic tests in mammals. In *Mutagenicity Testing. A Practical Approach*. S. Venitt and J.M. Parry (Editors). IRL Press, Oxford (1984), pp. 275-306.

Aguirrezabalaga, I, Santamaria, I., and Commendador, M.A. The w/wt SMART is a useful tool for the evaluation of pesticides. *Mutagenesis* 9: 341-346 (1994).

Al-Sabti, K. and Hardig, J. Micrunucleus test in fish for monitoring the genotoxic effects of industrial waste products in the Baltic Sea, Sweden. *Comp. Biochem. Physiol.* 97C: 179-182 (1990).

Amacher, D.E. and Turner, G.N. The L5178Y/TK gene mutation assay for the detection of chemical mutagens. *Ann. N.Y. Acad. Scis.* 407: 239-252 (1983).

Ames, B.N. Identifying environmental chemicals causing mutations and cancer. *Science* 204: 587-593 (1979).

Ames, B.N. Dietary carcinogens and anticarcinogens. *Science* 221: 1256-1264 (1983).

Ames, B.N., Durston, W.E., Yamasaki, E., and Lee, F.D. Carcinogens are mutagens: a simple test system combining liver homogenates for activation and bacteria for detection. Proc. Natl. Acad. Sci. U.S.A. 70: 2281-2285 (1973a).

Ames, B.N. and Gold, L.S. Too many rodent carcinogens: mito-genesis increases mutagenesis. *Science* 249: 970-971 (1990).

Ames, B.N., Gold, L.S., and Willett, W.C. The causes and prevention of cancer. *Proc. Natl. Acad. Sci. U.S.A.* 92: 5258-5265 (1995).

Ames, B.N., Gurney, E.G., Miller, J.A., and Bartsch, H. Carcinogens as frameshift mutagens: metabolites and derivatives of 2-acetylaminofluorene and other aromatic amine carcinogens. *Proc. Natl. Acad. Sci. U.S.A.* 69: 3128-3132 (1972a).

Ames, B.N., Kamen, H.O., and Yamasaki, E. Hair dyes are mutagenic: identification of a variety of mutagenic ingredients. *Proc. Natl. Acad. Sci. U.S.A.* 72: 2423-2427 (1975a).

Ames, B.N., Lee, F.D., and Durston, W.E. An improved bacterial test system for the detection and classification of mutagens and carcinogens. *Proc. Natl. Acad. Sci. U.S.A.* 70: 782-786 (1973b).

Ames, B.N., McCann, J., and Yamasaki, E. Methods for detecting carcinogens and mutagens with the *salmonella*/mammalian microsome mutagenicity test. *Mutat. Res.* 31: 347-364 (1975b).

Ames, B.N., Sims, P., and Grover, P.L. Epoxides of carcinogenic polycyclic hydrocarbons as frameshift mutagens. *Science* 176: 47-49 (1972b).

Ashby, J. and Purchase, I.F.H. Nongenotoxic carcinogens: an extension of the perspective provided by Perera. *Environ. Health Perspect.* 98: 223-226 (1992).

Bishop, J.M. Oncogenes. *Sci. Am.* 246: #3, 80-92 (1982).

Brusick, D.J., Simmons, V.F., Rosenkranz, H.S., Ray, V.A., and Stafford, R.S. An evaluation of *Escherichia coli* WP$_2$ and WP$_2$ uvrA reverse mutation assay. *Mutat. Res.* 76: 169-190 (1980).

Bull, R.J. and Pereira, M.A. Development of a short-term testing matrix for estimating relative carcinogenic risk. *J. Am. Coll. Toxicol.* 1: 1-15 (1982).

Bursch, W., Oberhammer, F., and Schulte-Hermann, R. Cell death by apoptosis and its protective role against disease. *Trends in Pharmacol. Scis.* 13: 245-251 (1992).

Carr, C.J. and Kolbye, Jr., A.C. A critique of the use of the Maximum Tolerated Dose in bioassays to assess cancer risks from chemicals. *Reg. Toxicol. Pharmacol.* 14: 78-87 (1991).

Carthew, P., Martin, E.A., White, I.N.H., DeMatteis, F., Edwards, R.E., Dorman, B.M., Heydon, R.T., and Smith, L.L. Tamoxifen induces short-term cumulative DNA damage and liver tumors in rats: promotion by phenobarbital. *Cancer Res.* 55: 544-547 (1995).

Cayama, E., Tsuda, H., Sarma, D.S.R., and Farber, E. Initiation of chemical carcinogenesis requires cell proliferation. *Nature* 275: 60-62 (1978).

Cohen, S.M. and Ellwein, L.B. Cell proliferation in carcino-genesis. *Science* 249: 1007-1011 (1990).

Cohen, S.M. and Ellwein, L.B. Genetic errors, cell proliferation, and carcinogenesis. *Cancer Res.* 51: 6493-6505 (1991).

Cole, R.J., Cole, J., Henderson, L., Taylor, N.A., Arlett, C.F., and Regan, T. A comparison of sister-chromatid exchanges and the micronucleus test in mouse foetal liver erythroblasts. *Mutat. Res.* 113: 61-75 (1983).

Dean, B.J. and Danford, N. Assays for the detection of chemically-induced chromosome damage in cultured mammalian cells. In *Mutagenicity Testing. A Practical Approach.* S. Venitt and J.M. Parry (Editors). IRL Press, Oxford (1984), pp. 187-232.

DeSerres, F.J. and Kolmark, H.G. A direct method for deter-mination of forward-mutation rates in *Neurospora crassa. Nature* 182: 1249-1250 (1958).

DeSerres, F.J. and Malling, H.V. Measurement of recessive lethal damage over the entire genome and at two specific loci in the ad-3 region of a two-component heterokaryon of *Neurospora crassa.* In *Chemical Mutagens: Principles and Methods for Their Detection.* A. Hollaender (Editor). Plenum Press, N.Y. (1971), pp. 311-342.

DeSerres, G.J. and Malling, H.V. The role of *Neurospora* in evaluating environmental chemicals for mutagenic activity. *Ann. N.Y. Acad. Scis.* 407: 177-185 (1983).

Druckery, H. Specific carcinogenic and teratogenic effects of indirect alkylating methyl and ethyl compounds, and their dependency on stages of ontogenic developments. *Xenobiotica* 3: 271-303 (1973).

Ecobichon, D.J. and Comeau, A.M. Comparative effects of commercial Aroclors on rat liver enzyme activities. *Chem.-Biol. Interactions* 9: 341-350 (1974).

Ennever, F.K., Andreano, G., and Rosenkrantz, H.S. The ability of plant genotoxicity assays to predict carcinogenicity. *Mutation Res.* 205: 99-105 (1988).

Expert Panel Report on Carcinogenicity of 2,4-D. Canadian Centre for Toxicology, Guelph, Ontario, Canada. March 23, 1987.

Farber, E. Possible etiologic mechanisms in chemical carcinogens. *Environ. Health Perspect.* 75: 65-70 (1987).

Fenech, M. The cytokinesis-block micronucleus technique. A detailed description of the method and its application to genotoxicity studies in human populations. *Mutation Res.* 285: 35-44 (1993).

Fucic, A., Horvat, D., and Dimitrovic, B. Mutagenicity of vinyl chloride in man: comparison of chromosome aberrations with micronucleus and sister-chromatid exchange frequencies. *Mutat. Res.* 242: 265-270 (1990).

Garner, R.C., Miller, E.C., and Miller, J.A. Liver microsomal metabolism of aflatoxin B$_1$ to a reactive derivative toxic to *Salmonella typhimurium* TA1530. *Cancer Res.* 32: 2058-2066 (1972).

Grant, W.F. The present status of higher plant bioassays for the detection of environmental mutagens. *Mutation Res.* 310: 175-185 (1994).

Grant, W.F. and Salamone, M.F. Comparative mutagenicity of chemicals selected for test in the International Program on Chemical Safety collaborative study on plant systems for the detection of environmental mutagens. *Mutation Res.* 310: 187-209 (1994).

Gregory, A.R. Species comparisons in evaluating carcinogenicity in humans. *Reg. Toxicol. Pharmacol.* 8: 160-190 (1988).

Heddle, J.A. A rapid *in vivo* test for chromosomal damage. *Mutat. Res.* 18: 307-317 (1973).

Higginson, J. Present trends in cancer epidemiology. *Can. Cancer Conf.* 8: 40-75 (1968).

Higginson, J. Rethinking the environmental causation of human cancer. *Food Cosmet. Toxicol.* 19: 539-548 (1981).

Hollstein, M., Sidransky, D., Vogelstein, B., and Harris, C.C. p53 mutations in human cancers. *Science* 253: 49-53 (1991).

Jones, G. Toxicity requirements of the U.K. and EEC. In *Testing for Toxicity.* Gorrod, J.E., Ed., Taylor and Francis Ltd., London (1981), pp. 1-10.

Kavlock, R.J. Symposium on application of pharmacokinetics in developmental toxicity risk assessments. *Fundam. Appl. Toxicol.* 16: 213-232 (1991).

Kier, L.D., Yamasaki, E., and Ames, B.N. Detection of mutagenic activity in cigarette smoke condensates. *Proc. Natl. Acad. Sci. U.S.A.* 71: 4159-4163 (1974).

Kipling, M.D. and Waldron, H.A. Percivall Pott and cancer scroti. *Br. J. Indust. Med.* 32: 244-250 (1975).

Kolmark, H.G. Differential responses to mutagens as studied by the *neurospora* reverse-mutation test. *Genetics* 39: 270-276 (1953).

Kolmark, H.G. and Westergaard, M. Induced back-mutations in a specific gene of *Neurospora crassa*. *Hereditas* 35: 490-506 (1949).

Kornburst, D. and Barfknecht, T. Testing of 24 food, drug and cosmetic and fabric dyes in the *in vitro* and the *in vivo/in vitro* rat hepatocyte primary culture DNA repair assay. *Environ. Mutagen.* 7: 101-120 (1985).

Krahn, D.F. Chinese hamster cell mutagenesis: a comparison of the CHO and V79 systems. *Ann. N.Y. Acad. Scis.* 407: 231-238 (1983).

LeCurieux, F., Marzin, D., and Erb, F. Study of the genotoxicity of five chlorinated propanones using the SOS chromotest, the Ames-fluctuation test and the new micronucleus test. *Mutation Res.* 341: 1-15 (1994).

Lee, W.R., Abrahamson, S., Valencia, R., Von Halle, E., Wurgler, F.E., and Zimmering, S. The sex-linked recessive lethal test for mutagenesis in *Drosophila melanogaster*. A report of the U.S. Environmental Protection Agency Gene-Tox Program. *Mutat. Res.* 123: 183-279 (1983).

Malling, H.V. Dimethylnitrosamine: formation of mutagenic compounds by interaction with mouse liver microsomes. *Mutat. Res.* 13: 425-429 (1971).

Maron, D.M. and Ames, B.N. Revised methods for the Salmonella mutagenicity test. *Mutat. Res.* 113: 173-215 (1983).

Maugh II, T.H. Cancer and the environment: Higginson speaks out. *Science* 205: 1363-1366 (1979).

McCann, J. and Ames, B.N. A simple method for detecting environmental carcinogens as mutagens. *Ann. N.Y. Acad. Scis.* 271: 5-13 (1976).

McCann, J., Choi, E., Yamasaki, E., and Ames, B.N. Detection of carcinogens as mutagens in the Salmonella/microsome test: assay of 300 chemicals. *Proc. Natl. Acad. Sci. U.S.A.* 72: 5135-5139 (1975a).

McCann, J., Spingarn, N.E., Kobori, J., and Ames, B.N. Detection of carcinogens as mutagens: bacterial tester strains with R factor plasmids. *Proc. Natl. Acad. Sci. U.S.A.* 72: 979-983 (1975b).

Metcalf, C.D. Induction of micronuclei and nuclear abnormalities in the erythrocytes of mudminnows (*Umbra limi*) and brown bullheads (*Ictalurus nebulosus*). *Bull. Environ. Contam. Toxicol.* 40: 489-495 (1988).

Mohtashamipur, E., Mohtashamipur, A., Germann, P.-G., Ernst, H., Norpoth, K., and Mohr, U. Comparative carcinogenicity of cigarette mainstream and sidestream smoke condensates on the mouse skin. *J. Can. Res. Clin. Oncol.* 116: 604-608 (1990).

Moody, D.E. Peroxisome proliferation and nongenotoxic carcinogenesis. Commentary on a symposium. *Fundam. Appl. Toxicol.* 16: 233-248 (1991).

Moolgavkar, S.H. and Knudson, A.G. Mutation and cancer: a model for human carcinogenesis. *J. Natl. Cancer Inst.* 66: 1037-1052 (1981).

Oestreicher, U., Stephan, G., and Glatzel, M. Chromosome and SCE analysis in peripheral lymphocytes of persons occupationally exposed to cytostatic drugs handled with or without use of safety covers. *Mutat. Res.* 242: 271-277 (1990).

Organization for Economic Cooperation and Development. OECD Guidelines for Testing Chemicals. OECD Publications and Information Center, Washington, D.C. (1983-1984).

Organization for Economic Cooperation and Development. OECD Draft Record of the Sixth Meeting of the National Co-ordinators of the Test Guidelines Programme, December 4-5, Paris (1995).

Page, N.P. Concepts of a bioassay program in environmental carcinogenesis. In *Environmental Cancer*. Kraybill, N.F. and Mehlman, Eds., Hemisphere Publishing Corp., Washington, D.C. (1977), pp. 87-171.

Parry, E.M. and Parry, J.M. The assay of genotoxicity of chemicals using the budding yeast *Saccharomyces cerevisiae*. In *Mutagenicity Testing. A Practical Approach*. Venitt, S. and Parry, J.M., Eds., IRL Press, Oxford (1984), pp. 119-147.

Parry, J.M., Parry, E.M., and Barrett, J.C. Tumor promoters induce mitotic aneuploidy yeast. *Nature* (London) 294: 263-265 (1981).

Pelclova, D., Rossner, P., and Pickova, J. Chromosome aberrations in rotogravure printing plant workers. *Mutat. Res.* 245: 299-303 (1990).

Pereira, M.A. Mouse skin bioassay for chemical carcinogens. *J. Am. Coll. Toxicol.* 1: 47-82 (1982a).

Pereira, M.A. Rat liver foci bioassay. *J. Am. Coll. Toxicol.* 1: 101-117 (1982b).

Perera, F.P. Perspectives on the risk assessment of nongenotoxic carcinogens and tumor promotors. *Environ. Health Perspect.* 94: 231-235 (1991).

Pickett-Heaps, J.D., Tippit, D.H., and Porter, K.R. Rethinking mitosis. *Cell.* 29: 729-744 (1982).

Purchase, I.F.H. and Ashby, J. Alternative tests for carcinogens. *Trends in Pharmacol. Sci. August* (1982), pp. 316-322.

Randerath, K., Randerath, E., Danna, T.F., van Golen, K.L., and Putman, K.L. A new sensitive ^{32}P-postlabeling assay based on specific enzymatic conversion of bulky DNA lesions to radiolabeled dinucleotides and nucleoside-5-monophosphates. *Carcinogenesis* 10: 1231-1239 (1989).

Rao, G.N. and Huff, J. Refinement of long-term toxicity and carcinogenicity studies. *Fundam. Appl. Toxicol.* 15: 33-43 (1990).

Roe, F.J.C. Testing *in vivo* for general chronic toxicity and carcinogenicity. In *Testing For Toxicity.* J.W. Gorrod (Editor). Taylor and Francis, London (1981), pp. 29-43.

Saffioti, U. and Wagoner, J.K. (Eds). Occupational Carcinogenesis. *Ann. N.Y. Acad. Scis.* 271: 1-516 (1976).

Sahu, K. and Das, R.K. Micronucleus assay in pulmonary alveolar macrophages, a simple model to detect genotoxicity of environmental agents entering through the inhalation route. *Mutat. Res.* 347: 61-65 (1995).

Schmid, W. The micronucleus test. *Mutat. Res.* 31: 9-15 (1975).

Schmitt, F.C.L., Estevao, D., Kobayashi, S., Curi, P., and DeCamargo, J.L.V. Altered foci of hepatocytes in rats initiated with diethylnitrosamine after prolonged fasting. *Food Chem. Toxicol.* 31: 629-636 (1993).

Schubert, I. and Rieger, R. Sister-chromatid exchanges in *Picea abies* — a test for genotoxicity in forest trees. *Mutation Res.* 323: 137-142 (1994).

Scott, R.E., Wille, J.J., and Wier, M.L. Mechanisms for the initiation and promotion of carcinogenesis: A review and a new concept. *Mayo Clin. Proc.* 59: 107-117 (1984).

Shields, P.G. and Harris, C.C. Environmental causes of cancer. In *Environmental Medicine. The Medical Clinics of North America.* A.C. Upton, Guest Ed., W.B. Saunders Company, Philadelphia. Vol.74, March (1990), pp. 263-277.

Shukla, V., Baqar, S.M., and Mehrotra, N.K. Carcinogenic and co-carcinogenic studies of thiram on mouse skin. *Food Chem. Toxicol.* 34: 283-289 (1996).

Simmon, V.F., Rosenkranz, H.S., Zeiger, E., and Poirier, L.A. Mutagenic activity of chemical carcinogens and related compounds in the intraperitoneal host-mediated assay. *J. Nat. Canc. Inst.* 62: 911-916 (1979).

Stowers, S.J., Maronpot, R.R., Reynolds, S.H., and Anderson, M.W. The role of oncogenes in chemical carcinogenesis. *Environ. Health Perspect.* 75: 81-86 (1987).

Styles, J.A. Other short-term tests in carcinogenesis studies. In *Testing for Toxicity.* J.W. Gorrod, Ed., Taylor and Francis, London (1981), pp. 331-336.

Takayama, S., Hasegawa, H., and Ohgaki, H. Combination effects of forty carcinogens administered at low doses to male rats. *Jap. J. Cancer Res.* 80: 732-736 (1989).

U.S. Environmental Protection Agency. Mutagenicity Testing in Pesticide Programs. Fed. Reg. 40: (163) (1978), pp.37388-37394.

Valencia, R. A cytogenetic study of radiation damage in entire genomes of *Drosophila. Mutat. Res.* 10: 207-219 (1970).

Valencia, R. The versatility of *Drosophila melanogaster* for mutagenicity testing. *Ann. N.Y. Acad. Sci.* 407: 197-207 (1983).

Vaux, D.L. and Strasser, A. The molecular biology of apoptosis. *Proc. Natl. Acad. Sci. U.S.A.* 93: 2239-2244 (1996).

Venitt, S. Microbial tests in carcinogenesis. In *Testing For Toxicity.* J.W. Gorrod, Ed., Taylor and Francis, London (1981), pp. 317-330.

Vogel, E.W. Approaches to comparative mutagenesis in higher eukaryotes: significance of DNA modifications with alkylating agents in *Drosophila melanogaster. Ann. N.Y. Acad. Scis.* 407: 208-220 (1983).

Vogel, E.W. Tests for recombinagens in somatic cells of *Drosophila. Mutat. Res.* 284: 159-175 (1992).

Vogel, E.W. and Nivard, M.J.M. Performance of 181 chemicals in a *Drosophila* assay predominantly monitoring interchromosomal mitotic recombination. *Mutagenesis* 8: 57-81 (1993).

Watanabe, P.G. and Gehring, P.J. Dose-dependent fate of vinyl chloride and its possible relationship to oncogenicity in rats. *Environ. Health Perspect.* 17: 145-152 (1976).

Weinstein, I.B. Mitogenesis is only one factor in carcinogenesis. *Science* 251: 387-388 (1991).

Weisburger, J.H. Does the Delaney Clause of the U.S. Food and Drug Laws prevent human cancers? *Fundam. Appl. Toxicol.* 22: 483-493 (1994).

Weisburger, J.H. and Williams, G.M. Carcinogen testing: Current problems and new approaches. *Science* 214: 401-407 (1981).

Weisburger, J.H. and Williams, G.M. Critical effective methods to detect genotoxic carcinogens and neoplasm promoting agents. *Environ. Health Perspect.* 90: 121-126 (1991).

Wilbourn, J., Haroun, L., Haseltine, E., Kaldor, J., Partensky, C., and Vainio, H. Response of experimental animals to human carcinogens: an analysis based upon the IARC Monographs program. *Carcinogenesis* 7: 1853-1863 (1986).

Williams, G.M. Detection of chemical carcinogens by unscheduled DNA synthesis in rat liver primary cell cultures. *Cancer Res.* 37: 1845-1851 (1977).

Williams, G.M. Methods for evaluating chemical genotoxicity. In *Annual Review of Pharmacology and Toxicology.* George, R., Okun, R. and Cho, A.K., Eds., Annual Reviews Inc., Palo Alto, CA. 29: 189-211 (1989).

Williams, G.M. Screening procedures for evaluating the potential carcinogenicity of food-packaging chemicals. *Reg. Toxicol. Pharmacol.* 12: 30-40 (1990).

Williams, G.M., Laspia, M.F., and Dunkel, V.C. Reliability of the hepatocyte primary culture/DNA repair test in testing for coded carcinogens and noncarcinogens. *Mutat. Res.* 97: 359-370 (1982).

Williams, G.M. and Weisburger, J.H. Systematic carcinogen testing through the decision point approach. In *Annual Review of Pharmacology and Toxicology.* George, R., Okun, R. and Cho, A.K., Eds., Annual Reviews Inc., Palo Alto, CA. 21: 393-416 (1981).

Wolff, S. Sister chromatid exchange as a test for mutagenic carcinogens. *Ann. N.Y. Acad. Scis.* 407: 142-153 (1983).

Yamagiwa, K. and Itchikawa, K. Experimental study of the pathogenesis of carcinoma. *J. Cancer Res.* 3: 1-21 (1918).

Yunis, J.J. The chromosomal basis of human neoplasia. *Science* 221: 227-236 (1983).

Zeiger, E. Carcinogenicity of mutagens: Predictive capability of the *Salmonella* mutagenicity assay for rodent carcinogenicity. *Cancer Res.* 47: 1287-1296 (1987).

Zimmerman, F.K. Screening with fungal systems. *Ann. N.Y. Acad. Scis.* 407: 186-196 (1983).

Zimmerman, F.K., Mayer, V.W., and Parry, J.M. Genetic toxicology studies using *Saccharomyces cerevisiae.* *J. Appl. Toxicol.* 2: 1-10 (1982).

Chapter 7

RISK ASSESSMENT

I. INTRODUCTION

The public is aware that it is exposed to a myriad of anthropogenic and natural "chemicals" in food, air, and water accidentally and/or by design as well as from sources arising from voluntary lifestyle activities (therapeutic agents, drugs of abuse, alcohol, tobacco products, etc.) throughout a "lifetime." What people want to know is how hazardous to their health is this lifetime "potpourri." To the toxicologist, "hazard" means the qualitative description of harmful effects. How much is enough? How little is too much? How safe is safe enough? These questions haunt the public who are constantly bombarded by media hype touting the toxic chemical of the week. Any mention of the word "chemicals" conjures up images of devastating diseases, cancer, and birth defects, giving rise to the syndrome "chemophobia." The entire situation is reduced to the public's understanding (perception) of what constitutes risk (Slovic, 1987). In the public's perception, if it is bad, more is worse!

As defined in any dictionary, **risk** is usually associated with the "chance of injury, damage, or loss." However, this definition has no quantifiable boundaries. To the toxicologist, "risk" means a quantitative measure of the probability for certain harmful effects occurring to a group of people as a result of exposure to a given agent. How large or small is this risk? Taking risks is a part of life but humans are unique in the sense that we frequently ignore high risks taken voluntarily but become terribly concerned, agitated, hostile, and even totally irrational about small, seemingly insignificant risks, particularly if these are being imposed upon us by some other group, frequently a regulatory agency (Starr and Whipple, 1980; Zeckhauser and Viscusi, 1990). "Acceptable risks" — acceptable to whom? Since the decision(s) of such regulatory groups are usually based upon research — animal and/or human — the validity of this research is examined closely by other groups, frequently having a prejudiced mindset. Conflict is inevitable when any group imposes a risk upon others.

Quantitative risk assessment is defined as the estimation of levels of exposure to a toxic substance which leads to specific increases in lifetime incidence rates or in the probable occurrence of a given undesirable consequence (Van Ryzin, 1980). However, in a more practical sense, according to Gots (1992) and others, risk assessment is "an instrument of social compromise, providing numerical answers in the face of vast scientific uncertainties. What it is not is science." It is not designed to reflect scientific truths, but to bring a semblance of order to chaos, permitting regulatory agencies to ease the tension between popular demands and scientific uncertainties. Risk assessment is "the use of the factual base to define health effects of exposure of individuals or populations to hazardous materials and situations" (Center for Risk Analysis, 1994). The methods used and the subsequent predictions are limited by the quality of biological knowledge, being capable to describe known biological effects but being unable to predict effects that are scientifically unknown (Gots, 1992). Risk assessment reflects a lack of data for a toxicant rather than any direct evidence that the agent induced harm at the exposures encountered (Bull et al., 1993). Better modeling can never improve the results, but better (more extensive and/or complete) will reduce or eliminate sources of uncertainty and error. Perhaps, a better definition of risk assessment is that it is a scientific process by which one attempts to characterize in as quantitative manner as data permits, the dose (exposure)-response curve in humans to provide scientific support for management decisions designed to decrease risks from exposures to agents (Becker, 1996a).

It is important to appreciate that research cannot demonstrate that a risk does not exist. Research can establish probabilistic bounds on possible risks and, if those bounds are sufficiently "low," the risk should be acceptable (Morgan, 1986). Research may not show that a hazard exists, but it may demonstrate that, under certain specific circumstances, injury, damage, or loss can be produced in living systems. How then, does a regulatory agency, a politician, a toxicologist, etc., justify to the public that enough research has been done and that additional research is unlikely to identify any new or different toxic properties that can be used to make a better assessment of the risk inherent in using a chemical, physical agent, or some form of energy. All of the questions frequently distill into one pertinent question: how good are the predictions on risk from existing toxicity data bases for chemicals that all of us come into contact with daily? The U.S. National Research Council (NRC) report in 1984 demonstrated that, overall, the toxicity data base for chemicals was poor (NRC, 1984). A complete health hazard assessment could be done for 6.8% and a partial assessment was possible for 16.4% of the 17,202 chemicals listed. There was a paucity of toxicity data for commercial chemicals. Certainly, this is not encouraging news.

Risk assessment reveals the type(s) of injury that might be associated with the unintended acquisition of a body burden of a chemical, physical agent, or form of energy. Who must risk estimates be determined for? As is shown in Figure 7.1, several populations of individuals may be identified as having possible exposure to a range of concentrations of a particular agent, including accidental and suicidal poisonings, occupationally exposed workers, bystanders (workers nearby, dwellers adjacent to a factory emitting a chemical or other "sources"), and the general public. The shape of the dose-effect relationship is dependent on sufficiently detailed knowledge of the amount of exposure received by each of these subpopulations. Frequently, exposure evaluations begin at the highest dosage where a narrow range of dosage always elicits easily identified signs and symptoms of toxicity. If no discernible adverse health effects are seen at high levels of exposure, it is unlikely that anything will be observed at lower levels of exposure. Although this hypothesis may be true for acute, possibly life-threatening effects, it is not applicable to chronic toxicity (subtle alterations in organ function, mutagenicity, teratogenicity, carcinogenicity) that may develop after some latent period of time following a single, high level exposure, repeated moderate or high level exposure, or annual exposure to low levels of the potential toxicant for decades. The annual, intermittent exposure of healthy workers, males and females, to a broader range of concentrations of the agent may result in quantifiable, toxicological signs and symptoms, hence the establishment of threshold limit values (TLVs or what are now call time-weighted averages, TWAs) and short-time exposure levels (STELs) for chemicals in ambient air to protect workers. Frequently, these values are based on considerable human exposure data in addition to

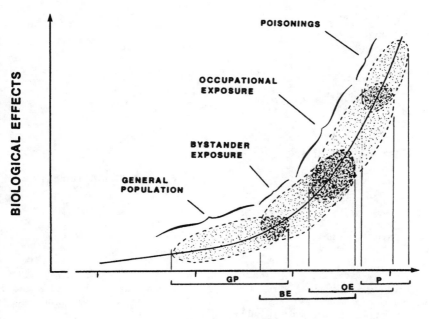

FIGURE 7.1
A theoretical dose-response relationship indicating the range of dosage (mg/kg of body weight) of a toxicant to which representative human populations might be exposed. Poisonings (P) tend to occur over a relatively narrow range, while in occupational exposures (OE), the range would be somewhat broader. Overlapping with occupational exposure, the dosage range to which bystanders would be exposed (BE) would be broader still, while the general population (GP) would encounter a dosage range of possibly one to three orders of magnitude.

recent animal studies demonstrating (or verifying) additional, chronic toxicity, i.e., teratogenicity or carcinogenicity. Bystander exposure is much more difficult to assess; frequently, the dosage ranges over one or two orders of magnitude and is often accompanied by spurious, ill-defined signs and symptoms not identified with the known toxicity associated with high level exposure(s). The general population — characterized by an age range from the very young to the elderly, a range in health status from good to poor, and inherent susceptibilities to certain chemicals as a consequence of altered physiological and biochemical function throughout life — is exposed to a broad range of low levels of the potential toxicant in food, air, and water. Few well-defined signs and symptoms of toxicity are observed, other than those (birth defects, fertility and reproductive outcomes, carcinogenicity) which appear to have a background incidence of occurrence within populations for no readily apparent reasons. This is where the difficulty arises in risk assesment: the utilization of the best available toxicity data base to predict any risk to the health of the general population. This is the crux of the entire risk assessment process. Is the data base for the chemical the best available? Is the interpretation of the results correct? Is the assessment of the risk carried out in an appropriate and convincing manner? Is the public cognizant of the infrequency with which the risk occurs? It is important to remember that single events govern political and public responses, not the probabilities of that single event being rare (Starr and Whipple, 1980).

The generic approach to quantitative risk assessment has evolved into a process of determining: (1) if a hazard exists, (2) the dose-response relationship, (3) the

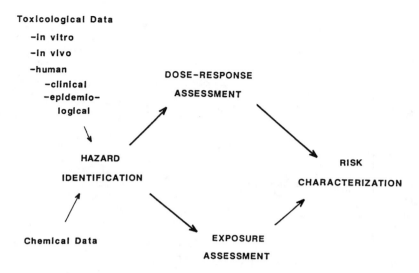

FIGURE 7.2
A schematic diagram depicting the process of risk characterization utilizing dose-response and exposure assessment information as well as hazard identification data obtained from physical and chemical properties of the agent plus relevant toxicological information.

potential for exposure, and (4) the characterization of the risk (Figure 7.2). The components of a health risk assessment have been described many times, and the reader is referred to the following sources for a more in-depth review: Tardiff and Youngren (1986), Hallenbeck and Cunningham (1987), Cothern et al.(1988), Paustenbach (1990), and Center for Risk Assessment (1993).

II. HAZARD IDENTIFICATION

A potential hazard to human health may come to light in a number of ways — a comment of a worker who notices a pungent, offensive odor, the opportune detection of a chemical in the environment (air, water), the presence of certain ingredients in foods that are required in the processing procedure or as preservatives, etc., concerns raised over a detectable contaminant (industrial chemicals, pesticides, etc.) or natural component in a food source, or a chemical-related hypersensitivity of a subpopulation of individuals. Whatever the trigger mechanism, the risk assessor must now develop a rational approach to address these concerns.

Hazard identification involves the qualitative evaluation of the adverse health effects of a substance in animals or humans. The literature should be searched for relevant epidemiological studies, case reports, and even unconfirmed anecdotal information relevant to the chemical. However, given the previously mentioned problems of estimating exposure in human studies as well as limited study design, it may be more advantageous to consider animal studies, the advantages of which are uniformity of the species, stringent control over the exposure, and route of administration, while the disadvantages include the interspecies relevance of signs and symptoms of toxicity and subsequent extrapolation of the results to the human. Factors that should be kept in mind include: (1) the route of exposure should, ideally, be the same as that by which the human could acquire the agent, (2) the problems of multiple target organ toxicity associated with all chemicals at different dosages, and (3) the relative seriousness and dose-associated relationship of each form of toxicity (Tardiff and Youngren, 1986). This does not preclude the use of *in vitro* test system results as predictors of certain types of toxicity, i.e., teratogenicity, carcinogenicity. Ideally, the animal studies should address the issues of:

1. The suitability of the test species as a surrogate for the human
2. The numbers of animals (each sex), age, and study groups
3. The types of observations made and the methods of quantitative analysis
4. The nature of all pathological changes observed
5. Alterations in metabolic responses (species- and sex-related)

Evaluation of the various studies should include objective endpoints for the assessor, including specific endpoints of toxicity (including delayed effects), use of species most predictive of human responses, and the determination of a dose-effect relationship capable of quantifying the adverse health effects (Tardiff and Youngren, 1986). The risk assessor should select studies utilizing the most sensitive species (greatest response per unit dose) in the dosage range of concern. At this stage, it is important to consider all of the evidence in terms of quality, strength of the results, and confidence that the toxicity observed in one biological system will pertain to another system.

III. DOSE-RESPONSE ASSESSMENT

Having gathered and examined the relevant studies of the potential toxicant in humans and/or animals, one can turn to the development of relationships between the dose of the test agent and the various adverse health effects. Three types of dose-response relationships can be identified (Tardiff and Youngren, 1986):

1. The *quantal* relationship in which the number of responding individuals in a population varies with the concentration of agent administered
2. The *graded* relationship in which the severity of the lesion within the individuals is a function of dose
3. The *continuous* response relationship in which some biological parameter (body weight, tissue weight, etc.) is changed by the dosage regimen

Regardless of the shape of the dose-response relationship (linear, convex, concave, or sigmoid-shaped), the intensity (or frequency) of response is generally increased with dosage, the response(s) essentially beginning at zero, or at least at an unquantifiable level, and rising to measurable changes as the dosage is increased. Tardiff and Youngren (1986) make a cogent point concerning experimental thresholds for a chemical in animal studies and comparable population thresholds in humans being dependent upon the breadth and distribution of sensitivities among all members of a population (the highly sensitive, the highly resistant, competing and modulating factors that govern the degree of biological response). While the dosage range used in an animal study may not reflect that encountered by the "exposed" humans, this should not be considered detrimental to the assessment. As was stated earlier in the text, the number of times that the same biological response(s) can be elicited in different species, the better is the chance that at some dosage the same effect may be elicited in humans. Theoretically, one might measure the same biological response in three species of test animal over a 1000-fold range of concentrations. With no reliable human data from accidental exposures to the test agent, one would initiate the risk assessment by selecting the results from the most susceptible species and would assess the risk based on low-dose extrapolation to some acceptable (safe) concentration.

IV. EXPOSURE ASSESSMENT

This component has been characterized as the "process of measuring (or estimating) the intensity, frequency, and duration of human exposures to an agent present in the environment or of estimating hypothetical exposures that might arise from the release of new chemicals into the environment. It describes the magnitude, duration, schedule, and route of exposure; the size, nature, and classes of the human populations exposed; and the uncertainties in all the estimates" (NRC, 1983). The completeness and the deficiencies in the available toxicity/exposure data are examined, the amounts in the environment (air, water, food) are determined, and measurements of human intake by various media are studied; all these parameters providing a historical data base in an attempt to reduce the magnitude of the uncertainties. Techniques by which exposure could be reduced would also be examined.

V. RISK CHARACTERIZATION

This component of the risk assessment package may be defined as the process of estimating the probable incidence of an adverse health effect to humans under various conditions of exposure. Human-based data should be used if at all possible, but frequently, good information is lacking, incomplete, or fragmented, and the assessor has to fall back on better controlled, chronic, animal studies for an adequate toxicity data base. The dose-response relationships developed from appropriate animal studies are introduced into model systems. One of the first considerations to be addressed is whether or not the dose-response relationships are *threshold* (non-zero threshold) — there is a level below which adverse health effects are unlikely to occur — or *non-threshold* (zero threshold) where, theoretically, there is always some response regardless of how small the exposure level is, i.e., one molecule of the chemical might induce an adverse health effect (Hallenbeck and Cunningham, 1987). One can see the derivation of the non-threshold concept from the theories of carcinogenesis where there is an irreversible, self-replicating lesion arising possibly from a mutation in a single somatic cell following exposure to a single dose (Lu, 1983; Munro and Krewski, 1981). Examples of threshold-type relationships include organ/tissue effects (neuro-, hepato-, nephrotoxicity, etc.) germ-cell mutations, and developmental effects, all of which can be studied in highly susceptible animal models by sensitive analytical techniques. Of the non-threshold relationship, the most frequently cited examples are mutagenesis (somatic mutations) and carcinogenesis, although recently there appear to be shifts in carcinogenesis theories that may accomodate the threshold concept (Weisburger, 1990). Acceptable concentrations for threshold chemicals are estimated using the *safety (uncertainty) factor* method while those for non-threshold chemicals are determined by the *risk analysis* method (Hallenbeck and Cunningham, 1987).

A. Threshold Relationships

All too frequently, the exact shape of the lower end of the dose-response relationship is obscured by the facts that low enough dosages were not used in the study or that, while the level of exposure can be measured by sensitive analytical techniques, comparable sensitivity is not available to measure minute biological effects. Therefore, one has no idea whether the low-dose relationship is curvilinear or linear. Prior to conducting a chronic toxicity study, it is extremely difficult to preselect a three-level range of appropriate dosages from a subchronic (90-d) study that will result in a span of toxicological effects from overt toxicity (the highest dosage), some intermediate expression of toxicity (the moderate dosage), and at the lowest dosage, no toxicity. The results obtained after 1 or 2 years of continuous administration are usually less than ideal, the variability being observed at the lower end of the dose-response relationship, with either no adverse biological effects being detected at the lowest and/or the moderate dosage or, conversely, some toxicity being measured at all levels in a dose-dependent manner. The threshold concept is important to regulatory agencies because it signifies that a range of exposures from zero to some finite value can be tolerated by any individual with essentially no chance of an adverse health effect (Becker, 1996).

As is shown in Figure 7.3, there are a number of effect-related "endpoints" at the lower end of the dose-response curve representing positive or negative effects in terms of exposure (Dourson and Stara, 1983). The first, the *lowest observed adverse effect level* (LOAEL), refers to the dosage rate of chemical at which there are statistically or biologically significant differences in the frequency or severity of adverse health effects between the exposed and the control groups. The next, the *no observed adverse effect level* (NOAEL), refers to that dose rate at which there are no statistically or biologically significant increases in frequency or severity of effects between the exposed and the control groups. There may be some effects observed, i.e., a reduction in body weight, etc., reflecting some test agent-related influence on well-being, but there are no measurable adverse health effects. The last, the *no observed effect level* (NOEL), refers to that dose rate of test agent at which the exposed animals appear identical to controls in all respects. One or more of these values may be obtained from a carefully conducted study using an appropriate preselected range of dosages. All of these values must be defined in terms of the duration of the exposure and the period of observation from first to last exposure. Invariably, these values are derived from long-term (chronic, lifetime) studies in the most susceptible species, the biological effects being measured by the most sensitive analytical techniques (Brown et al., 1988; Gregory, 1988).

In a practical sense, regulatory agencies can arbitrarily apply a series of safety, uncertainty, or modifying factors (SF, UF, MF) to the NOEL, NOAEL, and LOAEL, in order of preference, to determine *acceptable concentrations* variously described, depending on the agency, as a reference dose (RfD), a virtually safe dose (VSD), an estimated population threshold for humans (EPT-H), an acceptable daily intake (ADI), a maximum allowable concentration (MAC), etc. The mathematics associated with the calculation of a human dose from the results of animal studies have been addressed by Hallenbeck and Cunningham (1987) and U.S. EPA (1985). If the NOEL, the most suitable number, can be determined from the study results, this value may be divided by a factor of 100 (tenfold factor for intraspecies variability in response(s) and another tenfold factor to account for interspecies differences) to yield an acceptable concentration equal to NOEL/100. In a routine first analysis of toxicity data, a

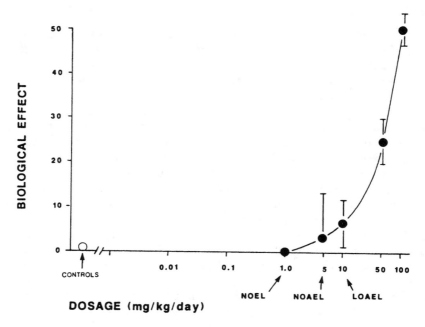

DOSAGE (mg/kg/day)

FIGURE 7.3

A theoretical dose-response relationship showing demonstrable dose-related toxicity over a range of 1.0 to 100 mg/kg/d. Also identified are the *lowest observed adverse effect level* (LOAEL), the *no observed adverse effect level* (NOAEL), and the *no observed effect level* (NOEL), all dosage reference points that can be used to derive acceptable concentration values with the arbitrary safety (uncertainty) factor approach.

risk assessor would usually apply the 100-fold UF to the NOEL. While the reasons for this factor were stated above, another way of looking at this uncertainty factor is that it takes into consideration the possibility that the human may be up to tenfold more sensitive than the animal species tested and allows for a tenfold variability in sensitivity within the human population. Additional safety factors may be applied to the lowest effect level, depending upon the confidence expressed in the study design, number of animals, the strength and quality of the data, etc. (Figure 7.4). Given the fact that the study results only yield a reliable NOAEL, an assessor may want to increase the UF five- or tenfold to address the problem that, while no adverse health effects were observed, there were still detectable differences between the exposed and control groups. The acceptable concentration may become the NOAEL/500 or NOAEL/1000. If only a LOAEL was obtainable from the study results, a risk assessor would have some reservations about the study design, the results, the fact that the lowest dosage used caused some toxicity (frequency or severity of effects), and the paucity of information at lower dosages. These concerns would be reflected in the application of a higher UF, the acceptable concentration becoming the LOAEL/1000 at least. A safety factor of 5000 has been used to arrive at acceptable concentrations of carcinogenic substances but has been abandoned in favor of the use of low-dose extrapolation models thought to be more scientifically sound (Weil, 1972). These will be discussed in the next section.

Despite the obvious arbitrary and subjective nature of applying various numerical UFs to a toxicity data base, and the concerns voiced that this does not appear to be very scientific, this system functions reasonably well. Obviously, the acceptable

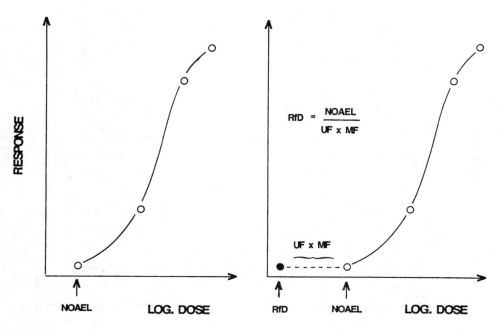

FIGURE 7.4
A theoretical dose-response relationship (left panel) with the identification of a no observable adverse effect level (NAOEL) and showing how this value is utilized to determine a reference dose (RfD) or acceptable daily intake (ADI) by dividing the NOAEL by uncertainty factors (UF) and modifying factors (MF), the magnitude of these factors being determined by the adequacy of the study design, the quality of the toxicity data, the nature of the toxic effect(s), the duration of exposure in the animal study in relation to the expected exposure of the human population at risk and data concerning sensitivity and specificity in various species and subpopulations.

concentration (mg/kg body wt/day) for a human cannot be taken directly from the results of animal studies adjusted by an appropriate UF. The proportion of the chemical acquired via air, water, or food must be considered, i.e., multimedia exposure for environmental contaminants, to ascertain what amounts the average human would obtain per day, week, year, or lifetime.

In attempting to address the paucity of definitive data on biological effects at dosages lower than those used in appropriate chronic animal studies, and to derive as conservative an estimate of an acceptable concentration as possible, other theoretical approaches are used to extrapolate for biological effects below the lowest dosage. Figure 7.5 shows several of these attempts. The first, drawing a straight line from the experimental threshold dose to the "zero" value gives an estimate of effects at substantially lower doses. The second, producing a more conservative estimate, takes into account the upper confidence limit of the variability in the population response to the experimental threshold dosage rather than the mean value (x) and consists of drawing a straight line from the upper confidence limit (x ± 2SD) to the "zero" value (Gaylor and Kodell, 1980). The larger the group of animals used at the experimental threshold level, the more normal the distribution will be, and the better (more narrow) the confidence limits will be. With this technique, the risk assessor anticipates that the aberrant, sensitive individuals in a population, if they could be identified, might respond to dosages lower than the experimental threshold level.

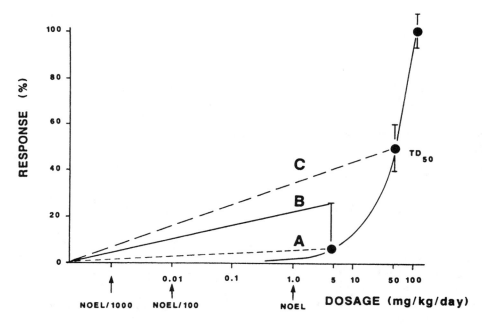

FIGURE 7.5

A theoretical dose-response relationship depicting three different methods of linear extrapolation from experimental data points to "zero" dosage. In A, a straight line is drawn from the lowest experimental value. In B, the line is drawn from the upper portion of the 95% confidence limit of the lowest experimental value (X ± 2SD), this technique accomodating for the highly sensitive individuals in the "population" who might respond to lower concentrations of the test agent (Gaylor and Kodell, 1980). In C, a technique used frequently in carcinogenic risk assessment to determine risk-specific doses (RSDs), the linear extrapolation begins at the TD_{50} (the dosage that produces tumors in 50% of the test animals) (Munro and Krewski, 1981).

B. Non-Threshold Relationships

The public phobia about cancer has had a marked influence on the regulatory philosophy for the determination of permissible levels of carcinogenic chemicals in air, water, and foods. The focus was sharpened in 1958 with the passage of the so-called Delaney clause (FDC Act, Section 409) which flatly prohibited approval of a food additive (including pesticides) found to induce cancer in humans and animals and introduced a *zero tolerance* approach to additives/contaminants. A value of zero is entirely dependent upon the sensitivity of the analytical methods used to detect and quantitate the chemical. Even in 1958, U.S. regulatory agencies were facing the problem of DDT, designated as a carcinogen, albeit falsely, which could be found almost everywhere one looked for it, since the analytical technique of gas-liquid chromatography was capable of detecting low parts-per-million (ppm, micrograms/g of sample) levels. Presently, there is no such thing as a *zero level* for any chemical, traces down into the parts-per-trillion (ppt, picograms/g of sample) being readily detected. The regulatory approaches to handling such vexing problems as trace levels of potential carcinogens have been described (NRC, 1987). How then does a risk assessor arrive at an acceptable concentration, balanced between the public's demand for a zero tolerance and state-of-the-art techniques capable of quantitating trace levels of possible carcinogens in media (air, water, food) acquired by the public involuntarily each and every day?

   If acceptable concentrations of carcinogens are determined by the application of a maximum UF approach, i.e., 5000, it is important to recognize that this method of determining a population threshold level does not take into account the slope of the dose-response curve. The application of a moderate UF may result in an adequate margin of safety for the chemical if the slope is steep but may be insufficient if the slope of the dose-response relationship is shallow (Munro and Krewski, 1981). The risk assessor is left in a quandary since, invariably, there is a poor visual picture of the lower end of the dose-response relationship, made even more difficult by the fact that the dosage range of concern for carcinogens may be several orders of magnitude below those known to elicit any carcinogenic response (occupational exposure, epidemiological studies, animal studies). Historically, the rejection of a population threshold concept for carcinogens has been based on the facts that: (1) thresholds will vary considerably between individuals, (2) extremely low concentrations of agents may produce a mutation in a single somatic cell, altering the genome sufficiently to initiate a cancer — the one-hit, one cancer theory, (3) cancers arise from single mutated cells and with survival, development, and progression, cause metastases in other organs, and (4) the original theories on carcinogenesis were based on the apparent, linear dose-response relationship for radiation-induced cancers, with the ability to measure low levels of radiation being technically feasible since the early 1900s. However, the non-threshold concept is contrary to observations. While everyone is exposed to trace amounts of numerous carcinogens daily, not everyone develops cancer in their lifetime, suggesting that in most cases the exposure was low enough that there was no response. Perhaps a practical threshold does exist for the actions of carcinogens. The basis for a population threshold level or acceptable concentration approach to carcinogens has been eloquently described (Mastromatteo, 1981; Truhaut, 1980; Weisburger, 1990).
   Before examining the various risk assessment models in current use, one should look closely at the tenet stating that cancer risk is always proportional to dose, no matter how small *or* that all exposures, no matter what the amount, carry an associated cancer risk — the one-hit (or molecule) one cancer theory. The reliance on these models has been eloquently challenged by Goldman (1996) who brings to light early data on mutations in fruit flies exposed to doses of x-irradiation in which the relationship was not linear with dose but with the square root of the dose (Muller, 1927). The linearity concept was introduced into cancer risk assessment during the era of nuclear weapons (atmospheric) testing and was adopted for chemicals when the Delaney Amendment was introduced in 1958. Cancer risk assessments are extrapolated from experiments involving exposure to high levels of agent as is shown in Figure 7.6. A conservative approach generally draws a straight line through the experimental data points and the zero intercept, describing the slope of the line as a risk coefficient, e.g., the fatal cancers per unit dose (Becker, 1996b; Goldman, 1996). The fallacy of this approach has been suggested by recent studies in which rats, exposed to low doses of 49 carcinogens, revealed damage to hepatic DNA, assuming that this is a mechanism involved in hepatic carcinoma, the relationship being curvilinear rather than linear with "very low" doses (Kitchin and Brown, 1994) (Figure 7.7). These results have generated considerable controversy pro and con the assumption that changes in alkaline-labile sites in hepatic DNA signify genotoxicity or DNA damaging/mutagenic activity as determined in short-term, *in vivo* genotoxicity assays (BELLE Newsletter, 1995). As investigators work down to molecular mechanisms rather than studying tumorigenicity in the intact animal, more curvilinear, and even threshold relationships will be established between some subcellular effect and low levels of exposure. This has been seen even for the dioxin receptor

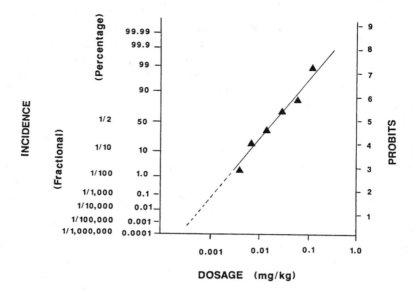

FIGURE 7.6
A hypothetical dose-response relationship of the incidence of tumors in groups of animals receiving different doses of a carcinogen, showing the linear extrapolation from the observed values to determine the dose required to achieve the excess lifetime risk level of one cancer per million of population.

model and levels of dioxin between 10^{-12} and 10^{-9}g (Roberts, 1991). The universal cancer risk curve may yet prove to be more of a sigmoidal than a linear relationship, with perhaps even a threshold level (Goldman, 1996).

A second point of consideration has to do with the origins of the units of expression, the numbers of cancers in excess of a background, and lifetime incidence of cancer of one cancer per million (10^6). Historically, where did this number come from? Kelly and Cardon (1994) claim that it arose in conjunction with drug residues in animal tissues, once again at the time of the Delaney Amendment. It came from a definition of a "safe" level of a carcinogen being equal to one chance in 100,000,000 (1×10^{-8}) of developing cancer. Rather unscientifically, the number was picked, sort of arbitrarily "out of a hat" by Mantel and Bryan (1961). The U.S. FDA adopted this original value for 1973 legislation but changed it to 1×10^{-6} for the final ruling in 1977 (U.S. FDA, 1973), hence, the need to extrapolate far below the actual experimental values as is shown in Figure 7.6. The 1×10^{-6} value is used by regulatory agencies for residues of various chemicals in foods, part of the "de minimus" risk approach, and also for hazardous waste sites. Does it represent a realistic acceptable (negligible) risk level?

The reliance, or perhaps misplaced loyalty, to the linear model, whatever form it takes, is illustrated by many ludicrous examples in the literature. Goldman (1996) illustrates the problem by relating cosmic radiation with an increased incidence of cancer worldwide if every person increased their height by one inch by wearing lifts of that height under their shoes for one year. Gots (1993) has a more humorous model, stating that if one million people jumped from a building 300 ft high, 900,000 would die. Assuming that for each one tenth the height is reduced that one tenth the number of people will die (the risk coefficient), then at 30 ft, it is assumed that 90,000 will die, at 3 ft some 9000 will die, etc. The model would predict 900 deaths at a jumping height of 0.3 ft and 90 deaths at a height of 0.03 ft. Caution must be exercised when using linear models for fear of reaching the level of the old theological argument of how many angels can dance on the head of a pin.

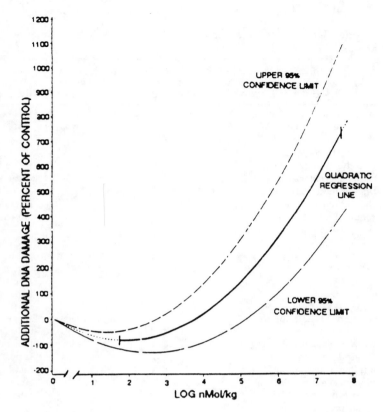

FIGURE 7.7

The dose-response relationship for alkaline-labile alterations in female rat hepatic DNA caused by an "average DNA-damaging carcinogen" as determined from the experimental results with ll chemical carcinogens. The solid line is the quadratic regression line from the experimental results, the dashed lines being the upper and lower 95% confidence limits. The nonlinear relationship suggests a lack of adherence to the non-threshold dogma currently used in models to assess low-dose response relationships for potential carcinogens. (From Kitchin and Brown (1994). With permission.)

The overall goal of the risk assessor is not to underestimate human risk. The issue of threshold vs. non-threshold approaches in terms of risk analysis resolves itself around the shape of the dose-response relationship in the subexperimental dose range and the manner by which an estimate of that shape is attained. A number of mathematical models have been used to achieve this end. Three types of models have been proposed: *tolerance distribution models* (probit, logit, Weibull); *mechanistic models* (one-hit, multihit, multistage); and *time-to-tumor occurrence models* (lognormal, Weibull) (Hallenbeck and Cunningham, 1987). The utility of these various models has been compared (Van Ryzin, 1980; Van Ryzin and Rai, 1980; Altshuler, 1981; Munro and Krewski, 1981). A summary of the cogent points for selected models is presented in Table 7.1. The main application of these models is for data obtained from appropriate chronic animal studies. Depending upon the mathematically derived, low dose-response curve obtained from experimental data, the curve may be linear, supralinear (convex and above the linear relationship), or sublinear (concave and below the linear relationship) (Munro and Krewski, 1981). Having chosen an acceptable level of risk, usually one extra cancer in a population of 100,000 or of 1,000,000 (mathematical risks based on scientific assumptions used in risk assessment) and

TABLE 7.1

Mathematical Models Used in the Determination of Low-Dose Response Relationships for
Potentially Carcinogenic Agents

Model	Description	Probability of a test animal responding at dose level "d"	Shape of parameter	Low-dose response
One-hit	Based on the concept that a response will occur after the target has been "hit" by a single biologically effective unit of dose	$1 - \exp^{-\beta d}$	$\beta > 0$	Linear at low doses
Multihit	Based on an extension of the one-hit model assuming that more than one hit is required to induce a response	$\int_0^{\beta d} \left(u^{k-1} e^{-u} / r(k) \right) du$	$k > 0$ $\beta > 0$	Linear at low doses *only* when the shape parameters are equal to unity
Weibull		$1 - \exp^{-\beta d^m}$	$m > 0$ $\beta > 0$	When shape parameters are curves approach zero at slower than linear or sublinear rate
Multistage	Based on the assumption that the induction of irreversible self-replicating toxic effects is the result of a number of random biological events, the time of each being in strict linear proportion to the dose rate	$1 - \exp{-\sum_{i=1}^{k} \alpha_i d^i}$	k, an integer $\alpha_i > 0$ $i = 1 \rightarrow k$	Linear at low doses only when the linear coefficient B_i is positive; the relationship is sublinear otherwise

Data from Van Ryzin (1980), Van Ryzin and Rai (1980), and Munro and Krewski (1981).

having acquired a suitable graphic expression of the dose-response curve, the risk
assessor can begin to estimate a virtually safe dose (VSD) for the chemical. Depending
upon the model used and the linearity, supra-, or sublinearity of the calculated
relationship, a wide range of VSD values may be obtained. Compared to the VSD,
based on a linear relationship, values from sublinear relationships would be much
higher, while values from supralinear relationships would be much lower. An examination of the figures for extrapolated relationships for nitrilotriacetic acid (NTA),
sodium saccharin, 2-acetylaminofluorene (2-AAF), and aflatoxin revealed that the
Weibull, logit, multihit, and probit models all had much steeper slopes than did the
multistage model or simple linear extrapolation and yielded much higher VSD values
(Krewski and Van Ryzin, 1981). The extrapolated relationships for aflatoxin, a known
carcinogen of natural origin, are shown in schematic form in Figure 7.8. As can be
seen, the aflatoxin dosage permitting an acceptable (negligible) risk of one cancer
per million population can vary markedly, over a million-fold concentration range,
depending upon the model used to extrapolate the available date. Conversely, as is
shown in Table 7.2, a particular level of exposure may give rise to very large estimates
of comparative risk, again depending upon the model used. The selection of a
preferred low dose model is more of a policy decision or assumption than a scientific
conclusion (Becker, 1996c).

Which is the best model to use? Obviously, other than the simple linear extrapolation, the multistage model produces the lowest estimate of VSD. In a recent study

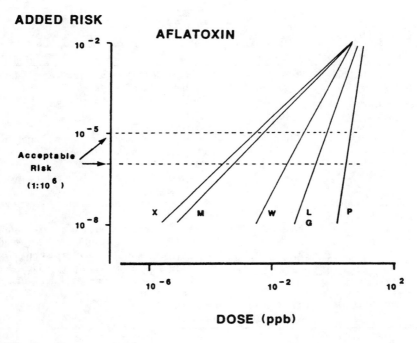

FIGURE 7.8

Linear low dose-response relationships for aflatoxin-induced tumorigenicity derived with the aid of several mathematical extrapolation models including: X, linear; M, multistage model; W, Weibull model; L, logit model; G, multihit model; and P, probit model. At the indicated levels of acceptable risk, i.e., one additional incidence of tumor per 100,000 or 1,000,000 population, the most conservative virtually safe dose (VSD) would be obtained from the multistage model or the simple linear extrapolation. (Modified from Krewski and Van Ryzin, 1981).

TABLE 7.2

Comparative Risk Estimates for a
Hypothetical Data Set

Model Used	Risk Estimates[a]	
One-hit	6×10^{-5}	1 in 17,000
Multi-stage	6×10^{-6}	1 in 167,000
Multi-hit	4.4×10^{-7}	1 in 2.3 million
Weibull	1.7×10^{-8}	1 in 59 million

From Rodericks and Taylor (1983).
[a] Values represent excess lifetime risk estimates.

of 585 chemical carcinogenesis experiments selected from the Carcinogenic Potency Data Base established by Gold et al. (1984), risk-specific doses (RSDs) were obtained from a simple linear extrapolation from the TD_{50} (dosage eliciting tumors in 50% of animals) to zero (see Figure 7.5) and yielded values that were generally within a factor of 5 or 10 of the values derived from the linearized multistage model (Krewski et al., 1990). A practical exercise on model-derived health risk estimates for 2,3,7,8-tetrachlorodibenzodioxin has been conducted (Fishbein, 1987). The multistage model is believed to be the most biologically plausible, since it incorporates contemporary understanding of chemical carcinogenesis, assumes no threshold for cancer

TABLE 7.3

Regulatory Classification of Carcinogens Based on the "Weight of the Evidence" Approach

Organization	Rating	Description
Environmental Protection Agency (EPA)	A	Sufficient evidence from epidemiological studies to support a causal association
	B1 (probable)	Limited evidence in humans from epidemiologic studies
	B2 (probable)	Sufficient evidence from animal studies but limited evidence in humans
	C (possible)	Limited or equivocal evidence from animal studies and inadequate or no data in humans
	D	Inadequate evidence in animals
	E	No evidence of carcinogenicity in at least two adequate animal tests in different species
International Agency for Research on Cancer (IARC)	1	Sufficient epidemiological evidence for carcinogenicity in humans
	2A	*Probably* carcinogenic in humans based on limited evidence in humans and sufficient evidence in animals
	2B	*Possibly* carcinogenic in humans based on sufficient evidence in animals but inadequate evidence in humans or limited evidence in humans with insufficient evidence in animals
	3	Not classifiable
	4	Not carcinogenic

initiation, and allows for the use and "best" fit of the full range of experimental data (Tardiff and Youngren, 1986).

In a simplified non-mathematical manner, this discussion presents some of the problems of low dose extrapolation to accomodate the non-threshold theory of carcinogenesis prevalent at present. Hopefully, a more realistic approach will be developed, one which will take into account the fact that, while many individuals are exposed daily to an array of carcinogens, only 20 to 25% of these develop cancer. These afflicted individuals come from two sources: (1) those exposed to a high dosage of carcinogen(s), and (2) those who are aberrant, highly sensitive members of a population. How do the models, threshold or otherwise, propose to estimate risks for these individuals? At present, there is no acceptable manner in which to reliably determine a threshold for a carcinogen, one fact that is agreed upon by all regulatory agencies.

VI. CARCINOGEN CLASSIFICATION

The above discussion of risk characterization goes hand-in-hand with an evaluation of the published data from both human and animal studies and interspecies comparisons of tumor type, tumor site, metabolism/pharmacokinetics, etc. (Brown et al., 1988; Gregory, 1988). Depending upon the national or international agencies involved, guidelines have been proposed for carcinogen classification on the basis of a "weight-of-the-evidence" approach. Earlier classifications had been based on "strength-of-the-evidence" concepts whereby an animal tumorigen should be deemed as identifying a potential human risk (Barnard, 1991). A summary of two such classifications in present use are shown in Table 7.3. The importance of having definitive data from human epidemiological studies is fully appreciated, thereby allowing the risk assessor to extrapolate from moderate-to-high dose, long-term occupational exposure, etc., to the general population exposed to much lower concentrations.

However, such a data base is usually lacking or, at best, is weak and risk assessment becomes dependent upon appropriate animal studies. It is crucial to recognize the category "*mammalian carcinogen*" and its interpretation found in International Agency for Research on Cancer (IARC) documents. As stated, "in the absence of adequate data on humans, it is biologically plausible and prudent to regard agents for which there is sufficient evidence of carcinogenicity in experimental animals as if they presented a carcinogenic risk to humans (IARC, 1987). Hence, the "probable" and "possible" categories (2A, 2B), shown in Table 7.3, are based on the weight-of-the-evidence. While only 45 of some 350 to 400 mammalian carcinogens have proven to be carcinogenic in the human (Upton, 1988), positive results in two or more species and/or in different strains of the same species are considered to be indicative that the agent, at some dosage and duration of exposure, might cause cancer(s) in the human. A major problem arises when the test chemical causes cancers in only one species or in one sex of one strain of one species, negative results being observed in all other well-conducted studies. Such a situation suggests a species (strain or sex) specificity — possibly involving some biochemical (biotransformation rate) and/or physiological (enhanced absorption, altered disposition, and/or elimination) function unique to the animal and should be investigated further to ascertain the mechanism of action.

A recent hypothesis suggested that chemicals inducing multiple site tumors in both mice and rats were less influenced by the genetic variability among different species than were chemicals that induced tumors in only one target site of one species (Tennant, 1993). The hypothesis was confirmed by examining a number of carcinogens already categorized according to the IARC classification (Table 7.3). The author strongly suggested that trans-species carcinogens should be a first priority of attention for human health risk.

Whether the above, in the context of the discussion in the previous chapter, a high proportion of both mutagens and nonmutagens induce tumors in rodent bioassays at the MTD, mitogenesis being important for cell proliferation. Mutagens are (1) more likely to be carcinogenic, (2) more likely to induce tumors at multiple target sites, and (3) more likely to be carcinogenic in two species (Gold et al., 1993). An examination of data for rodent carcinogens revealed that, of carcinogens inducing tumors at multiple sites in both mice and rats, 81% were mutagens. Of those carcinogens positive at only a single site in one species and negative in the other species, 42% were mutagenic. The analysis did not support the idea that mutagens and nonmutagens induced tumors in different target organs, both types of chemicals inducing tumors in a variety of sites, most organs being target sites for both categories. Ashby and Paton (1993) concluded that putative genotoxic rodent carcinogenesis could be correlated with chemical structure, the extent and the nature of the induced effect, whereas putative nongenotoxic carcinogenesis was more closely related to the test species than to the test chemical.

Whether by the use of a safety (uncertainty) factor approach based on a threshold dose-response relationship or by a risk analysis method to accomodate a non-threshold dose-response relationship, the risk assessment goal is to arrive at an acceptable concentration or VSD that does not underestimate human risk to the chemical. Although newer techniques of predicting absolute human risk(s) of cancer are being developed (Ames et al., 1987), they are controversial to say the least and have not yet received any official regulatory sanction as alternative methods to the chronic, lifetime animal bioassay for carcinogenicity. No doubt, significant advances will be made in this area in the next decade.

Using a linearized, multistage model, the U.S. EPA extrapolated the data of Kociba et al. (1978) to arrive at a risk-specific dose (RSD) for 2,3,7,8-tetrachlorodibenzo-*p*-dioxin (TCDD) of 0.006 pg/kg/day, an upper-bound confidence limit of a lifetime cancer risk of one per million population (EPA, 1985). More recently, an attempt was made to develop a threshold dose-response relationship for TCDD at a Banbury Center meeting at the Cold Spring Harbor Laboratory in November 1990 (Gallo et al., 1991; Roberts, 1991). The hypothesis being tested was that, before TCDD could cause any of its biological effects (chloracne, immunosuppression, birth defects, cancer), it had to bind to and activate a certain number of arylhydrocarbon (AH) receptors. This suggested that there might be a practical "threshold" for TCDD exposure below which no biological effect(s) occurred. While epidemiological studies have indicated that TCDD is a human carcinogen at high doses, as was seen in animal studies, other animal data have shown an absence of tumors at low doses (Fingerhut et al., 1991; Kociba, 1991). TCDD is one example of early attempts to develop mechanistic models for risk assessment (Lucier et al., 1993). While considerable insight has been gained into the complex events associated with TCDD binding to a receptor, nothing has been finalized for the biologically based, dose-response model (EPA, 1991b). An argument has been made that the current EPA reassessment overstates TCDD risk at low levels of exposure (Conolly, 1994). Can models be developed, modified, and applied to other (all) carcinogens? Toxicologists, oncologists, and risk evaluators eagerly await such models. Challenges to the old cancer risk assessment paradigm have appeared in the literature, generating a healthy debate on whether or not a new paradigm is needed and what form it should take. The positions were summarized succinctly by investigators in a recent publication (BELLE Newsletter, 1996). No doubt, the issues of a new model, a harmonization of cancer and non-cancer models, fine-tuning of the present model, etc., will be explored for years to come.

REFERENCES

Altschuler, B. Modeling of dose-response relationships. *Environ. Health Perspect.* 42: 23-27 (1981).

Ames, B.N., Magaw, R., and Gold, L.S. Ranking possible carcinogenic hazards. *Science* 236: 271-280 (1987).

Ashby, J. and Paton, D. The influence of chemical structure on the extent and sites of carcinogenesis for 522 rodent carcinogens and 55 different human carcinogen exposures. *Mutat. Res.* 286: 3-74 (1993).

Barnard, R.C. Presentation: Distinguished Fellow Awardee. *The Toxicology Forum.* Feb. 18-20 (1991), pp. 80-88.

Becker, R.A. Risk assessment. Human health risk assessment — the process. In *Environmental Toxicology.* Vol. 3. Ruchirawat, M. and Shank, R.C., Eds., Chulabhorn Research Institute, Bangkok, Thailand (1996a), pp. 457-503.

Becker, R.A. Risk estimation of chemical carcinogens. In *Environmental Toxicology.* Vol. 3. Ruchirawat, M. and Shank, R.C., Eds., Chulabhorn Research Institute, Bangkok, Thailand (1996b), pp. 505-531.

Becker, R.A. Factors affecting the risk assessment process. In *Environmental Toxicology.* Vol. 3. Ruchirawat, M. and Shank, R.C., Eds., Chulabhorn Research Institute, Bangkok, Thailand (1996c), pp. 533-548.

BELLE Newsletter. Dose-response studies of genotoxic rodent carcinogens: thresholds, hockey sticks, hormesis or straight lines. Vol. 3., #3, February (1995).

BELLE Newsletter. Is there a need for a new cancer risk assessment paradigm? BELLE Newsletter 5: #2/3, Nov. (1996).

Brown, S.L., Brett, S.M., Gough, M., Rodricks, J.V., Tardiff, R.G., and Turnbull, D. Review of interspecies risk comparisons. *Reg. Toxicol. Pharmacol.* 8: 191-206 (1988).

Bull, R.J., Conolly, R.B., DeMarini, D.M., McPhail, R.C., Ohanian, E.V., and Swenberg, J.A. Incorporating biologically based models into assessment of risk from chemical contaminants. *J. Am. Water Works Assoc.* 85: 49-52 (1993).

Centre for Risk Analysis. A Historical Perspective on Risk Assessment in the Federal Government. Harvard School of Public Health, March (1994).

Conolly, R.B. U.S. EPA Reassessment of the Health Risks of 2,3,7,8-Tetrachlorodibenzo-p-dioxin (TCDD). CIIT Activities 14: #12 (1994), pp. 1-8.

Cothern, C.R., Mehlman, M.A., and Marcus, W.L. (Editors). *Risk Assessment and Risk Management of Industrial and Environmental Chemicals.* Princeton Scientific Publishing Co., Inc., Princeton, NJ. (1988).

Dourson, M.L. and Stara, J.F. Regulatory history and experimental support for uncertainty (safety) factors. *Reg. Toxicol. Pharmacol.* 3: 224-238 (1983).

EPA. Health Risk Assessment for Polychlorinated Dibenzo-p-dioxin. U.S. Environmental Protection Agency, Washington, D.C., EPA/600/8-84/0146 (1985).

EPA. *Health Advisories for Drinking Water Contaminants.* Lewis Publishers, Boca Raton, FL. (1993).

EPA. Estimating Exposure to Dioxin-like Compounds. U.S. Environmental Protection Agency, Washington, D.C., EPA/600/6-88/005 Ca-c (1994a).

EPA. Health Assessment Document for 2,3,7,8-Tetrachlorodibenzo-p-dioxin (TCDD) and Related Compounds. U.S. Environmental Protection Agency, Washington, D.C. EPA/600/BP-92/001 a-c (1994b).

Fingerhut, M.A., Halperin, W.E., Marlow, D.A., Piacitelli, L.A., Honchar, P.A., Sweeney, M.H., Greife, A.L., Dill, P.A., Steenland, K., and Suruda, A.J. Cancer mortality in workers exposed to 2,3,7,8-tetrachlorodibenzo-p-dioxin. *New Eng. J. Med.* 324: 212-218 (1991).

Fishbein, L. Health-risk estimates for 2,3,7,8-tetrachloro-dibenzodioxin. An overview. *Toxicol. Ind. Health* 3: 91-134 (1987).

Gallo, M.A., Scheuplein, R.J., and Van Der Heijden, K., Eds. *Banbury Report 35: Biological Basis for Risk Assessment of Dioxins and Related Compounds,* Cold Spring Harbor Laboratory Press (1991).

Gaylor, D.W. and Kodell, R.L. Linear interpolation algorithm for low dose risk assessment of toxic substances. *J. Environ. Pathol. Toxicol.* 4: 305-312 (1980).

Gold, L.S., Slone, T.H., Stern, B.R., and Bernstein, L. Comparison of target organs of carcinogenicity for mutagenic and non-mutagenic chemicals. *Mutat. Res.* 286: 75-100 (1993).

Gold, L.S., Sawyer, C.B., Magaw, R., Backman, G.M., DeVeciana, M., Levinson, R., Hooper, N.K., Havender, W.R., Bernstein, L., Peto, R., Pike, M.C., and Ames, B.N. A carcinogenic potency database of the standardized results of animal bioassays. *Environ. Health Perspect.* 58: 9-322 (1984).

Goldman, M. Cancer risk of low-level exposure. *Science* 271: 1821-1822 (1996).

Gots, R.E. Quantitative risk assessment: an attempt to link science to cancer policy. In *Toxic Risks. Science, Regulation and Perception.* Lewis Publishers, Boca Raton, FL., Ch.10, pp. 143-152 (1993).

Gregory, A.R. Species comparisons in evaluating carcinogens in humans. *Reg. Toxicol. Pharmacol.* 8: 160-190 (1988).

Hallenbeck, W.H. and Cunningham, K.M. *Quantitative Risk Assessment for Environmental and Occupational Health.* Lewis Publishers Inc., Chelsea MI (1987).

International Agency for Research on Cancer (IARC). Overall Evaluations of Carcinogenicity: An Updating of IARC Monographs. Vols. 1-42, Suppl. 7. IARC, Lyon, France (1987).

Kelly, K.A. and Cardon, N.C. The myth of 10^{-6} as a definition of acceptable risk. *EPA Watch* 3: #17, 4-8 (1994).

Kitchin, K.T. and Brown, J.L. Dose-response relationship for rat liver DNA damage caused by 49 rodent carcinogens. *Toxicology* 88: 31-49 (1994).

Kociba, R. Rodent bioassays for assessing chronic toxicity and carcinogenic potential of TCDD. In *Banbury Report 35: Biological Basis for Risk Assessment of Dioxins and Related Compounds,* Gallo, M.A., Scheuplein, R.J., and VanDer Heijden, K., Eds., Cold Spring Harbor Press (1991), Ch. 1. pp. 3-26.

Kociba, R.J., Keyes, D.J., Beyer, J.E., Carreon, R.M., Wade, C.E., Dittenber, D.A., Kalnins, R.P., Frauson, L.E., Park, C.N., Barnard, S.D., Hummel, R.A., and Humiston, C.G. Results of a two-year chronic toxicity and oncogenicity study of 2,3 7,8-tetrachlorodibenzo-p-dioxin in rats. *Toxicol. Appl. Pharmacol.* 46: 279-303 (1978).

Krewski, D., Szyskowicz, M., and Rosenkranz, H. Quantitative factors in chemical carcinogenesis: variation in carcinogenic potency. *Reg. Toxicol. Pharmacol.* 12: 13-29 (1990).

Krewski, D. and Van Ryzin, J. Dose response models for quantal response toxicity data. In *Statistical and Related Topics.* J. Csorgo, D. Dawson, J.N.K. Rao, and E. Shaleh (Editors). North Holland, New York (1981), pp. 201-231.

Lu, F.C. Toxicological evaluations of carcinogens and noncarcinogens: pros and cons of different approaches. *Reg. Toxicol. Pharmacol.* 3: 121-132 (1983).

Lucier, G.W., Portier, C.J., and Gallo, M.A. Receptor mechanisms and dose-response models for the effects of dioxins. *Environ. Health Perspect.* 101: 36-43 (1993).

Mantel, N. and Bryan, W.R. Safety testing of carcinogenic agents. *J. Natl. Cancer Inst.* 42: 455-461 (1961).

Mastromatteo, E. On the concept of threshold. *Am. Ind. Hyg. Assoc. J.* 42: 763-776 (1981).

Morgan, M.G. Risk research: when should we say "enough"? *Science* 232: 917 (1986).

Muller, H.J. Artificial transmutation of the gene. *Science*, 66: 84-87 (1927).

Munro, I.C. and Krewski, D.R. Risk assessment and regulatory decision making. *Food Cosmet. Toxicol.* 19: 549-560 (1981).

National Research Council. Risk Assessment in the Federal Government. A report of the Committee on the Institutional Means for Assessment of Risks to Public Health. National Academy Press, Washington, D.C. (1983).

National Research Council. Toxicity Testing. Strategies to Determine Needs and Priorities. National Academy Press, Washington, D.C. (1984).

National Research Council (NRC). Regulating Pesticides in Food. The Delaney Paradox. National Academy Press, Washington, D.C. (1987).

Paustenbach, D.J. Health risk assessment and the practice of industrial hygiene. *Am. Ind. Hyg. Assoc. J.* 51: 339-351 (1990).

Roberts, L. Dioxin risks revisited. *Science* 251: 624-626 (1991).

Rodricks, J. and Taylor, M.R. Application of risk assessment to food safety decision making. *Reg. Toxicol. Pharmacol.* 3: 275-307 (1983).

Slovic, P. Perception of risk. *Science* 236: 280-285 (1987).

Stara, J.F. and Erdreich, L.S. (Editors). Advances in Health Risk Assessment for Systemic Toxicants and Chemical Mixtures. *Toxicol. Ind. Health* 1: 1-333 (1985).

Starr, C. and Whipple, C. Risks of risk decisions. *Science* 208: 1114-1119 (1980).

Tardiff, R.G. and Youngren, S.H. Public health significance of organic substances in drinking water. In *Organic Carcinogens in Drinking Water.* N.M. Ram, E.J. Calabrese, and R.F. Christman, Eds., Wiley Interscience, New York (1986), pp. 405-436.

Tennant, R.W. Stratification of rodent carcinogenicity bioassay results to reflect relative human hazard. *Mutat. Res.* 286: 111-118 (1993).

Truhaut, R. The problem of thresholds for chemical carcinogens — its importance in industrial hygiene, especially in the field of permissible limits for occupational exposure. *Am. Ind. Hyg. Assoc. J.* 41: 685-692 (1980).

Upton, A.C. Carcinogenic risk assessment in proper perspective. *Toxicol. Ind. Health* 4: 443-452 (1988).

Van Ryzin, J. Quantitative risk assessment. *J. Occup. Med.* 22: 321-326 (1980).

Van Ryzin, J. and Rai, K. The use of quantal response data to make predictions. In *The Scientific Basis of Toxicity Assessment.* H.R. Witschi (Editor). Elseview/North-Holland, New York (1980), pp. 273-290.

Weil, C.S. Statistics vs. safety factors and scientific judgment in the evaluation of safety for man. *Toxicol. Appl. Pharmacol.* 21: 454-463 (1972).

Weisburger, E.K. Mechanistic considerations in chemical carcinogenesis. *Reg. Toxicol. Pharmacol.* 12: 41-52 (1990).

Zeckhauser, R.J. and Viscusi, W.K. Risk within reason. *Science* 248: 559-564 (1990).

INDEX